DATE			

THE ALIEN DOCTORS

HEALTH, MEDICINE, AND SOCIETY:
A WILEY-INTERSCIENCE SERIES
DAVID MECHANIC, Editor

Evaluating Treatment Environments: A Social Ecological Approach
by Rudolf H. Moos

Human Subjects in Medical Experimentation: A Sociological Study of the Conduct and Regulation of Clinical Research
by **Bradford H. Gray**

Child Health and the Community
by **Robert J. Haggerty, Klaus J. Roghmann, and Ivan B. Pless**

Health Insurance Plans: Promise and Performance
by **Robert W. Hetherington, Carl E. Hopkins, and Milton I. Roemer**

The End of Medicine
by **Rick J. Carlson**

Humanizing Health Care
by **Jan Howard** and **Anselm Strauss**, Volume Editors

The Growth of Bureaucratic Medicine: An Inquiry into the Dynamics of Patient Behavior and the Organization of Medical Care
by **David Mechanic**

The Post-Physician Era: Medicine in the Twenty-First Century
by **Jerrold S. Maxmen**

A Right to Health: The Problem of Access to Primary Medical Care
by **Charles E. Lewis, Rashi Fein, and David Mechanic**

Gift of Life: The Social and Psychological Impact of Organ Transplantation
by **Roberta G. Simmons, Susan D. Klein, and Richard L. Simmons**

Mentally Ill in Community-Based Sheltered Care: A Study of Community Care and Social Integration
by **Steven P. Segal** and **Uri Aviram**

The Alien Doctors: Foreign Medical Graduates in American Hospitals
by **Rosemary Stevens, Louis Wolf Goodman, and Stephen S. Mick**

THE ALIEN DOCTORS

FOREIGN MEDICAL GRADUATES IN AMERICAN HOSPITALS

Rosemary Stevens

Tulane University
New Orleans, Louisiana

Louis Wolf Goodman

Social Science Research Council
New York, New York

Stephen S. Mick

Yale University
New Haven, Connecticut

A WILEY-INTERSCIENCE PUBLICATION

JOHN WILEY & SONS
New York · Chichester · Brisbane · Toronto

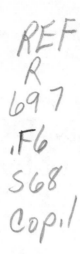
Library of Congress Cataloging in Publication Data:

Stevens, Rosemary.
  The alien doctors.

  (Health, medicine, and society)
  "A Wiley-Interscience publication."
  Includes index.
  1. Physicians, Foreign—United States. I. Goodman, Louis Wolf, joint author. II. Mick,
Stephen S., joint author. III. Title.

R697.F6S68   331.11   77-12934
ISBN 0-471-82455-0

Printed in the United States of America
10 9 8 7 6 5 4 3 2 1

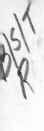

FOR ROSE

ACKNOWLEDGMENTS

Survey research of the magnitude of this study requires the unstinting efforts of many individuals and institutions. We have been unusually fortunate in this respect.

First and foremost, our thanks go to the 865 physicians in hospitals throughout the United States who took time from their house staff schedules and off-duty hours to answer our battery of interview questions. Their courtesy, willingness to respond, and interest in the survey form the single most important element in this study. We hope this book justifies their efforts and those of the many other physicians who participated at different stages as the study developed.

Staff of the National Opinion Research Center administered the survey for us in the field and were constantly available for consultation. Robert Banacki of the New York office helped coordinate our early field research efforts and was a rigorous critic of the interview schedule as it developed. Other NORC staff who consulted on the survey development were Paul Sheatsley, Gertrude Peterson, Eve Weinberg, Margit Gerow, Wendy Kreitman, and Yvonne Johnson. Martin Frankel advised us on NORC sampling procedures. We thank them all for their invaluable assistance.

At the American Medical Association, we are indebted in particular to Gene Roback, and also to Kenneth Monroe and Chris Theodore, all of the Association's Center for Health Services Research and Development. All were available for discussion, suggestions, and information. By no means least, they provided us with the critical sampling frames we needed.

James Haug, now with the American College of Surgeons, was another early supporter of our efforts.

David Fitch, the project officer at the National Center for Health Services Research, Health Resources Administration, U.S. Department of Health Education and Welfare, advised and aided us throughout the lengthy endeavor, 1972 through 1976. Among other staff who were working at HEW on related investigations during the project's development, we thank in particular Betty Lockett, Kathleen Williams, and Thomas Dublin.

Many fellow investigators from other universities were generous in sharing their work with us and supportive in ideas and encouragement. Our thanks go to Roland Knobel, Irene Butter, John Colombotos, and Donald Yett. David Mechanic read the whole book in draft, and made detailed and cogent suggestions on the text.

Those closest to the work as it progressed, and essential to its completion, were the staff of the Yale National House Staff Survey in New Haven, appointed for various periods as the study progressed. We thank all who participated at different stages. Special thanks are due to three superb staff associates, who acted as research methodologists, programmers, coding supervisors, and data analysts: Susanne Harris, June G. Darge, and Marcia Richardson. Ms. Richardson served on the project from its earliest glimmerings. All were rigorous and constructive critics of the work as it progressed.

Richard Wilson, our data manager and computation consultant at the Yale Computer Center, enabled us to organize and to retrieve efficiently the enormous body of information gleaned through the survey interview. Paul Pastor, Arthur Frank, Graves Enck, Bruce Grogan, Arlene Goldblatt, and Gary Sax provided valuable materials and ideas through pilot studies of physicians in hospitals and other studies during the planning period.

We are grateful to the staff secretaries for putting up with endless drafts, scribbled notes, and messy tables. Thank you for your good humor: Marie Young, Nancy Okie, Eileen Hoffman, and Diane Clemmons.

Finally, we thank, in memory, Rose McAree, who died in 1975 and to whom this book is dedicated. No large-scale project can work well without a skillful office manager. Rose McAree acted as the immovable mainstay of the project, coordinating work, developing data-tracking procedures, insisting that these procedures be followed properly, and generally organizing all of us.

In dedicating this book to Rose, we acknowledge how much research such as this depends on the activities of those whose names do not appear on the title page. As those who do, we must take the customary blame (however reluctantly) for all the remaining deficiencies in the text.

This study was supported by grant USPHS 1-R01-HS-00767 from the National Center for Health Services Research, Health Resources Administration (formerly the National Center for Health Services Research and Development, Health Services and Mental Health Administration), U.S. Department of Health, Education and Welfare.

R.A.S.
L.W.G.
S.S.M.

CONTENTS ————————————————

TABLES

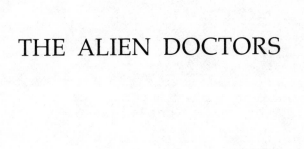

THE ALIEN DOCTORS

1

INTRODUCTION _____

In the decade 1965–1974, 75,000 foreign physicians entered the United States intending to stay for at least a temporary period of work. Most are still here; the more recent arrivals are completing specialist training in United States hospitals; others are established in more permanent positions as fulltime hospital staff or private practitioners.[1] By the academic year 1973–74, when this study was undertaken, foreign medical graduates comprised one-fifth of physicians in the United States and one-third of physicians in graduate training as interns or residents.

This migration has been little short of spectacular. In an era—1950 through the 1960s—in which enrollments of medical students in the United States remained virtually stationary, circumstances combined to enable physicians trained in other nations to flock to the United States to fill an expanding supply of internship and residency positions. Now the situation is reversed. In the last few years, new medical schools have been built and old ones expanded in the United States, increasing the supply of American-trained physicians. The job market for house staff is tightening up, leaving fewer vacancies available for immigrants. Because there are fewer jobs, it is not as easy as it was a few years ago for foreign doctors to

1

gain the necessary United States visas, and changes in visa requirements promise further restrictions. Nevertheless, immigrant physicians continue to be a major factor in medicine in the United States.

Our aim in this book is to describe and document the characteristics of this physician migration through the eyes and experiences of those migrating. Who has come to the United States, and why do they come? What do foreign physicians, as individuals, expect to achieve with their United States education? How are these expectations translated into reality? What is it like to make a substantial career shift after several years of postgraduate training or work in a different country? What contributions do foreign physicians make to medical practice in this country during the time that they are here, and how do they perceive their roles in comparison to United States graduates in similar positions?

A number of studies have examined the gross, structural elements of migration—notably, the development of United States policies that have facilitated migration into this country, and aggregate numbers and trends.[2] However, such studies have shed little light on the *process* of physician migration, from the first decision through adjustment to the United States. This is the first nationwide study that asks foreign physicians, through personal interviews, why and how they decided to come to the United States, what they are doing, and what are their career expectations. The result is a data set that can be aggregated to describe national trends and can also be disaggregated to reflect the heterogeneity of individual experiences.

WHY ARE FOREIGN MEDICAL GRADUATES IMPORTANT? THREE CONTEXTS

Information about physician migrants has been lacking in part because official statistics gloss over differences. Whatever his or her status in the homeland—new graduate, experienced teacher, or seasoned practitioner —the foreign physician who enters the United States immediately relinquishes all distinctions and becomes the "FMG" (foreign medical graduate). The FMG, in turn, is labeled "alien" or "stranger," an element in the continuing debates about the "FMG Problem" in Congress and within the United States medical profession.

Yet a better understanding of migration is important to developing health policy in the United States. For practical purposes, it makes little sense for United States government agencies, the American Medical Association, and other national organizations to devise programs, attempting to expand or contract the supply of physicians *unless* the reasons physicians come to the United States are elucidated, their experiences documented, and their future expectations are explained. Without such information, policies cannot be developed that satisfy (1) United States interests in the domestic supply of physicians, (2) United States interests in encouraging doctor migration for the exchange of specialist knowledge and education and (3) the individual interests of thousands of potential migrant physicians.

A second context is the international marketplace. The presence here of 18,000 FMGs in specialist training, working as house staff in American hospitals, inevitably triggers questions about the balance sheets of international exchange. Few American physicians go abroad for training; the flow of migration is virtually one way. The United States is not alone in being a recipient in the widespread migration of highly skilled talent, yet this country is perhaps unique in what it has offered to migrant physicians and what it has, in turn, received. Meanwhile, certain basic assumptions have become inherent in physician migration as a phenomenon and must color any specific debates.

Terms such as "brain drain" and "overflow" have passed into general circulation. The first may have an implicit connotation that affluent nations lure graduates from poorer countries to their domains for economic gain. Under the second, it is the so-called donor nations who are to blame; it is argued that some countries train too many professionals (or the wrong kind) for their own needs and must pass on an excess. Studies of institutional factors involved in migration have thus, not surprisingly, produced a "push-pull" model of migration that attempts to show how individual decisions are affected by conditions in both the donor and recipient nations. The argument goes that there are certain factors in a specific country that may "push" a physician to emigrate (for example, a lack of desirable jobs) and others that may "pull" him or her to countries such as Britain, Canada, or the United States (such as higher salaries). All these assumptions are mechanistic; they assume that immigrants are relatively passive participants in the process of migration, affected by national considerations beyond their control. Although we do not find the push-pull model helpful and instead cast our analysis in terms of the migrant physician's career, the strategic and macroeconomic elements implicit in such terms as brain drain, overflow, or push–pull provide an underlying context to current debates.

Physicians may not be the helpless pawns on an international chessboard that some debates suggest. Nevertheless, those who migrate and continue to consider migration as a future option in their careers clearly do so within limitations that result from institutional and governmental policies as well as cultural, political, and economic factors. However, these policies set parameters for individual decisions—they do not completely determine these decisions. Inevitably, then, there is a moral or ethical undercurrent in interpreting any individual decision to migrate. For example, should the United States continue to have visa procedures that make it relatively simple for physicians to enter for training and remain? Given the fact that most entrants come from developing nations that often have relatively few physicians and have invested substantially in the migrants' education, ought the United States to encourage such "reverse foreign aid"? What policies should donor nations adopt? Should they attempt to prevent their physicians from migrating? If so, how can they get them to practice in poor and rural areas? What might be the role for international organizations?

United States domestic policy and international policies toward physician migration provide two important contextual elements in considering the process of migration. In this regard we hope our findings will interest policy makers at both the national and international levels.

There is another level on which the study of physician migrants to the United States in the 1970s has importance. These physicians are a special group of migrants in terms of interest to scholars building social science theories. This interest derives both from the fact that physicians play important roles in society, and because they are a group on which there is a relatively large amount of data already available. As members of society, physician migrants can be seen as part of the phenomenon of migration of talent to this country in the mid-twentieth century, as major contributors to the pool of physician manpower in the United States, as professionals whose experiences and careers provide insights into more general processes of occupational behavior and socialization, and as individuals caught in the dilemma of having "modern" expectations in developing nations.

FMGS AS MIGRANTS, AS MANPOWER, AND AS PROFESSIONALS: INTER-LOCKING ELEMENTS IN A COMPLEX SYSTEM

As *migrants*, FMGs are leading representatives of the "new" migration:[3] the unprecedented movement of professionals to the United States and other New World countries in the mid-twentieth century. Although the international migration of professionals is not a new phenomenon, this movement is characterized by the large proportion of professionals relative to other migrants and the sheer numbers of professionals involved. In the decade 1901–1910, for example, only 1% of all immigrants to the United States were trained in one of the professions; in fiscal year 1974, 23 percent of the immigrant visas given to those reporting an occupation were classified as "professional, technical or kindred workers." Of the total 151,268 immigrants reporting occupations (i.e., excluding dependents with no occupation), 35,483 were such "professionals"; of these, 4537 were physicians.[4]

When entrants on exchange visitor and other temporary visas are included, the proportion of physicians rises. However, the figures are less important than the characteristics of the migrants. Instead of a flow of immigrants drawn from the working classes of specific countries at specific times, the "new" migration is distinguished by a flow of immigrants from many different countries, who are bound together by common skills. Whereas the "old" patterns of immigration led to the development of identifiable ethnic groups in American life, new migrants being helped in America by fellow nationals, the modern professional migrants, with internationally recognized occupations, are less dependent on cultural ties than their unskilled predecessors, but they are more dependent on professional networks.

Among the various implications of this phenomenon is the difficulty of developing any single foreign or international policy toward the migration of professionals, including physicians. The international context is not bilateral but multilateral: it is no longer a question of how many individuals the United States should admit from, say, Eire, Taiwan, or Italy, but how many nurses, physicians, engineers, or accountants should be admitted, irrespective of country. One rather curious result is that the international elements of physician migration tend *either* to be diffused into broad ethical or economic judgments rather than into focused policies between the United States and specific nations *or* to be narrowed into purely domestic United States issues: for example how many physicians (or nurses or accountants) does the United States want?

The largest groups of physician migrants are alumni of medical schools in a small heterogeneous set of countries: the Philippines, whose graduates represented 9500 of the 72,000 foreign-trained physicians in the United States at the beginning of 1974; India, with 7000; Italy, West Germany, South Korea, and Cuba, each with more than 3000 medical alumni in this country; the United Kingdom, Switzerland, Iran, Mexico, and Spain, each with 2000 or more graduates.[5] Physicians, individually, have been drawn to the United States from countries and schools all over the world. For one reason or another, at some point in their careers these men and women made a decision to come to the United States, at least for a limited period of training. Once here, they are irrevocably linked together. Whatever their national origins or experiences, they are all physicians. To United States physicians, they are all aliens.

As health *manpower*, FMGs have made substantial contributions to the United States health care system, while playing an uncertain and ambivalent role in it: uncertain because many FMGs come to the United States undecided about their career plans or with the expectation of a temporary stay that may change at some point during training in the United States; ambivalent because FMGs, as foreigners, are "strangers" in the United States system. In some respects the system treats FMGs as a tactical reserve—a useful addition to manpower where shortages exist, but a potential competitive threat in times of surplus.

The cumulative effect of migration is substantial. In 1974, FMGs comprised 40 percent of all physicians receiving their first license to practice in the United States. Foreign medical graduates in private practice numbered 27,000 by the end of 1973. Concentrated in certain states and in cities such as New York, Chicago, Baltimore, Philadelphia, and Newark, these FMGs provide services to thousands of members of the United States population; many offer invaluable services to the poor through state Medicaid programs. Together with the FMGs who have joined fulltime hospital staffs or are still in training, FMGs now represent more than half of all physicians in some states. They represent, therefore, a major source of physician manpower in the United States.

A discussion of the decisions, expectations, and experiences of individual FMGs thus inevitably impinges on the nature and peculiarities of the United States health care system. The presence of FMGs is, indeed, an established part of the health care system. If FMGs were suddenly removed from specialist training in New Jersey, for example, United States graduates, who represent only one-fourth of all house staff in the state, would presumably have their work substantially extended. Or, possibly, alternative forms of medical care delivery might arise to fill the gap, including extensive use of physician substitutes. However, the behaviour of the system toward FMGs is an important element in their experience in the United States. Where FMGs are trained and how they are otherwise accommodated by, and assimilated into, United States hospitals may affect the individual behavior of FMGs—and thus may rebound on the health care system in the United States.

From an economic point of view, the migrants may be seen as responding in market terms of demand and supply. Jobs are offered; physicians are available; migration follows. Hospitals that might not otherwise have house staff benefit from the availability of these physicians, and the medical staff of these hospitals is able to delegate and teach rather than shoulder the full burden of providing medical services.

These manpower aspects of migration revolve around demands made by the United States system for physicians, particularly interns and residents. As in all aspects of migration, however, the rationale for decision making cannot solely be understood by focusing on a single hypothesis or simple factors. To study FMGs is to study complexity. For, in the terms used here, FMGs are not just "manpower." They are, at one and the same time, "migrants" who may be responding to more subtle factors of migration than sheer job availability and "professionals" for whom United States training may be a logical step in a planned career.

As *professionals*, FMGs coming to positions as interns and residents in the United States are socialized to a greater or lesser extent into the medical care system they have just left. Usually they have left the professional system of their own countries with a medical degree but without the period of graduate education that has become essential for modern specialists. Half-trained, the FMG enters the United States for final training, joining graduates of United States schools who are also part-way through their training. For some this is a difficult transition.

FMGs bring with them to the United States a package of assumptions about medicine and their roles as physicians and expectations that may be realized in the United States socioprofessional system. The assimilation of strangers into an alien professional system, the coping mechanisms used by different individuals with greater or lesser success, and the timing of decisions at different career stages are themes that fall squarely into studies of the sociology of occupations. Yet, with a few notable exceptions, the behavior of FMGs as professionals has barely been touched in the sociological literature.[6]

This study provides a partial addition to the literature. We investigate the assimilation (or lack of assimilation) of FMGs into United States hospitals and social life, analyzing the data not in terms of socialization of a group of professionals into their careers, but as part of an on-going process of migration. We are aware that there are both costs and benefits in this approach, but this is not an uncommon dilemma in social research. In analyzing the process of migration through the investigation of individual careers, we do not attempt to make a detailed theoretical contribution to the literature of professionalization. Rather, by concentrating on the process of migration and viewing FMGs continuously in their three basic dimension—as migrants, manpower, and professionals—we seek to portray the decision-making frame in which our actors make their decisions.

Indeed, each dimension overlaps the others. As a special group of migrants linked by common skills as much as (or rather than) nationality, FMGs may be particularly susceptible to pressures for developing a professional identity in the United States. Working hard to belong to the adopted professional culture, even if the adoption is supposedly temporary, the FMG may be successfully socialized. Such a process may make it difficult for the FMG, in an ambiguous role at the best of times, to decide on his or her future career. Thus the process of professionalization is inextricably linked with the FMG's role as a potential member of the long-term manpower pool of physicians in the United States and with his or her future direction as a migrant. Each dimension is connected to the next.

THE STUDY: FROM GENERAL TO SPECIFIC

In planning this study, we were quite clear from the beginning that our investigation would span the individual FMG's career from his or her early background to the time of training in an internship or residency position in the United States. To look at the FMGs as migrants, we needed to know, in particular, the FMG's background characteristics, motivations, and expectations in coming to the United States. As an element in United States manpower, the FMG's experiences and work-loads are naturally relevant, as are his or her future career expectations. We also had to know how far the FMG experience is like that of United States graduates in house staff positions. In terms of professional assimi-lation, we examined the type of hospital and program an FMG entered, the FMG's mobility within the system and the FMG's reports of, and attitudes toward, life in the United States, including those related to decisions to stay here or leave.

Three major research questions are addressed:

1.   What have been the patterns of *recruitment and the expectations of foreign medical graduates* in coming to the United States, and how have these expectations been translated into reality?
2.   What are the primary *roles of FMGs in training in American hospitals?*
3.   How do foreign medical graduates expect to *utilize their American education* in terms of their subsequent location and careers?

Schematically, the data required to answer these three questions fall into the chronological elements of a career. Systematically, our findings span three linked but independent ideas: how FMGs are recruited and recruit themselves into the United States specialist training system; how the relative roles of FMGs and United States graduates are established in the evolving structure of medicine in the United States; and to what extent FMGs are assimilated as permanent additions to the United States medical profession.

To gather our information, personal interviews were conducted with 865 physicians in training as interns and residents in hospitals in the United States in April–May, 1974. The study methodology and the reasoning and planning studies that preceded it are presented in Appendix A; the interview schedule is presented in Appendix B. It may be helpful to remark here on three specific aspects of the methodology.

First, the study is designed to produce a stratified representative sample of all FMGs in the United States, including FMGs from all countries and in all specialties; thus we could generalize from our findings to all FMGs in training in the United States. This consideration was important for drawing inferences and conclusions that would be relevant to current policy debates.

Second, the personal interview approach was chosen after experience with other techniques as the only means of developing sufficient and valid information (particularly with respect to attitudinal questions) from a group of busy physicians who, as part of the "FMG situation" were sometimes concerned or skeptical about being questioned. Although very expensive, this method is successful. It provides both a high response rate (89.8 percent) and valid responses. In addition, personal interviews allow for the incorporation into the schedules of additional, unsolicited materials that are valuable in providing anecdotal materials.

Third, the sample contains information on graduates of both foreign and United States schools. Our completed returns include 690 foreign medical graduates who were foreign nationals at the time of graduation from medical school (the FMGs), an additional 42 physicians who graduated from foreign schools but were United States citizens at the time of graduation (almost all were United States citizens from birth and are designated USFMGs), and 133 graduates of United States schools (USMGs). In order not to confuse the comparisons between FMG experiences and those of USMGs, we do not analyze in detail the experiences of the 42 USFMGs. However, we do present statistical data in the tables for all groups; thus readers who are particularly interested in USFMGs may draw their own conclusions.

RATIONALE, LIMITATIONS, PRESENTATION

Although the three of us had not worked together before, each of us had undertaken work that was directly relevant to the theoretical, methodological, or policy questions inherent in a study of migration. Rosemary Stevens, a social historian interested in the development of public and private policy toward the supply, distribution, and role of physicians in the United States (and an immigrant) had analyzed the institutional elements involved in physician migration and areas for policy decisions, but was concerned that there was virtually no information available about decision making from the migrant's point of view. Louis Wolf Goodman, a sociologist interested in the dynamics of international relations, had worked on various aspects of social change in the Third World and the role of multinational corporations and was drawn to the study of migration as an element of his wider concerns about international stratification. Stephen S. Mick, a sociologist interested in occupations and career mobility, had undertaken studies of the behavior of industrial workers in the United States and was attracted by the opportunity to explore these issues in the context of the migration of professionals.

From a more general point of view, we were linked by our developing common interests in the study of complex social systems and policy analysis. All of us brought to the study considerable skepticism toward several of the assumptions about foreign medical graduates that had pervaded discussions on physician migration at Congressional hearings, professional meetings, and, to some extent, in the research literature.

The assumptions included reliance on the "push–pull" model of migration, with the usual finding that FMGs come to the United States because of "pull" factors here, rather than factors that "push" them from their own countries; that FMGs fill "shortage" areas in the United States geographically, by specialty, and by institution; that the United States diverts physicians who might otherwise work in needed areas (such as government hospitals or organizing preventive care) in other countries into superspecialist training that is inappropriate outside major university centers or cities in highly developed nations; that FMGs have a generally inferior medical educational background compared to United States graduates and may thus be less "competent"; that FMGs enter and remain in United States hospital training positions that are "least desirable" in terms of the expectations of United States graduates; and that FMGs come to the United States with the intention of remaining. Our concern is not that such assumptions are necessarily wrong, but that they were unsubstantiated.

These and other largely untested assumptions created a mosaic of myths and stereotypes about FMGs. In some discussions FMGs were presented as if they were all non-English speaking, poorly trained graduates of a school somewhere in Asia, with little previous clinical experience, working in United States hospitals with little or no university affiliation and were struck there for all their training. In fact, as we show here, FMGs are an extraordinarily heterogeneous group; the great majority speak fluent English; most come with at least some postgraduate clinical experience; they are quite mobile in the United States hospital training system; and most receive training in university-affiliated institutions. As migrants, FMGs are, indeed, a gifted and resourceful group. We began our study with a strong desire to test stereotypes and debunk myths.

This motivation was not, however, an end in itself. As investigators concerned with policy analysis and development, we were concerned about the uses of myths in policy formation at a time at which the United States postures toward migration promised radical change. This concern is being borne out. The migration of FMGs appear to have passed its peak, apparently because of near-saturation in a constricting job market for FMGs and the tightening of United States visa procedures. However, in limiting numbers, questions of priorities must be raised. The need for reliable and precise information became more acute as the study progressed. What types of physicians should be encouraged to come to the United States for training? Which physicians should be denied entry? There are no criteria generally acceptable to government agencies or spokesmen for United States hospitals and professional agencies regarding which physicians (or other professionals) should be selected for training that might be invaluable for their home countries or should be given priority among other immigrants. Such criteria, to be effective, should rest on hard, reliable information; this we attempt to gather and present.

In its simplest form, this study is descriptive. It is designed to develop information about foreign medical graduates to provide a definitive profile of FMGs and to compare their backgrounds, outlooks, and responsibilities with those of graduates of the United States schools (USMGs). The results of the findings of any large-scale survey can, however, be treated in a variety of ways. We chose to present our findings in terms of the chronology of the physician's career. The book begins by analyzing the physicians' backgrounds and experiences before coming to the United States (Chapter 2), moves to the decision and mechanics involved in migration (Chapters 3 and 4), arrival and adjustment (Chapters 5 through 7), experiences in the United States (Chapters 8 through 10), and the decision as to whether to return or remain (Chapter 11). The last chapter (chapter 12) presents our conclusions.

This book is for a general audience: we try to avoid being too technical and to eschew the jargon of the social sciences. We hope it will be read, in particular, by members and their staff of Congressional Committees dealing with health services development, immigration policy, and international relations, by staff in the federal agencies concerned with migration (the Departments of State, Justice, Labor, HEW), by policymakers at the state level considering professional regulation and manpower planning, and by representatives of the major professional associations of medicine, as well as social scientists and physicians. Although foreign-trained physicians can be seen in the context of domestic and international events and as migrants, manpower, or professionals, this study is about individuals. It is about individuals whose lives—or the lives of those like them—may be changed for better or worse by decisions made in America in the next decades.

NOTES

1. In the interest of readability, we attempt throughout this book to keep footnotes to a minimum. As a general guide, we include footnotes that refer readers to source materials (as this footnote), to the work of others that has been helpful to us in formulating our ideas, and to work to which readers may wish to turn for additional perspectives or materials.

    The figure of 75,000 entering physicians is drawn from two sources. An analysis of migration figures for the years 1965–1973 was presented in Rosemary Stevens, Louis Wolf Goodman, Stephen Smith Mick, and June G. Darge, "Physician Migration Reexamined," *Science* (1975), *190*: 439–442. These were updated to 1974 by unpublished figures supplied by the U.S. Department of Justice, Immigration and Naturalization Service and by the National Science Foundation.

    Estimates of how many physicians, once here, actually stay in the United States, rely largely on two other studies our research group has undertaken. A follow-up study of a sample of FMG interns and residents in training in Connecticut in 1964 found 67 percent of the sample and 71 percent of those reporting, to be in the United States in 1971–1972, long after training should have been completed. A second study matched the American Medical Association's computer file of all FMGs known to be in specialist training in 1963 with the names of all physicians in the United States in 1971; this produced an estimated "stay-rate" of 75 percent of those reported. For various reasons detailed in the publications these figures cannot be generalized into a numerical probability that, on average, a given FMG entering the United States will stay permanently. Nevertheless, given the general situation we have observed in our series of studies of FMGs over the last seven years, it seems likely that, conservatively, at least half—and probably more than 70 percent—of all FMGs who completed their specialist training in this period elected to remain in the United States. See Rosemary A. Stevens, Louis Wolf Goodman, and Stephen S. Mick, "What Happens to Foreign-Trained Doctors Who Come to the United States?" *Inquiry* (1974), *11*: 112–124; James N. Haug and Rosemary Stevens, "Foreign Medical Graduates in the U.S. in 1963 and 1971," *Inquiry* (1973), *10*: 26–32.

2. For analysis of United States policy making towards physician migration, see Rosemary Stevens and Joan Vermeulen, *Foreign Medical Graduates and American Medicine*, DHEW Publication No. (NIH) 73–325, Washington, D.C., 1972; Thomas D. Dublin, "The Migration of Physicians to the U.S.," *New England Journal of Medicine* (1972), *286*: 870; Betty A. Lockett and Kathleen N. Williams, *Foreign Medical Graduates and Physician Manpower in the United States*, DHEW Publication No. (HRA) 74–30, Washington, D.C., 1974; Joseph G. Wheelan, *Brain Drain: A Study of the Persistent Issue of International Scientific Mobility*, Committee Print prepared for the Subcommittee on National Sec-

urity Policy and Scientific Development of the Committee on Foreign Affairs, U.S. House of Representatives by the Foreign Affairs Division, Library of Congress, Washington, D.C., 1974; Stephen S. Mick, "The Foreign Medical Graduate, *Scientific American* (February 1975), 232: 14.

3. See Edward P. Hutchinson, Ed., "The New Immigration," *The Annals of the American Academy of Political and Social Science* (September 1966), 367; Gregory Henderson, *The Emigration of Highly Skilled Manpower from the Developing Countries*, New York: United Nations Institute for Training and Research (UNITAR), 1970; Judith A. Fortney, "International Migration of Professionals," *Population Studies* (1970), 24: 217.

4. *Historical Statistics of the United States Colonial Times to 1957*, U.S. Department of Justice, Immigration and Naturalization Service, *Annual Report for Fy 1974*, Washington, D.C., 1974, p. 39.

5. Figures on FMGs by country of medical education and as a proportion of all United States physicians can be found in Judith Warner and Phil Aherne, Eds., *Profile of Medical Practice '74*, Center for Health Services Research and Development, American Medical Association, 1974.

6. Notable exceptions are Barbara Harrison, *Foreign Doctors in American Hospitals: A Sociological Analysis of Graduate Medical Education*, Columbia University Ph. D., 1968 (University Microfilms), Ann Arbor, Michigan, 1969; Emily Mumford, *Interns: From Students to Physicians*, Harvard University Press, Cambridge, 1970.

2

WHO COMES TO
THE UNITED STATES? _____

INTRODUCTION

Ordinarily the description of a study group is a cut and dried affair. This is
not so in the case of foreign medical graduates in the United States. First
and foremost, FMGs are not "average" immigrants, if any immigrant
group can be characterized as such. In contrast to immigrants of earlier
periods, the men and women whom we in the United States have labeled
FMGs are distinct in their high educational attainment, their middle to
upper class origins, and their fundamentally voluntary decisions to come
here.

In the case of their educational backgrounds, men and women in this
group have unusually high expectations of what United States society
generally, and graduate education specifically, have to offer them. Their
high expectations are not necessarily fulfilled when they get here, a factor
often leading to disappointment or bitterness.

Their socioeconomic background, often reflecting privileged statuses
in their home societies, suggests that their move into United States

society may be accompanied by some misgivings, given the pace of change here and the breakdown of conventional (and worldwide) distinctions based on gender, race, and religion. More generally, their move into United States society is a move into cultural unknowns with a myriad of status distinctions and other cultural trappings that must be learned from the bottom. Finally, except in a few cases, most FMG migration is voluntary. Few postwar FMGs are political refugees as were pre-World War II physicians.[1]

Not only are most FMGs voluntary participants in this wide-scale immigration, they are men and women in important formative years of their profession. On one hand they are not medical students undergoing the full weight of medical professionalization and socialization; on the other hand, they are not people who have successfully established their professional lives and are merely changing their permanent international addresses. They are physicians in mid-career, half-way through their training, who have willingly subjected themselves to an alien culture and society and have elected to undergo a sometimes impossibly hectic occupational life, a frequently frustrating sense of discrimination, and at times an incomprehensible system of advanced training and service geared to the graduates of its own medical schools.

These themes suggest that it is essential to identify these migrants, to sketch in relief the characteristics of participants in one of the most important immigrant phenomena in United States history, and perhaps among physicians in all history. Besides these historical and intellectual reasons for knowing who these men and women are, there are other more immediate considerations.

Knowing which FMGs come to the United States is important in at least three practical respects. First, such knowledge provides the neccessary context within which to situate the specific findings of our study. The contrasts between FMGs and USMGs establish the sources of the many differences that emerge as both groups progress through the graduate medical educational system. Data from the 42 United States citizens in our study group who went abroad for medical degrees, the so-called United States foreign medical graduates (USFMGs), provide additional comparisons. They act as a "natural" control group, simultaneously having a medical education similar to bona fide FMGs and a familiarity with United States culture and language shared by USMGs.

Second, a description of the study sample enables us to delineate the sheer manpower contributions of FMGs to United States hospitals. Such things as specialty choice, level of training position, and amount of experience prior to entry into the United States hospital system are critical to an understanding of the role FMGs play in the delivery of medical care in hospitals.

Third, knowing who the FMGs are who come to this country sheds light on discussions in progress among health planners about who should and should not come to the United States for graduate medical education. We do not presume to answer this one way or the other; rather, we show that somewhat discrete and separable groups of FMGs are represented in the study cohort and thus, since our sample is representative, in the FMG population. This observation inevitably raises the question, whether one group or another should be subjected to similar restrictions and constraints with respect to United States visa requirements, or enter similar educational programs.

The purpose of this chapter, then, is descriptive. It shows that FMGs are as heterogeneous—different from one another—as USMGs are homogeneous—alike one another. However, despite the variation among groups of FMGs, the gap between USMGs and FMGs reveals a "foreignness" that other researchers have emphasized among exchange students as a group.[2]

CHARACTERISTICS OF THE 1973–1974 HOUSE STAFF COHORT

The 865 physicians were drawn from the total population of physicians in approved house staff positions in 1973–1974. Seven hundred and thirty-two were graduates of foreign medical schools, and 133 received their medical education in the United States. Among the FMGs were 36 native-born United States citizens and six naturalized United States citizens who studied medicine abroad. For the purpose of this study, a naturalized United States citizen is defined as a USFMG (United States foreign medical graduate) when the date of naturalization is prior to entrance to medical school.[3]

Among FMGs, all regions of the world are represented by a total of 73 countries. Table 2.1 compares the combined distribution of FMGs and USFMGs in the study sample with published data from the American Medical Association (AMA). Our sample overrepresents Asian nations by 3.3 percent and underrepresents Middle East and African nations by 2.6 percent. Otherwise the fit of the study sample with an independent population data set is almost perfect. Our ability to generalize is allowed through procedures described in Appendix A; the comparison in Table 2.1 is merely presented to show that our sample is not out of line with published statistics.

Canadian medical graduates are excluded from Table 2.1 because the

TABLE 2.1 SAMPLE AND POPULATION DISTRIBUTIONS OF FMGS AND USFMGS GROUPED BY MAJOR GEO-POLITICAL REGIONS OF THE WORLD[a]

Region	1973–1974 Study sample	AMA data[b] Jan. 31, 1973
United Kingdom, Europe, former Commonwealth Nations	16.2	16.4
Asia, Far East	59.9	56.6
Middle East, Africa	8.6	11.2
Central, North America[c]	5.8	6.3
South America	9.4	9.4
Total	100.0% (716)[d]	100.0% (18,221)

[a] Data include USFMGs (*N* = 42 in our sample), with the exception noted in footnote [c].
[b] Computed from Table 1–c, American Medical Association, *Directory of Approved Residencies, 1974—75*, Chicago.
[c] Excludes 14 Canadian FMGs and 2 USFMGs who went to medical school in Canada.
[d] Percentages are weighted; *N* is unweighted. In this and other tables, percentages may not add to 100.0%, due to rounding.

AMA treats United States and Canadian graduates equally with respect to medical education and graduate work; consequently, Canadian graduates are not included in AMA statistics on FMGs but are added into USMG tabulations.

We take the view, in presenting our data in all other tables, that Canadians, as foreign nationals, are FMGs. USFMGs are not treated separately in AMA statistics; thus, for comparative purposes, we include them among the FMGs only for Table 2.1. USFMGs in our study sample were trained almost exclusively in Western Europe, the United Kingdom, and Canada (92.3 percent), with a few in Central America (6.5 percent) and South America (1.2 percent).

The Asian nations, not suprisingly, given past documentation,[4] contributed the largest proportion of FMGs, with 59.9 percent of the population. They are followed by the United Kingdom, Europe, and former Commonwealth nations like South Africa (16.2 percent), South American nations (9.4 percent), the Near Eastern and African countries (8.6 percent), and Central American and Caribbean nations (5.8 percent). Black

African nations (other than the Arab states) provide less than 1 percent of the total of FMGs in United States house staff positions. The distribution of regional contributions, as well as single-country contributions, is one that has been prevalent for the last decade.

The medical school backgrounds of FMGs and USMGs are alike in that a vast number of medical schools is represented in both groups. The 690 FMGs in our sample attended 229 different medical schools in 73 countries. The 133 USMGs attended 72 medical schools all over the United States. Our sample thus included, on average, about two graduates per United States medical school and three graduates from each represented foreign school.

Ten foreign medical schools located in six countries trained over one-quarter (27.0 percent) of all the 1973–1974 FMG house staff. The largest contributing schools are located in the Philippines, with the Faculty of Medicine and Surgery of the University of Santo Tomas leading the list with 4.1 percent of all house staff. Two other Filipino schools accounted for another 6.6 percent. Iran's Faculty of Medicine of the University of Teheran was the second largest school, with 3.4 percent of the total. India was represented by three schools including the University of Bombay. South Korea's College of Medicine at the National University of Seoul was another major institution of FMG medical education. The largest United States colleges of medicine were the Ohio State University College of Medicine (6.2 percent), Tufts University Medical College (4.6 percent), and Cornell University Medical College (4.0 percent). The statistical similarity of different medical schools between the two groups should not, however, be pushed too far. United States medical schools are generally regarded as relatively uniform, and they certainly are more culturally similar than one would expect the different foreign medical schools to be, underlining once again the cultural diversity among FMGs.

Table 2.2 summarizes personal, familial, and demographic variables used to compare the three groups of medical graduates. On the whole, FMGs come from earlier graduating classes than USMGs. (The USFMGs fall somewhere in between.) Almost four out of five USMGs in house staff training in 1974 graduated between 1970 and 1973; in contrast, only a fourth of the FMGs graduated during the same period. Therefore when one speaks of an FMG house officer, one is usually talking about a person who has been out of medical school at least three years.

FMGs are also older, on average, than USMGs: only 31.2 percent were born in the postwar years (after 1945), whereas over half (53.3 percent) of the USMGs were born during this period. As we see later, most FMGs did not migrate to the United States until at least a year after their medical school graduation, a factor that helps to account for their slightly higher age. This in itself is important because FMGs have spent more time out of medical school in medically related employment, usually the practice of medicine.

Yet another important distinguishing characteristic of FMGs is the proportion of women among their number. At a time in the history of United States medical education when much emphasis is placed on the admission of women into the medical profession, it is interesting to note that female FMGs are twice as numerous, relatively speaking, as female USMGs (15.2 versus 7.2 percent). Although these patterns may change by the late 1970s, as women now in training graduate from United States schools, the addition of FMG women into the supply of physicians has been one of the major ways in which the profession has been "feminized." This change has gone almost unnoticed because most of the attention has centered on the admission of women to United States medical schools and the career problems of women physicians in practice.[5]

Women who are FMGs comprise a group whose characteristics underline the theme of FMG heterogeneity. For example, they come from a concentrated number of countries: Philippines, Thailand, India, Pakistan, and Iran. Over half ($N = 55$) of the 101 women FMGs in our study group graduated from schools in these five countries. Women represented 40 percent of the Filipino FMGs, 36 percent of the Thais, 22 percent of the Indian graduates, 19 percent of the Pakistanis, and 12 percent of the Iranian FMGs.

The majority of these are married women who followed their husbands to the United States. Their careers are characterized by unusual travel, dislocation, and mobility. In contrast to both single and married male FMGs (as well as unmarried female FMGs), whose careers are orderly, predictable, and lacking in extensive international mobility (aside from the trip to the United States), married women appear to have gone through enormous disruptions in their careers. Data in Chapter 4 attest to this when the circumstances surrounding their passing the United States medical qualifying test, the ECFMG examination, are examined. They are characterized by multiple sittings for the exam and the sittings usually taking place in this country rather than the more usual foreign sites. (The ECFMG examination is usually a requirement of a United States visa, but not for migrants who come in as dependents.)

Finally, the women tend to train in different medical specialties. The great majority of the male Filipino graduates, for example, held positions in general surgery and internal medicine in the United States; the great majority of female Filipino graduates were in pediatrics and pathology. In part, the specialty difference reflects a deliberate choice by married women of fields compatible with their husbands' location and/or with

TABLE 2.2 CHARACTERISTICS OF 1973–1974 FOREIGN- AND UNITED STATES-TRAINED HOUSE STAFF

| | Type of medical graduate | | |
Characteristic	FMG	USMG	USFMG
Year of medical school graduation			
1949 and earlier	7.2	1.7	2.4
1950–1964	12.0	—	9.4
1965–1969	54.3	20.3	28.5
1970–1973	26.5	78.0	59.7
Total	100.0% (690)[a]	100.0% (133)	100.0% (42)
Gender			
Male	84.8	92.8	93.5
Female	15.2	7.2	6.5
Total	100.0% (690)	100.0% (133)	100.0% (42)
Size of the community in which the respondent grew up			
Large city (100,000 or more population)	71.8	57.1	72.3
Medium city (10,000 to 99,999)	20.6	27.5	24.1
Town or village	7.2	12.2	3.7
Rural area	0.5	3.2	—
Total	100.0% (685) NA = 5	100.0% (133)	100.0% (41) NA = 1
Mother's education			
Some college or more	26.8	55.6	40.2
High school graduate or less	73.2	44.4	59.8
Total	100.0% (689) NA = 1	100.0% (132) NA = 1	100.0% (42)
Father's education			
Some college or more	50.1	64.7	55.6
High school graduate or less	49.9	35.3	44.4
Total	100.0% (690)	100.0% (133)	100.0% (42)
Mother's occupation			
Professional, administrative	20.0	31.5	24.8
Other	80.0	68.5	75.2
Total	100.0% (687) NA = 3	100.0% (133)	100.0% (42)
Father's occupation			
Professional, administrative	78.2	69.3	65.3
Other	21.8	30.7	34.7
Total	100.0% (687) NA = 3	100.0% (133)	100.0% (41) NA = 1

Table 2.2 (*Continued*)

Characteristic	Type of medical graduate		
	FMG	USMG	USFMG
Relatives who are MDs			
Yes	70.6	42.2	46.7
No	29.4	57.8	53.3
Total	100.0% (686)	100.0% (133)	100.0% (42)
	NA = 4		
Religious affiliation			
Jewish	2.5	22.9	28.4
Roman Catholic	36.6	18.6	47.9
Protestant	9.5	38.0	13.0
Non-Western	32.9	2.4	—
No religion	18.6	18.1	10.7
Total	100.0% (690)	100.0% (129)	100.0% (42)
		NA = 4	
Racial background			
White (light)	18.5	71.4	76.3
White (dark)	17.3	24.1	23.7
Black	3.6	2.8	—
Oriental	34.5	1.7	—
Indian	26.1	1.7	—
Total	100.0% (690)	100.0% (133)	100.0% (42)

[a] Percentages are weighted; *N* is unweighted.

rearing children in a society in which domestic help is unavailable. Thus 14 of the 19 Filipino women in our sample were in the United States with their husbands, and 13 of these women had dependent children. (Eight of the husbands were also physicians; others were accountants, lawyers, and businessmen.)

Typical of the disruptions and complex career patterns of the women physicians is Dr. D, a Filipino graduate married to another Filipino FMG. Dr. D grew up in urban Manila and graduated from medical school in 1969. She took a year off to have a child in the Philippines and then entered private practice there. Dr. D came to the United States in 1972 on a dependent visa and took no work for 16 months after her arrival ("I was just a dependent, I was pregnant, and I was not sure I was going to get a position.") After a while, in her own phrase, she "pulled herself together," adjusted her visa so that she could work, and found a convenient internship. At the time of interview she held a fellowship in pediatrics. The future promises more career changes for Dr. D. She and her husband are planning to return to the Philippines.

Coincidentally, both Dr. D and her husband were included as members of our sample. They typify the relatively simple career pattern of the average male FMG and the relatively complex pattern of the average married female FMG. Thus, in this couple, the male reported no break in his career since medical school; he was a surgical resident at the time of the survey. These differences in the careers of men (and single women) and married women apply to all FMGs irrespective of country of citizenship or education.

We have digressed somewhat on the female FMG, first to underscore the observation that FMGs are extremely varied. Second, we wish to alert the reader that, as a group, FMG women deserve special analysis, and possibly, particular attention from a policy standpoint. If it is true that, as a group, they are here because they have accompanied their husbands, that they enter on visas not commonly used by other FMGs, and that they tend to have children while they are here, often before reentering medicine, then women FMGs constitute a group with unique characteristics that stands outside the usual pool of physician resources. It should be stressed that women physicians who are here as dependents remain relatively unaffected by Federal (immigration) policy on physician supply. Generally, women FMGs tend to be underutilized in United States medicine, and in some respects their existence is totally bypassed.[6]

For both men and women, the FMGs in the survey sample come from backgrounds at least as elitist as those of USMGs. For example, whereas 57.1 percent of the USMGs grew up in large urban areas (more than 100,000 population), 71.8 percent of FMGs were raised in areas as large. USFMGs also tend to come from large metropolitan areas (72.3 percent). Growing up in a large city does not necessarily imply middle- to upper-class origins, but it does suggest that FMGs had more opportunities for acquiring urbane, sophisticated tendencies and tastes—and, perhaps, a disinclination for practice in rural areas. Furthermore, the predominantly urban background of FMGs is associated with other factors that corroborate the hypothesis of FMGs' privileged status.

The educational and occupational attainments of FMGs' parents is one such complex of factors. Although USMGs' mothers had, on the average, higher educational attainment than those of FMGs or USFMGs, paternal educational achievement of USMGs and FMGs showed great similarity (29.5 percent of the USMGs versus 36.3 percent of the FMGs reported fathers with graduate or professional education). In short the FMGs' fathers were an unusually well-educated group, whereas the FMGs' mothers appeared to follow traditional middle-class patterns of a lower educational attainment than males, with a large number involved in housework or the supervision of households. The mothers of USMGs were also more likely than the FMG mothers to hold professional, technical, managerial, and administrative positions. The FMGs' fathers, however, were more highly represented among these latter categories than those of the USMGs or USFMGs.

As a final, yet suggestive note, FMGs had substantially more relatives who were physicians than either group of United States citizens. Seven out of ten FMGs reported other physicians in the family. The FMG appears to be a person steeped in professionalism from the moment he or she is born. Well-educated parents with high positions in society, themselves part of a larger kinship network consisting of at least one physician, provided abundant role models and levels of aspiration probably greater than those available to young United States' men and women in medicine.

Certain attitudes of FMGs regarding medicine reflected a cosmopolitan and scientific outlook. All medical graduates were asked how strongly they agreed with a statement that "medicine is a science which can be practiced anywhere in the world regardless of social or cultural differences." Almost three–fourths of the FMGs strongly agreed with this statement (compared with a fourth of the USMGs). Nearly half of the FMGs agreed strongly with a statement that "medical care can be delivered best by teams of physicians trained in subspecialities"; less than a third of the USMGs expressed such sentiments (Table 2.3). It appears that

TABLE 2.3   ATTITUDES OF HOUSE STAFF TOWARD SELECTED ASPECTS OF MEDICINE

Percentage who agreed "strongly" with these statements	FMG	USMG	USFMG
In general, medicine is a science which can be practiced anywhere in the world regardless of social or cultural differences.	71.3%[a] (685) NA = 5	25.6% (126) NA = 7	48.5% (40) NA = 2
In general, medical care can be delivered best by teams of physicians trained in subspecialties.	49.8% (685) NA = 5	28.3% (125) NA = 8	62.8% (42)

[a] Percentages are weighted; *N* is unweighted.

FMGs see themselves as possessors of a transferrable, acultural body of knowledge and skills. Although they would clearly have interest in expressing such attitudes in an interview conducted in an alien culture where denial might draw into question their right to be here in medical roles, one cannot rule out the possibility that their earliest backgrounds and the act of migrating instilled a sense of medical professionalism more highly developed than that of our own graduates.

The racial background of the medical graduates was frequently difficult to assess. Rather than attempting to force standard categories of racial characteristics on the respondents, we merely coded individuals according to skin color based on the judgments of the interviewers. The result was a five-category scheme consisting of light-skinned Whites, dark-skinned Whites, Blacks, Orientals, and Indians, the latter group encompassing more than those FMGs from India. Even with this gross approximation, it is clear from Table 2.2 that, whereas USMGs and USFMGs were almost exclusively white skinned, the majority of FMGs (64.2 percent) were not. This important difference is discussed in later chapters; it suffices here to underscore yet another differentiating characteristic possessed by FMGs, setting them apart socially from the nearly exclusively white United States-born and/or -trained house officer.

Finally, religious affiliation gives one more clue about the differences among FMGs and the wider differences between FMGs and USMGs. There are very few Jews among FMGs, but they make up large proportions of the USMG and USFMG groups. Roman Catholics constitute the largest single category of FMGs, but the relative size of this religious group is half that for USMGs. On the other hand, nearly half of the USFMGs are Roman Catholic, underlining the ethnic groupings, such as Italian- or Spanish-speaking Americans, from which many USFMGs come. Protestants constitute less than 10 percent of FMGs and only 12 percent of USFMGs, but, not surprisingly, 38 percent of USMGs. Members of non-western religions like Buddhism and Hinduism make up 32.9 percent of declared affiliations of FMGs, only a minor proportion (2.4 percent) for USMGs, and virtually none for USFMGs.

To sum up, the typical USMG in a house staff position in 1974 was a male physician working in a heavily populated state, such as California or New York, or in one of a host of less urbanized, noncoastal areas such as Missouri, Colorado, or Minnesota. He is white, unmarried, and was born between 1945 and 1949. His studies in medical school ended between 1970 and 1973. Most often he was a resident in internal medicine who anticipated joining a private group practice after completing graduate medical education. His home while growing up was probably a large city, although quite a few of his counterparts came from smaller cities spread around the United States; he was Jewish or Protestant. He already possessed one state license to practice medicine, the first of which he probably obtained in California.

This simplistic description is useful as a rough approximation in contrasting the even rougher one that might be constructed for the "average" FMG who, in the first place is an Oriental married male. There is also some chance that she is an unmarried Latin American female. The FMG was most likely found in New York, New Jersey, Illinois, or Massachusetts, usually in large metropolitan areas. The FMG, usually nonwhite, is older than the average USMG and graduated from medical school between 1965 and 1969, an average of four or five years before the USMGs. Before arrival in the United States, the FMG will have had at least 1 year of medical experience of some sort, again making for an important difference between FMG and USMG. Most often, the FMG was a resident in a medical or surgical specialty, but he or she might also have been in a hospital-based specialty like pathology. The FMG has a wide range of preferences for future work, but there is a trend towards academic pursuits of medicine: research and teaching. FMGs typically did not report a United States license to practice medicine; for those who did, it was most likely to have been granted by New York State. Despite the country in which they received the MD degree, FMGs came from the larger cities, had more relatives who were physicians than did USMGs, and were immersed in a professional, medical milieu.

There were also characteristic patterns for the United States citizen educated abroad. The USFMG is a white male, substantially older than either his FMG or USMG counterparts (39 percent were born before 1940). He graduated from a foreign medical school in the years between those of FMGs and USMGs. USFMGs tend to be older on graduation than either of the other groups. When we interviewed them, they had positions in surgery, medicine, and obstetrics-gynecology, and expressed an interest in a career in private group practice, much the same as USMGs. They had about the same proportion of MD relatives as USMGs, but fewer than FMGs. They were predominantly from large urban areas in proportions similar to those of FMGs, but much greater than the average USMG. They also were born in eastern states in the United States and, judging from the original sample of surnames of physicians identified as USFMGs, came predominantly from families with a recent immigrant heritage. Additionally, the USFMG was very likely to have been Roman Catholic or Jewish, and not likely to have been Protestant as was the case with the USMGs.

PATTERNS OF INTERNATIONAL MOBILITY

Aside from the obvious fact that FMGs are "foreigners," stress should be placed on the extent of their geographic mobility. The FMG is necessarily peripatetic, some only to the extent that they migrated from their home countries to the United States; others, veritable nomads, move from one country to another, to the point where one is hard pressed to speak of the "home" country. Minimally, however, mobility is an essential occupational characteristic of many of these men and women. As we shall see, this movement is not random, but patterned in rather clear ways.

The issue of migration is complicated because there are a variety of ways in which migrant physicians can be categorized. Country of birth, country of primary residence, country of medical education, and country of last permanent residence, are valid ways of classifying mobility patterns. For our purposes much is gained by examining FMGs as they move from one point to another, stressing the dynamic view of their career development. Indeed, anticipating a major point in Chapter 3, the progression of an FMG through his or her whole career is a fruitful way of understanding why FMGs come to the United States. This approach contrasts with the more static way of classifying FMGs by trying to single out one major factor associated with patterns of migration, such as where an FMG received medical instruction.

Static explanations can be misleading because they give incomplete information. The country in which a student attends medical school need not be his or her country of birth, or his country of citizenship, Analyzing migration patterns solely by country of medical education (CME) takes no account of the cosmopolitan characteristics of these student populations—as evidenced by mobility before and after graduating. One basic preprofessional form of geographic mobility we sought to understand was the movement—its size and direction—of FMGs from their countries of birth to their countries of medical education. Another was their experience in countries other than the CME before coming to the United States.

We calculate that slightly over 85 percent of all FMGs received their MD degree in the countries in which they were born. Thus, although global mobility of a greater or lesser degree exists for a minority, the great majority of FMGs display geographical stability (within national boundaries) up to the period of medical school graduation.

Mobility after medical school graduation is not extensive and tends, as well, to be confined to a few countries. Many Egyptian, Lebanese, and Cuban medical graduates had lived in other countries before coming to the United States, but medical graduates from countries like the Philippines, Taiwan, Argentina, Thailand and Iran tended to come directly to the United States.

To illustrate and provide some flesh for numbers like these, let us examine three major nations from which a total of 119 of 150 Asian medical graduates originated: Pakistan, the Philippines, and India.

In the cases of the Pakistanis, there was some history of apparent mobility of respondents between Pakistan and India, but this reflected, no doubt, both the proximity of national boundaries and changes in political jurisdictions during the respondents' lives. Altogether, 15 of the mothers and 14 of the fathers of the 31 Pakistani physicians were born in India. Thirteen of the FMGs themselves were born in India, whereas all but one reported growing up in Pakistan, most (22) of them in the largest cities, mainly Lahore and Karachi. International mobility after medical school and before arrival in the United States was limited to eight of the 31 medical graduates. England figures in the mobility patterns exclusively in six cases, and in the other two cases it was one of the countries involved. Only one individual had extensive mobility before coming to the United States: beginning in England, this physician went to Scotland and then Wales for graduate education. He returned to Pakistan and worked as an internist for 5 years and spent the next 6 years as a consulting physician in Libya. He passed the ECFMG examination there and arrived in the United States in 1971 to become at the same time a resident in internal medicine and fellow in cardiology.

This kind of mobility is rare for Pakistani medical graduates. Typically, the mobility consists of the trip to the United States. However, as we noted more generally in an earlier section, the female pattern differed from that of the males. Of the six female Pakistani medical graduates, four came to the United States after sojourns in other countries. This figure represents one-half of those who did experience international mobility other than the trip to the United States.

The picture of international mobility of Filipino medical graduates is much the same. Of the 47 Filipino medical graduates interviewed, every one was born and grew up in the Philippines. Most lived in and around Manila. Even more striking is the fact that none of the 47 reported any international mobility after medical school graduation except the trip to the United States. They were even less inclined to roam around the world than the Pakistanis.

As for the Indians, the impression here, too, is simplicity of movement. Thirty-three of the 41 Indian medical graduates migrated directly to the United States. Of the other eight, five spent some time in England before their entry into the United States; others had gone to Canada, another to Saudi Arabia, and another to Uganda and then Kenya.

In fact, for only a few countries—the People's Republic of China, Cuba, Malaysia, and Peru—were there substantial proportions of medical students who left their homelands for other countries before coming on to the United States. From the perspective of the group of FMGs in the United States, we see that China "lost" all its medical students, Cuba 46.7 percent, Malaysia 87.0 percent, Peru 20 percent. Of these, two—China and Cuba—were socialist societies, and the FMGs essentially constituted a refugee population. Thus, FMGs born in China attended medical school in Taiwan, Cuban refugees went to medical school in Spain.

POSTGRADUATE TRAINING EXPERIENCE

The fact that some FMGs did not migrate directly to the United States raises the issue of what they did prior to their arrival. Actually, the question is germane to all FMGs, regardless of migratory experience, since, as will be seen, some FMGs have had consideration postgraduate experience in their own countries of medical education.

The activities of FMGs between medical school graduation and arrival in the United States have escaped the attention of FMG researchers.[7] As Table 2.4 shows, FMGs had extensive medical training and practice even before coming to the United States. Among FMGs, only 8 percent who were in house-staff positions in 1973–1974 came here immediately after graduation. Over 60 percent had at least 1 year of experience, and nearly 30 percent had a minimum of 2 years. In contrast, the foreign physicians' peer group of USMGs had none of this background.

The roles of foreign medical graduates as they entered their first postgraduate positions are more diverse when compared to the standard

TABLE 2.4   DISTRIBUTION OF FOREIGN MEDICAL TRAINING
EXPERIENCE AMONG FMGS

Years in foreign training and practice	Percentage
None	36.8
One	33.8
Two to four	10.2
Five or more	19.2
Total	100.0% (690)[a]

[a] Percentages are weighted; *N* is unweighted.

pattern of the USMGs' careers. The first position of FMGs was widely distributed across an array of roles, ranging from a high of 51.6 percent who were engaged in internship duties to a low of 1.0 percent in research activity (Table 2.5). Other areas of employment in which FMGs focused their medical training skills included residencies (13.1 percent), military service (11.2 percent), and hospital physician posts (6.7 percent). Five percent were engaged in "other" medical work, and 2.7 percent were involved in employment unrelated to their training. It is entirely possible that many of the FMGs reporting "resident" or "hospital physician" duties were actually engaged in internship-level graduate training.

TABLE 2.5   DISTRIBUTION OF TYPES OF POSITIONS TAKEN BY FOREIGN MEDICAL GRADUATES UPON GRADUATION FROM MEDICAL SCHOOL

Type of position	Percentage
Nonmedical	2.7
Intern	51.6
Resident	13.1
Research, postdoctoral	1.0
Hospital physician	6.8
Medical school faculty	2.2
Private practice	2.7
Student	3.6
Military	11.2
Other	5.0
Total	100.0% (690)[a]

[a] Percentages are weighted; *N* is unweighted.

Of those FMGs who began their first postgraduate activity here, that is, those who came to the United States immediately after medical school graduation, the proportion entering internship positions resembled that of USMGs. Nevertheless, USMGs entered internships in a greater proportion (94.5 percent) than did FMGs (51.6 percent). If the percentage in residencies is added to this, it can be said that almost all United States-educated physicians moved directly from medical school into graduate medical education. USFMGs display an intermediate position, with 74.0 percent entering internships and 8.3 percent entering residencies.

Additionally, USFMGs eschew postgraduate activity outside the United States, reflecting the absence of medical activity by United States citizens abroad. However, no matter where the first position was held, more than 60 percent of each group apparently began their graduate education without a clear idea of future specialty choice. Those who did enter specialties showed similar choices whether they were USMGs, USFMGs, or FMGs. Of all FMGs in their first activity, 36.5 percent declared a specialty area. For USFMGs the figure was 30.8 percent; for USMGs, 31.9 percent. Thus only a minority of the medical graduates rushed immediately into specialty training. Of those who did enter into specialty training, a rough approximation across the various specialty groupings was maintained (Table 2.6). Medical specialties ranked first in all three groups, followed by a unanimous second choice of surgical fields.

TABLE 2.6   SPECIALTY TRAINING OF HOUSE STAFF IN THEIR FIRST POSITION AFTER MEDICAL SCHOOL GRADUATION

Specialty area	FMG	USMG	USFMG
General practice	4.1	0.5	0.0
Medicine	13.4	18.0	10.6
Surgery	7.8	5.0	9.4
Ob-Gyn	1.4	0.5	5.3
Psychiatry	0.5	3.4	0.0
Hospital-based[a]	3.2	2.9	4.1
Pediatrics	0.9	1.7	0.0
Public health	1.9	0.0	0.0
Other specialties	3.3	0.0	1.2
Undetermined/undecided[b]	60.7	68.1	64.5
Nonmedical posts	2.7	0.0	4.7
Total	100.0% (690)[c]	100.0% (133)	100.0% (42)

[a] Anesthesiology, pathology and radiology.
[b] Includes general and rotating internships.
[c] Percentages are weighted; N is unweighted.

After this, the rankings break down somewhat, particularly in the case of general practice (4.1 percent of FMGs and only 0.5 percent of USMGs), but even here a rough correspondence is maintained; for example, 4.1 percent of the USFMGs and 2.9 percent of the USMGs were in hospital-based specialties. It appears that the first move of the newly graduated MDs is largely nonspecialty oriented.

Since we have no data on foreign-educated physicians who did *not* migrate to the United States, it is impossible to tell whether this group differed in specialty choice from those who did migrate. Yet, because the FMGs in our survey chose the same specialty areas as USMGs, we can state that FMGs attracted to the United States follow the established initial preferences for specialty training.

A mere 8 percent of the FMGs came directly from medical school graduation to house-staff positions in this country. Overwhelmingly, migration to the United States begins at least 1 year after medical school graduation. After this, the movement to the United States begins in earnest and is almost complete by the time FMGs begin their third or fourth career activity.

Perhaps the best way to appreciate the statistics on the foreign medical experience of FMGs is to examine the situations of some of the most experienced FMGs, that is, those with 10 or more years between medical school and arrival in the United States.

Take the example of Dr. P., a male Cuban, married with four children, who first entered the United States in May 1968. Prior to his arrival, he spent 19 years in surgical medicine, including an internship and residencies, in a Havana hospital. He entered private practice in the Cuban capital and was also a surgical instructor in a medical school in the same hospital. After his arrival in the United States, he spent several months at the University of Miami medical school training for the ECFMG examination. He passed the examination and spent the next 6 years in a variety of surgical internships and residencies. At the time of the interview, he was in the last stages of a third-year surgical residency.

A critical issue is whether this man's 19 years of experience in surgery proved to be of any value to him in his search for new work or to the host society in its quest for medical manpower. Was it necessary for him to retake internships and residencies? If remedial work was necessary, was a potpourri of residencies the best way to go about it? Whichever hypothesis proves to be true, that is, that his experience was squandered or that fundamental remedial education was necessary, in neither case did there appear to be an appropriate match between this FMG and the graduate education system available.

Less extreme examples are the cases of two Indian FMGs, one of whom came directly to the United States from India and the other indirectly. The first, Dr. F., a male and married pediatrician with two children, was, at the time of the survey, engaged in a pediatric residency in a Connecticut hospital. He entered the United States less than 1 year earlier in July 1973, and graduated from medical school 13 years earlier in 1960. During that period he trained in pediatrics and psychology and taught both subjects at his medical school hospital.

The situation of Dr. T., the second Indian, was somewhat different.

Graduating from medical school in 1962, Dr. T., married with no children, spent time in a rotating internship and residency in surgery in India, then 1 year as a lecturer in anatomy at his medical college. He left India and spent three years in England as a surgical resident and a senior surgical resident in Liverpool. Returning to India, he became a surgical research officer in a Bombay medical college. Only then did he come to the United States. He spent the next two years in surgical residencies and was in a third-year residency in a Philadelphia hospital at the time of the survey.

Both of these men brought a history not only of postgraduate training but also of experiences in teaching and responsibility. When they came to the United States, was this backlog of experience so irrelevant or so poor that they were unable to gain anything more than second-year training positions?

The biographies of 58 additional men and women in our study—people with 10 or more years of experience between medical school and arrival in the United States—show similar patterns. Previous experience was discounted on arrival in the United States system. These portraits suggest the desirability of examining what, indeed, ought to be recognized as "competence" in any future discussions of FMG migration. Is previous experience of medicine "good" or "bad"—or is it, even, to be regarded as irrelevant? The questions are important because, as we see in Chapter 4, FMGs with several years of experience tend to enter on immigrant visas (as permanent residents) more often than as exchange visitors. This means that they have every intention of staying in the United States and should be explicitly included in discussions about permanent additions to the United States manpower pool.

CONCLUSION

The debate about FMG migration has been confusing and confused in part because of a fundamental ambivalence by observers of the United States medical care system. On one hand, there is the feeling that foreigners should not be categorically barred from studying here. There are several reasons behind this. First, such restrictions would be philosophically and politically contrary to the notion of free movement across national boundaries, regardless of background. Second, few argue that the United States should curtail its role in advanced medical education for foreigners who otherwise would get little, if any advanced medical education. On the other hand, there is the feeling that foreign-educated physicians should neither be encouraged to remain permanently in large numbers nor become essential for delivering sub-stantial amounts of medical care. The reasons for these sentiments are complex and the subject of debate, and are discussed in other sections of this book and in other sources.[8]

Whatever the arguments for or against the FMGs' presence in the United States, some of these countervailing positions will probably define criteria to judge who should be encouraged to come to the United States.[9] This assumes that something is known about FMGs who have been and are coming to study and that values can be attributed to the resulting data. Are FMGs coming here who should not come? What are they like? Why do they come? How do they get here? Conversely, are there FMGs who would probably meet criteria of acceptable reasons for study? If so, why did they come and how did they arrive? This chapter demonstrates that FMGs are anything but homogeneous, a point made by many others but which nonetheless is frequently ignored in policy recommendations. FMGs are at once diverse and experienced; a minority are already well traveled. They are, in their social backgrounds and urban up-bringing, not unlike USMGs. They differ from USMGs in cultural background (symbolized by distinctive religious affiliations), in ethnic characteristics (symbolized by skin color), in greater professional experi-ence, and in age.

Attitudinally, too, FMGs and USMGs form different groups. Not only do FMGs take a more "technological" view of medicine than the average USMG, typified in the responses in Table 2.3, FMGs have different professional perspectives.[10] The USMG almost always expects to work in his country of medical education, the United States; his view of the world is both ethnocentric and relatively uncomplicated. The FMG is an island between two cultures. On one hand, there is the culture he or she brings with him and to which he may return; on the other, the United States, to which he has committed his career, at least temporarily. These con-siderations are not irrelevant in attempts to formulate United States policy for the training of foreign students and in considering the role of FMGs as long-term manpower for the United States.

NOTES

1. The composition of immigrant physicians admitted to the United States between 1933 and 1940 was largely Jewish. Of 5056 admitted, 3357 (66 percent) of the physicans were Jewish. Nearly half of the total emigrated from Germany. See David L. Edsall and Tracy J. Putnam, "The Emigré Physician in America, 1941," *Journal of the American Medical Association* (November 29, 1941), *117*: 1881–1888.

2. The social psychological literature contains a number of articles that stress the cultural separateness of foreign students in the United States. See for example, Rose K. Goldsen, Edward A. Suchman, and Robin M. Williams, Jr., "Factors Associated with the Development of Cross-Cultural Social Interaction," *Journal of Social Issues* (1956), 12: 26–32; Simon N. Herman and Erling O. Schild, "The Stranger Group in a Cross-Cultural Situation," *Sociometry* (June 1961), 24: 165–176; Gayle G. Marsh and Jacob L. Halberstam, "Personality Stereotypes of United States and Foreign Medical Residents," *Journal of Social Psychology* (April 1966), 68: 187–196; Erling O. Schild, "The Foreign Student as Stranger, Learning from the Norm of the Host-Culture," *Journal of Social Issues* (1962), 18: 41–54.

3. See Appendix A, pp. 292–295, for a more thorough discussion of the method of measurement employed in this study and for our rationale for using the country of medical education as the critical defining characteristic of foreign-educated physicians.

4. American Medical Association, *Directory of Approved Internships and Residencies*, selected years, contains the most extensive annual analyses of FMG statistics.

5. Some writings on women in medicine include Patricia H. Beshiri, *The Woman Doctor: Her Career in Modern Medicine*, New York: Cowles, 1969; Lillian K. Cartwright, "The Personality and Family Background of a Sample of Women Medical Students at the University of California," *Journal of the American Medical Women's Association* (May 1972), 27: 260–266; Mary A. Fruen, Arthur I. Rothman, and Jan W. Steiner, "Comparison of Characteristics of Male and Female Medical School Applicants," *Journal of Medical Education (February 1974)*, 49: 137–145; Arlene Goldblatt and Phillip B. Goldblatt, "The Status of Women Physicians: A Comparison of USMG Women, USMG Men, and FMGs," *Journal of the American Medical Women's Association* (to appear); Carol Lopate, *Women in Medicine*, Baltimore: Johns Hopkins Press, 1968; Special Report, "Results of Pilot Survey of Household Help Problems of Women Physicians in the United States," *Journal of the American Medical Women's Association* (June 1972), 27: 324–327. Little, if any, reference is made in any of this literature to foreign-educated women physicians.

6. Separate and comparative analyses of the woman FMG, based on this data set, are currently in the planning stages and will be reported in future publications.

7. An exception to this is Joel C. Kleinman, Ursula C. Brandt, and Robert J. Weiss, "Postgraduate Training and Work Experience of Non-ECFMG Certified Physicians in the U.S.," *Medical Care* (March 1975), 13: 205–208.

8. It could be argued that FMGs deprive, if only indirectly, American minority groups of the opportunity to attend United States medical schools. Internships and residencies that might be filled by American minorities, so the argument goes, are taken by FMGs. It is hard to find this a convincing argument, and it is one that appears to use FMGs as scapegoats for the simple reason that there has been an excess of available house staff positions ever since World War II, *despite* the influx of FMGs. The problem of minority admissions rests in the policies and procedures of United States medical schools.

    Others have strenuously argued that FMGs may be less competent than USMGs, and that the health of United States citizens is at undue risk by allowing FMGs to migrate. These and rebuttals are summarized in Aaron Lowin, *FMGs? An Evaluation of Policy-Related Research*, Minneapolis: Interstudy, 1975.

    Another argument is that by relying on FMGs, the United States health care system is unduly postponing the full-scale entry of paraprofessional health workers such as nurse practitioners, nurse midwives, physicians' assistants, and so on. There may be some truth to this; however, since the available research literature suggests that FMGs do little to improve either geographic or specialty maldistributions in the United States, the argument seems somewhat blunted. See, for example, Irene Butter and Richard Schaffner, "Foreign Medical Graduates and Equal Access to Medical Care," *Medical Care* (March–April 1971), 9: 136–141. At least as plausible an argument could be made that (1) legal restraints at the state level, (2) a general reluctance of physicians to employ middle-level professional "substitutes," and (3) increasing conflict among the various paraprofessional groups concerning roles and tasks, indeed, the essence of their professional identity, pose more of a barrier to the effective use of para-professionals than the inflow of FMGs.

9. In the text of the Health Professions Educational Assistance Act of 1976 (P.L. 94–484, Title VI), it appears that those opposed to FMG immigration carried the day. However, a closer reading of the bill leads one to suspect that, either intentionally or accidentally, the section amending the Immigration and Naturalization Act will have less effect than intended in restricting FMG supply. Other provisions of the Act, such as a strengthened National Health Services Corps, as well as processes unrelated to this legislation, such as a possible reduction in available house staff positions, may act to reduce the inflow of FMGs. In any case, none of the legislation with respect to FMGs appears to have attempted to differentiate among FMGs or to take into account their differing needs and skills.

10. Our findings also showed FMGs to be more liberal politically than USMGs, at least with respect to the role of government in providing health services: 77.7 percent of the FMGs agreed "strongly" that government should be responsible for providing medical care for the whole population, as opposed to 47.0 percent of the USMGs. This finding bears out a similar observation by John Colombotos, Corinne Kirchner, and Michael Millman, "Physicians View National Health Insurance: A National Study," *Medical Care* (1975), 13: 369.

3

THE DECISION TO MIGRATE_____

INTRODUCTION: THE PROBLEM

Ever since scholarly and policy-oriented attention has been directed to the reasons for FMG migration, the question, why do FMGs come to the United States? has been treated as obvious, simple-minded, or so complex that only exceedingly detailed and complicated analyses could produce useful knowledge. Simple answers to the question have ranged from "the financial and material benefits available in the United States" to "more specialization." Complicated analyses have not been done. As a result, despite wide interest in the presence of FMGs in the United States, there has been surprisingly little systematic empirical research on why FMGs migrate. Indeed, as one of the few serious analysts of migrant behavior, William A. Glaser, has noted, a "paucity of theory and of systematic research about persons' decisions characterizes the entire field of migration."[1]

Glaser's work has substantially improved the quality of systematic knowledge about elite migration. However, his work specifically excludes physicians, the result of divided constituencies among the international research sponsoring agencies.[2] Thus, although Glaser analyzes more fully than we do the overall pattern of migration throughout professionals' careers, there has been no way of knowing how far, and in what ways, the behavior of physicians is like or unlike that of other professions.

Other studies of migration, particularly the migration of doctors to the United States, have limitations in point of view, since much of the research has stemmed from the interests of organizations concerned with international relations and/or development. These interests typically lead to case studies that focus less on reasons for migration and more on particular structural forces conducive to migration, such as liberal immigration legislation or the availability of employment opportunities.[3] These are not unimportant concerns, but a fuller understanding can only be obtained by building on studies that portray FMGs' responses to multiple social phenomena and by attempting to depict the broad and complex personal process of migration.

Our aim is to develop a more coherent model for understanding the migration of physicians to the United States by focusing on the behavior of migrants and the process of migration, rather than the organization and institutions affecting that behavior. Using a slightly different vocabulary, our approach is to study what happens to members of a particular work group in a situation of given organizational processes and constraints. Most other studies have attempted to model the processes and constraints.

This distinction is of particular importance in looking at the reasons and motivations for physician migration. If one is looking at a worldwide system of interacting forces to explain migration—for example, at the demand for and supply of physicians in the international marketplace or at the relative attractiveness of countries ranked in some order of "development," political stability, and/or other attributes—the resulting study is inevitably one of macrosystems. The individual gets lost in the drama of events, a pawn on a gigantic checkerboard. If, on the other hand, one concentrates on the individual (as we do), on how that individual makes up his or her mind to leave one country and go to another, major events on the worldwide scene may have to be assumed without detailed description. Dr. Fernandez may decide to come to the United States from the Philippines for a host of personal reasons and will clearly not be disinterested in United States immigration policies that may encourage or discourage him from coming. However, the investigator cannot, as a general principle, study at the same time Dr. Fernandez's decision principles and the decision-making processes of the United States Government. Much of the work on why physicians migrate has been a study of the migration system rather than a study of individuals *in* the system. We tread warily over what is virtually new ground by looking at individual decision making in the framework of a personal career.

METAPHORS USED TO DESCRIBE MIGRATION

The principal metaphor used in the literature to describe the migration system is based on an analogy from the physical sciences. This is the "push-pull model." Worldwide migration sounds like a complex system of plumbing, with valves opening and shutting with measurable precision. Stated in its simplest form, a potential migrant is subjected to both "push" and "pull" factors. Push factors are forces in a potential migrant's current locale that push him or her to migrate. Pull factors originate in the country to which the individual is considering migrating and pull the migrant away from his or her current locale. When the combination of push factors and pull factors exert a stronger force on the potential migrant than do factors encouraging the individual to remain in his or her current locale, migration takes place.[4]

It should be noted that this model is not useful for explaining individual migration behavior. It provides no way for assessing when push and pull factors overwhelm the attraction of the current locale, independent of the simple fact of migration. The attraction of the model is that it enables researchers to evaluate reasons for migration in relation to their correspondence to aspects of the country from which a potential migrant is considering migrating or the country to which the potential migrant is considering migrating. Since this convenience is helpful when one is trying to characterize countries with respect to the strength of their push or pull factors, the push-pull model is a model whose main virtue is evaluating the attractiveness of migration locales and the political influence of national policy decisions (e.g., expansion or contraction in the number of medical students).

A very different metaphor is needed to describe the migration behavior of individuals. The model we develop here is that of the career. Everett C. Hughes has pointed out that in a rigidly structured society ". . . a career consists, objectively, of a series of statuses and clearly defined offices. . ." but that, in modern industrial society, ". . . the individual has more latitude for creating his own position or choosing from a number of existing ones."[5] For this study, we conceive of a career as a series of related positions occupied by an individual during his or her lifetime. Some portions of a person's career may follow a rigidly prescribed order, whereas other sections may be linked through individual decisions based on the meaning of specific job opportunities.

Our field studies showed the physician to be an individual attempting to maximize personal benefit and minimize inconvenience when evaluating personal career and migration alternatives. This conception makes the question, to migrate or not to migrate? a permanent question rather than one that is only considered once during a medical career. Indeed, as indicated by the table of contents of this book, we present our data as a natural history of FMG training, beginning, in this chapter, with the decision to migrate and ending with a discussion of the decision to stay in the United States or to return to one's host country. Throughout this natural history we document as a social process the career sequence of deciding to migrate to the United States, obtaining medical training here, and finally leaving the United States or deciding to stay after the training period. We describe this not as a single outcome to be "explained," but as a continuing stream of experience, options, and decisions confronting members of an exceedingly privileged occupational group.

Our examination of the decision to migrate to the United States for advanced medical training requires (1) that we describe the motivations of individual FMGs in making the decision to migrate, (2) that we indicate patterned differences, if any, among groups of these decision makers; for example, whether there are different bases for migration decisions at different stages of a medical career, or if the migration decision has different meanings for FMGs of different national backgrounds or different in other personal respects. We assume that when a migration decision is made by an FMG, it is made within the context of at least the individual's medical career and family situation; that it is made in an attempt to maximize the decision-maker's range of options and to minimize risk and inconvenience; and that migration alternatives were constantly available to these physicians, if only in their country of medical education.

One point must be stressed before we discuss findings drawn from the experience of actual migrants, that is, those who have made the decision to come to the United States and have carried out this decision. In the career of a physician trained outside the United States, it is unusual for him or her actually to migrate to the United States to receive advanced training or to take up medical practice. World Health Organization statistics show that it is highly unusual for more than 5 percent of a nation's stock of physicians to be located in the United States. This indicates that FMGs in the United States are normally a small proportion of physicians trained in their countries of medical education. Conversely, it indicates that the vast majority of physicians trained outside the United States do not migrate to the United States.

However, at least one study has shown that it is normal for such a physician to *consider* migrating to the United States.[6] Alejandro Portes has shown that, in Argentina, whether or not a recent medical school graduate planned to migrate to the United States, virtually all had considered migrating and had substantial knowledge of how to migrate. His respondents (1) knew they "had to take the Council"—pass the ECFMG examination to migrate; (2) knew at least one Argentine-trained physician who had migrated permanently and had discussed the mechanics of migration with that physician, and (3) had detailed knowledge of conditions for work and graduate study in the United States.

Argentina's extremely high proportion of physicians per capita makes it a country for which such findings are more likely than a more physician-scarce country such as Turkey, Peru, or Malaysia. However, Portes' findings are so clear and the structure of medicine and health care so similar in capitalist countries (although the provision of medical care varies)[7] that we feel confident concluding, as stated previously, that it is normal for a physician trained outside the United States to consider migrating to the United States.

If it is normal for a physician to consider migrating to the United States, but highly unusual for a physician actually to migrate, we suspect that there is no single point in a medical career at which a physician decides to come to the United States for advanced medical training.

STAGES IN THE MEDICAL CAREERS OF FOREIGN MEDICAL GRADUATES

The first step in depicting the process of medical migration is the identification of discrete phases in the career for which the migration decision is important. The medical career is not a single continuous process with each succeeding year echoing the experiences of the past.[8] The first-year medical student is different in outlook and experience from the graduate, the first-year intern from the last-year resident, and the younger from the old practitioner. One useful way to view the medical career is to separate it into a series of discrete periods corresponding to the chronological stages through which a physician passes to autonomous medical practitioner. This study focuses on the training received and the services provided by foreign medical graduates during the time they are in the United States for advanced medical training, as interns or residents in the United States health care system; thus our career stages stop at the period of graduate education.

Five stages precede the period of advanced medical training in the United States: (1) the period of time before entering undergraduate medical school, (2) early in undergraduate medical school (the first two years) (3) late in undergraduate medical school, (4) the time period within 1 year of the completion of medical school, and (5) later than 1 year after completing medical school.

The earliest part of a physician's career is divided into these five stages because they reflect different points at which a foreign-trained physician may decide to come to the United States for advanced training. As indicated in Table 3.1, 5 percent of the FMGs in our sample decided to come to the United States before beginning medical school. Thirty-nine percent of the sample decided to come to the United States during medical school. However, most FMGs decided to come to the United States for advanced training after they left medical school, 20 percent within 1 year of completing medical school and an additional 36 percent later than 1 year after medical school.

TABLE 3.1 STAGES IN THE MEDICAL CAREER AND MIGRATION DECISION

	Percentage deciding to come to US
Before medical school	5.1
Medical school (early)	17.0
Medical school (late)	22.1
Within 1 year of completing medical school	19.5
One year or more after medical school	36.2
	100.0 % (685)[a]
	NA = 5

[a] Percentages are weighted; *N* is unweighted.

These stages are indicated because they reflect important decision points regarding the migration of physicians to and from the United States. This periodization is extremely useful for indicating that different individuals in the group come to seemingly similar career decision points at different stages in their own medical careers. One interesting finding contained in Table 3.1, that only 5 percent of FMGs who decide to come to the United States make this decision before entering medical school, indicates that medical education is not generally used as a vehicle for migration. Individuals desiring to migrate do not choose medical school over other career options solely because of its international cachet.

A second important general finding is that, although there is clearly a high point in the timing of the decision to migrate, centering on graduation from medical school, the physicians in our sample made the decision to come to the United States for advanced medical training at points ranging from before beginning medical school to well after the completion of medical school. The finding that physicians can and do decide to migrate at virtually any point in their medical careers indicates that physician migration cannot be discussed in simple terms or explained by a few key factors. In the next section of this chapter, we present a discussion of the motivations for migration in which we treat separately each stage in the medical career presented in Table 3.1.

MIGRATION MOTIVATIONS AT DIFFERENT STAGES OF THE MEDICAL CAREER

Tables 3.2 and 3.3 show the motivations for medical migration at different stages of the medical careers of the FMGs in our sample.[9] Two major reasons for migrating are evident. *The desire for medical specialization in the United States* was of overwhelming predominance at every stage. This reason was cited as the predominant reason for migration by more than 76 percent of our FMG sample.

The attraction of high medical salaries in the United States stands out as the second most important migration motivation and was of roughly equal importance for FMGs migrating at all five career stages.

Although these two reasons are the most important migration motivations reported by our sample of FMGs, the desire for medical specialization in the United States is clearly the most important reason cited. Table 3.2 shows that it was mentioned by fully 10 percent more FMGs than was the attraction of high salaries. Moreover, it was cited as the "most important" migration motivation by 60 percent more respondents than any other motivation. In short, although there are many complex reasons why individual FMGs migrate to the United States, there does exist one overwhelmingly important reason for this migration. Physicians come because they want to be specialists.

A third relatively important factor in all five career stages is *the motivation to leave one's country of medical education because of poor medical employment prospects*. This reason was taken into account by over 50 percent of the FMG sample. Career opportunities in the FMGs' countries of medical education appear to have motivated not only migration decisions made by physicians attempting to practice medicine, but also the decisions made while an FMG had not yet completed medical school.

However, this motivation was far less important than the desire for advanced training or the attraction of high salaries.

Three other factors were of some importance at all five stages and of particular importance for decisions made in one or more stages. *Advice from medical school faculty in the FMG's country of medical education* was particularly important for decisions made early in medical school. Physicians who decided to migrate after medical school were particularly influenced by *the anticipation of missing family and friends* and were also concerned by *political and social problems in their countries of medical education.*

It is not surprising that particular career stages emphasize the importance of certain costs or benefits related to migration decisions. The frequency of contact and persuasive influence of faculty members make their advice particularly salient during the years spent in medical school. Similarly, the importance of family and friendship ties grows with age and career development. Apprehension at the prospect of reestablishing one's family or building a new network of friends increases from one career stage to the next. Political and social problems were felt most by FMGs who decided to migrate more than 1 year after medical school. Such problems were felt more acutely when individuals had moved beyond the training stages of their careers and were attempting to earn a living through the practice of medicine.

Five other reasons discouraging migration and two reasons encouraging migration were identified in our pretest and are reported in the final seven columns of Table 3.2. Although none was of major importance, most proved relatively more important for decisions made at certain stages of the medical career.

The desire to avoid military service was of minimal importance for the sample of FMGs. Only 4 percent attached any importance to it. However, it was most often mentioned during a time at which the physician was not protected by membership in an educational institution—right after medical school.

The other factor encouraging migration was *the feeling that the practice of medicine was restricted in the FMG's country of medical education.* This and *the fear of effectively taking oneself out of the medical job market in one's country of medical education* were more likely to be taken into consideration by FMGs who made the decision to migrate well after medical school. Such factors are more relevant for individuals making their own way in the world than for those whose work lives are structured by a formal institution such as a medical school.

Four other reasons suggested in our pretests reflected antipathetic feelings toward United States culture that might tip the balance in the

TABLE 3.2 MIGRATION MOTIVATIONS AT DIFFERENT STAGES IN MEDICAL CAREER[a]

Stages in medical career	More medical specialization in US	US salaries higher	Separation from friends and family*	Advice from professors in CME[b]	No positions in CME	Political and social problems in CME	Miss CME job market*	Fast pace of life in US*	Competitiveness in US*	English language problems*	Practice restricted in CME	Illegal drug use in US*	Avoid military service in CME	(N)
						(percent)								
Before Medical School	74.0[c]	59.1	31.5	42.5	46.9	22.6	24.3	13.3	5.5	22.1	8.3	5.5	3.9	(34)
Medical School (Early)	82.6	76.4	56.9	70.6	58.8	48.5	36.0	33.2	37.1	24.0	18.3	19.0	3.7	(118)
Medical School (Late)	77.2	69.3	53.7	49.6	49.0	44.8	49.1	41.2	36.7	35.3	20.7	6.9	2.8	(152)

Right After Medical School	76.1	62.3	65.3	53.3	48.8	36.0	30.4	28.0	26.3	20.8	18.2	8.1	6.1	(138)
One year or more After Medical School	73.6	62.8	65.3	53.8	48.4	55.4	48.1	35.0	32.5	30.3	26.8	20.5	3.7	(243)
Total	76.2	66.2	59.5	55.1	50.3	46.6	41.6	33.6	31.7	28.1	19.8	14.0	4.0	(685)
Rank Order	1	2	3	4	5	6	7	8	9	10	11	12	13	

[a] Motivations marked by an asterisk (*) are reasons against coming to United States. Those without an asterisk are reasons for coming to United States.

[b] Country of Medical Education.

[c] Percentages are weighted; N is unweighted.

TABLE 3.3 MIGRATION MOTIVATIONS AT DIFFERENT STAGES IN
MEDICAL CAREER

Stage of medical career at which decided to migrate	Reasons mentioned by more than 50% of sample in order of importance
Before medical school	1)Medical specialization in US (74.0%)[a] 2)US salaries (59.1%)
Medical school (early)	1)Medical specialization in US (82.6%) 2)US salaries (76.4%) 3)Advice from professors (70.6%) 4)No positions, CME[b] (58.8%) 5)Separation from family (56.9%)
Medical school (late)	1)Medical specialization in US (77.2%) 2)US salaries (69.3%) 3)Separation from family (53.7%)
Right after medical school	1)Medical specialization (76.1%) 2)Separation from family (65.3%) 3)US salaries (62.3%) 4)Advice from professors (53.3%)
One year or more after medical school	1)Medical specialization (73.6%) 2)Separation from family (65.3%) 3)US salaries (62.8%) 4)Political and social problems, CME (55.4%) 5)Advice from professors (52.5%)

[a] Percentages are weighted.
[b] Country of Medical Education.

decision to migrate. There were *apprehension at the fast pace of life in the United States, an antipathy to the competitiveness of the United States culture, a fear of having problems because of a lack of English language skills,* and *a fear of the effects of illegal drugs in the United States.*

In fact few FMGs mentioned these reasons as important elements in their decision. Indeed, 60 percent of those who did also reported a desire to stay in the United States to practice medicine. These responses may indicate an understandable concern about life in the United States held by students who lacked experience with the responsibilities of career or family and information about the United States.[10] However, when compared to the other factors, these apprehensions were of little consequence for those who decided to come to the United States.

These findings are summarized in Table 3.3. They show that three motivations were important for decisions made at all stages of the medical career—the desire for more medical specialization, the attraction of higher salaries, and the feeling that medical employment prospects were poor in the FMG's country of medical education.[11] Three other motivations were particularly important for decisions made at certain career stages. Advice from professors was the third most important motivation for decisions made early in medical school. Anxiety over separation from family and friends discouraged migration, especially after the completion of medical school, when it was the second most frequently cited reason. Pressure from political and social conditions in the country of medical education was also important for decisions made later in the medical career.

These findings indicate, in great detail, the nature of the individual decision processes that cause FMGs to come to the United States for advanced training. However, they do not answer the question raised by Portes' study—why, if all FMGs know how to migrate to the United States, do some decide to migrate and others not? Portes notes that "the only type of doctor who looks forward to migrating was one whose devotion to 'good medicine', indifference to social relations, and clear separation of work and non-work roles made the plan to study and locate in the United States even before he had graduated from Medical School."[12] In general, migration was perceived by Portes' sample as a viable but contingent alternative, one that would be carried out only if all hope for opportunities in Argentina was gone.[13] Portes summarizes his findings in a typology of seven responses of Argentine physicians to the possibility of migration:

1. Professionals who do not migrate because they have sufficient opportunity in Argentina.
2. Professionals who do not migrate for nationalistic reasons, who feel that they owe things to their home country (a small number in Portes' study).
3. Professionals who do not migrate because they have hopes that they will do well enough in the future in Argentina (the largest number in Portes' study).
4. Professionals who, for idiosyncratic reasons, cannot migrate even though they would like to.
5. Professionals who abandon the country because they cannot make

a minimal living there (what Portes calls migration based on absolute survival).

6.   Professionals who abandon the country because they cannot live as well as they would like to (what Portes calls migration for relative survival).

7.   Professionals who abandon the country to practice medicine with pay and work conditions that he or she deem personally appropriate (what Portes calls migration based on occupational realization).[14]

Although this typology was developed to describe permanent migration decisions, it puts our findings in a larger context. Most of our sample fall into Portes' seventh category with respect to their initial decision to come to the United States.[15] The "more appropriate conditions" sought by members of our sample were indicated by the motivations at different career decision points summarized in Table 3.3.

The clustering of our respondents in the category labeled "occupational realization" derives from the more tentative nature of the decision to seek advanced specialist training, compared to the decision to migrate to practice medicine. Futhermore, Portes' findings are similar to ours in that they indicate that coming to the United States for advanced training is one of many alternatives confronting FMGs and that the great majority of FMGs do not automatically link this decision with the intention to migrate permanently to the United States.

THE COUNTRY OF MEDICAL EDUCATION AND THE DECISION TO MIGRATE

Although migration is inherently an individual decision, the migration decision is also patterned by the nature of the country in which the FMG received medical education. Table 3.4 indicates that Western European countries have substantially more "early deciders" (i.e., FMGs deciding to come to the United States before medical school). Eastern Europeans, Central Americans and Caribbeans, and Asians constituted most of the "late deciders." FMGs from South America and the Near and Middle East were most likely to decide to migrate while in medical school. Although these data are inherently interesting, their main function here is to summarize the fact of a relationship between an FMG's country of medical education and the migration decision. This relationship can be examined more meaningfully when one analyzes the migration motivations for FMGs from distinct nations.

TABLE 3.4   STAGE IN MEDICAL CAREER OF MIGRATION DECISION FOR
DIFFERENT REGIONS OF THE WORLD (PERCENTAGE DECIDING)

	Before medical school	Early medical school	Late medical school	Right after medical school	Year or more after medical school	Total	N
Western Europe Canada and S. Africa	15.9	20.4	25.5	20.4	17.8	100.0	(110)[a]
Eastern Europe	11.4	22.6	15.9	9.1	41.0	100.0	(27)
South America	4.5	20.4	33.4	13.5	28.2	100.0	(95)
Central America and Caribbean	2.2	14.2	20.8	14.1	48.7	100.0	(56)
Near and Middle East	8.9	29.6	23.1	9.6	28.8	100.0	(82)
Asia and Far East	3.3	13.7	20.0	21.2	41.8	100.0	(307)
Total	6.4	18.0	23.0	17.5	34.9	100.0	(677)
							NA = 13

[a] Percentages are weighted; *N* is unweighted.

Although there are many dimensions on which one can compare nations, one global characterization is most relevant for an analysis of individual decisions. This is *the range of options* open to a physician as a result of receiving a medical education in a given nation. This refers both to the career alternatives open in a physician's country of medical education and the alternatives available to the physician in other nations.

This dimension is difficult to measure with precision, because, for each individual and country of medical education, it is determined by a wide variety of attributes. Medical career options within an FMG's country of medical education are strongly influenced by the effective demand for physicians in that country and whether political and social conditions there make a professional life style satisfactory. A low demand for physicians and a difficult political situation limit options, because they make the practice of medicine difficult. Three attributes that affect options outside an FMG's country of medical education are worldwide perceptions of the quality of medical training in that country, whether the country's culture is Western or non-Western, and whether English is the national language. FMGs trained in Western, English-speaking nations reputed to have excellent medical schools probably have the most options outside their country of medical education.

In table 3.5, 15 countries, beginning with Western Germany and ending with Cuba, are ordered to reflect, in a crude fashion, our judgment of the range of options open to the medical graduates of each of these countries. The countries represent the 15 nations that, in 1974, had the most medical graduates serving as interns or residents in United States-approved training hospitals. Graduates of West German medical schools are presumed to have more options than those of Spanish medical schools, who in turn have more options than those of Colombian medical schools, and so on. In the analysis that follows, the data for each country are analyzed separately in the order of the rows of Table 3.5.

West Germany

Compared to FMGs from other nations, West Germans were not overwhelmingly motivated by any particular reason for coming to the United States. Their only major concerns regarding migration reported in Table 3.5 were anxiety over separation from family and friends and concern over missing the job market in West Germany. West German-trained FMGs were not motivated by a desire for more medical specialization or the attraction of high salaries in the United States, as were the great majority of physicians from other nations. Presented with an open-ended question, four of the seven West Germans indicated that a desire to travel and "see the United States" was an important reason for migrating. FMGs of no other nation gave similar responses. As a supplier of foreign medical graduates to the United States medical system, West Germany represents an extreme case. Not only do its physicians return home in disproportionate numbers, but they are also not motivated to come to the United States for reasons that resemble those of FMGs of other nations. Their reasons are highly personal, and they are not pressured by a lack of opportunity either at home or in other nations.

Spain

Spanish FMGs as a whole were mildly attracted to the United States for its opportunities for medical specialization and higher salaries. Similarly, other migration motivations, such as advice from professors, a lack of positions, and political and social problems, were relatively less important for Spanish FMGs than for those of all other nations except West Germany. Spanish FMGs also showed little concern over separation from friends and family or missing the job market in their country of medical education. The only responses that were higher than average indicated a concern over restrictions on practice in Spain and a desire to avoid military service there.

One reason for this curious set of responses is that Spain is a training nation for Spanish speakers of other nations. Seven of the 15 physicians educated in Spain had actually been born in Cuba. The result is that the aggregate statistics presented in Table 3.5 for Spain are somewhat artifactual. Although the responses of the Cubans trained in Spain are not identical to those of Cubans who come to the United States directly from Cuba (reported in row 15 of Table 3.5), they were different from those of the Spanish nationals, whose responses were closer to those of the West German that those of any other nation. None of the Spaniards reported that they had come to the United States for touristic reasons. Their responses did follow the general pattern, although the proportions of physicians indicating given reasons were low. Opportunities for Spanish nationals, although not as good as those for West German nationals, were substantially higher both within and outside of Spain than they were for individuals trained in the other nations reported in Table 3.5.

Colombia and Peru

Colombia and Peru are both middle-sized Latin American countries. Neither has been characterized by marked urban political unrest or violence in the last 15 years, although Colombia has an earlier history of extreme rural violence, and Peru's rural areas, until recent years, have been dominated by an autocratic oligarchy. Physicians from both these countries came to the United States with a desire for advanced medical training and because of the attraction of higher salaries. In making the decision to migrate, physicians from both countries were influenced by advice from medical school professors and feared missing out on job opportunities at home while they were in the United States.

The migration motivations of physicians trained in these two nations appear to be straightforward. Both groups were influenced by medical school professors and sought advanced training and higher salaries. Although concerned about separation from family and friends and the job market in their countries of medical education, they were not overly apprehensive about American culture. The only important difference between the two countries is that 80 percent of Peruvian FMGs were influenced by a lack of positions in their country of medical education, whereas this factor influenced only 20 percent of Colombian FMGs.

These two cases are important comparisons for the Middle Eastern and Asian countries discussed later. They are useful because, of all the Western countries that provide substantial numbers of FMGs to the United States medical system, they are most similar to these Asian and Middle Eastern nations, in terms of level of socioeconomic development. This is

TABLE 3.5 MIGRATION MOTIVATIONS OF FMGS FROM DIFFERENT COUNTRIES OF MEDICAL EDUCATION

(percent)

	More medical specialization in US	US salaries higher	Separation from friends/family*	Advice from professor in CME	No positions in CME	Political and social problems in CME	Miss CME job market*	Fast pace of life in US*	Competitiveness in US*	English language problems*	Practice restricted in CME	Illegal drug use in US*	Avoid military service in CME
West Germany	24.1[a]	6.0	54.6	12.1	27.3	6.0	48.6	6.0	12.1	0.0	6.0	6.0	0.0
Spain	55.8	57.1	28.6	24.6	33.7	19.5	28.6	37.7	10.3	5.9	23.4	2.6	9.1
Colombia	88.3	74.5	52.9	96.1	19.6	51.0	66.7	23.5	11.7	2.3	0.0	7.8	3.9
Peru	75.0	70.5	79.5	84.1	79.5	34.1	59.1	13.6	33.4	34.1	0.0	4.5	0.0
Argentina	79.2	75.0	86.2	41.6	55.5	50.1	70.1	30.6	25.0	47.2	34.8	5.5	0.0
Brazil	68.6	55.7	71.4	74.3	47.2	28.6	28.6	47.2	18.6	47.2	28.6	10.7	0.0

United Kingdom	31.0	79.4	62.1	31.0	79.4	31.0	37.9	0.0	24.2	0.0	37.9	24.2	0.0
Thailand	90.5	82.0	50.6	69.0	64.3	74.4	22.0	27.3	26.1	40.4	15.5	11.4	5.4
Philippines	91.6	82.2	53.3	47.7	51.4	40.8	27.2	29.0	34.6	3.8	7.5	13.1	5.6
Egypt-UAR	84.2	57.9	61.4	22.8	45.6	57.9	31.6	50.9	35.1	7.0	30.1	15.8	0.0
Iran	80.7	53.4	71.4	62.6	59.0	37.9	42.2	37.7	41.1	34.1	10.5	13.7	5.6
Taiwan	87.9	72.8	61.9	73.2	78.7	65.3	37.4	38.9	46.8	59.8	14.6	19.2	11.3
South Korea	78.5	82.2	64.2	88.7	33.2	60.0	60.0	26.8	63.6	80.0	21.6	16.8	6.8
India	76.3	73.2	62.5	42.6	40.6	47.0	51.5	41.6	32.7	5.8	21.6	23.1	0.0
Cuba	34.4	34.4	62.6	34.6	0.0	100.0	12.5	0.0	6.2	18.7	87.5	22.0	12.5
All FMGs	76.2	66.2	59.5	55.1	50.3	46.6	41.0	33.6	31.7	28.1	19.8	14.0	4.0

Motivations marked by an asterisk (*) are reasons against coming to the United States. Those without an asterisk are reasons for coming to the United States.

[a] Percentages are weighted.

important because, despite similarities in levels of development, the cultural differences between the Western and non-Western nations limit the opportunities of physicians trained in non-Western nations.

Argentina

Argentina, a large nation in South America, has a ratio of physicians per capita even higher than that of the United States.[16] Among Latin American nations, Argentina has been at a relatively high level of development for the past 30 years, but it has not developed at high rates in recent years. The desire for more medical specialization and higher salaries attracted Argentine physicians as they did FMGs of most other nations. However, Argentine–trained physicians were more anxious than those of any other nation about their separation from their country of medical education, reporting the highest levels of anxiety over separation from family and friends and missing the job market in their country of medical education of any group of FMGs. Argentine physicians also reported slightly above average motivations for migration because of a lack of positions, political and social problems, and restrictions on medical practice in Argentina.

Argentine physicians are handicapped because of a lack of opportunities to practice in their country of medical education. However, they are probably favored because Argentina's situation as a Western nation makes it relatively easy for these physicians to assimilate in the United States, and because the quality of training in Argentina is generally perceived as adequate by physicians in the United States.

Argentine physicians do, however, have one very important characteristic that is discussed in greater detail for other countries, that is, they are in a double bind in making their career decisions. In this case, the double bind is the tension between not wanting to leave their country of medical education and feeling at the same time that it is difficult to practice medicine there. Physicians may be simultaneously attracted by some conditions in the United States while they are "turned off" by other elements, and repulsed by their country of medical education, while preferring to stay there. Although this double bind is not as strong for Argentine-trained FMGs as it is for FMGs from a nation such as South Korea, the process is clear. In contrast to physicians from non-Western cultures and the United Kingdom, Argentine-trained FMGs are not, however, markedly repulsed by the culture of the United States. (This is indicated by lower than average responses to concerns over the fast pace of life in the United States, competitiveness in the United States, and illegal drug use in the United States).

Brazil

Brazil is also a large country in Latin America. However, in contrast to Argentina, its national prestige and economic growth were rapid in the 10 years before our survey was conducted. The result is that Brazilian responses are similar to those of the Argentines but with somewhat less concern about a lack of positions and political and social problems in the country of medical education. Of all Latin FMGs, Brazilians seemed least attracted by United States salaries and medical specialization opportunities. This may be due, in part, to the nationalistic self-confidence generated by recent economic growth in Brazil and the burgeoning opportunities for medical practice there. However, career opportunities are not quite as broad as they are for West Germans. Overall, concerns reported by Brazilian-trained FMGs are more similar to those of other Latin-trained physicians than to those of European-trained physicians.

The United Kingdom

The pattern of responses given by FMGs trained in the United Kingdom is different from those of any other national group. This is the only group for whom the attraction of salaries in the United States was the most frequently mentioned migration motivation. United Kingdom-trained physicians attributed more importance to the attraction of high salaries, a lack of desirable positions at home, and restrictions on medical practice in their countries of medical education than any other national group (except for the Cubans, who reported more restrictions). It is fair to say that, compared to other groups of FMGs, United Kingdom-trained physicians came to the United States because of a perceived lack of career opportunities in their country of medical education.

A desire for medical specialization, advice from professors, and pressure from political and social problems were all markedly less important for United Kingdom-trained physicians than for other groups. FMGs from other nations usually indicated a desire for medical specialization as the most important migration motivation, with the attraction of high salaries second in importance. The relative unimportance of a desire for a greater medical specialization as a migration motivation makes United Kingdom-trained physicians distinct from all other principal suppliers of FMGs to the United States medical system. FMGs of other nations have two strong positive reasons for coming to the United States—increased medical specialization and higher salaries; United Kingdom-trained physicians had only one strong positive reason—the attraction of higher salaries. When the United Kingdom-trained physicians were confronted

with the decision of whether to return home after completing their training, earnings opportunities in the United States, combined with their
reaction to United States culture and their view of their home country as
presenting few opportunities, created a continuing tension.

Asian and Middle Eastern Countries

Seven Asian and Middle Eastern countries are listed in Table 3.5: Thailand, the Philippines, Egypt, Iran, Taiwan, South Korea, and India. Table
3.4 indicates that Asian FMGs tend to decide late in their careers to
migrate, whereas Middle Eastern FMGs tend to decide during medical
school. However, in terms of migration motivations, one can see broad
similarities among the migration motivations reported by the FMGs of the
seven nations. Compared to FMGs trained in other nations, these FMGs
attach greater importance to coming to the United States for more medical
specialization, and higher salaries, and are simultaneously more negative
about United States culture. They are apprehensive about the fast pace of
life in the United States, competitiveness in the United States, and the
illegal use of drugs in the United States (and for those who did not receive
medical training in English, they are apprehensive about language problems in the United States). Furthermore, they are somewhat negative
about their countries of medical education. Their response rates are
among the highest mentioning lack of positions in their countries of
medical education, political and social problems, and restrictions on
medical practice.

There are, of course, differences among these seven groups. FMGs
from Thailand and the Philippines tend to be more positive than FMGs
from the other five nations about obtaining medical specialization and
higher salaries, and they also appear to be less negative about United
States culture. South Koreans were in great conflict, because they were
highly motivated by the attraction of higher salaries and advice from
medical school professors, yet were concerned about competitiveness in
the United States and language problems. Taiwanese FMGs were highly
motivated by their perception of a lack of job opportunities in their
country of medical education. Iranians were relatively untroubled by
political and social problems or by restrictions on medical practice in their
country of medical education. Egyptians and Indians, because of their
English language medical training, did not exhibit language-based
anxieties, but reported the other concerns indicated by other Middle
Eastern and Asian FMGs.

In varying degrees, physicians from these nations are caught in the
double bind that we began to discuss previously. They see problems in

their countries of medical education, although they, like FMGs from all nations, express much anxiety over separation from family and friends; they are unusually attracted (perhaps as a result of perceived political and social problems in their country of medical education) to the opportunities for medical specialization and higher salaries in the United States. However, they were all trained in non-Western nations, and, perhaps because of differences between their cultural background and the Western culture of the United States, they express more concern about American culture than do other FMGs. We have already mentioned this double bind in a less extreme fashion in the cases of FMGs trained in the United Kingdom and Argentina. However, because of the apparent alienation of a substantial portion of Asian and Middle Eastern FMGs from United States culture, the bind of being attracted by professional advantages of the United States while simultaneously desiring contact with family members, yet despairing over professional opportunities in the country of medical education, is greatly exacerbated by this alienation from United States culture. This tension is not only in the minds of these FMGs but has great consequences for their lives in the United States, and for the way non-Western FMGs interact and learn within hospital settings.

To summarize, Asian and Middle Eastern-trained FMGs who come to the United States are not attracted by professional opportunities that are presented in their country of medical education and are greatly attracted by those of the United States, but a substantial portion of the Asian FMGs are simultaneously alienated from United States culture and lament a loss of contact with family and friends at home.

Cuba

FMGs trained in Cuba provided an extreme set of responses that are different from those of any other nation that has contributed substantial numbers of physicians to the United States medical system. The only other group that reported a similar pattern of responses were physicians who had been trained in Eastern European nations. Since both these and the Cubans tend to be political refugees, they gave substantial importance to political and social problems in their country of medical education and restrictions on medical practice in their country of medical education as motivations for migration. These reasons overwhelm all other motivations.

In terms of opportunities, the situation for Cuban FMGs is dramatically clear-cut. Having decided to leave Cuba and come to the United States, they saw absolutely no remaining opportunities for them in their country of medical education. Furthermore, the United States has extended unusual opportunities to Cubans leaving their homeland.[17] Other nations have not extended similar opportunities to Cubans. Therefore, opportunities for Cubans outside the United States were extremely limited, and they were promising in the United States. The patterns of responses of Cubans are unambiguous: FMGs trained in Cuba indicate their strong intention to stay in the United States and continue the practice of medicine here.

CONCLUSION

The decision to migrate to the United States for advanced medical training is not a one-shot decision. The option of migrating to the United States is an early and continuous consideration for many physicians, and physicians who do decide to come to the United States for advanced training do not make this decision at any single career point. The responses of the FMGs in our sample indicate that the decision to come to the United States for advanced medical training is not a single-minded and eager effort to leave one's country of medical education and come to the United States. Rather it is usually a reluctant decision to leave one's country of origin and family and friends in the face of professional frustration. When this decision is made, the primary motivation for coming to the United States is to obtain increased medical specialization. However, other considerations, such as the attraction of higher salaries in the United States, advice from medical school professors, and pressure from political and social problems, are also important.

Most physicians trained outside the United States consider migrating to the United States as one alternative among many. In varying degrees, these physicians make continual calculations regarding the frustrations and benefits of coming to the United States, and a relatively small number of physicians actually make the decision to migrate.

Once this decision has been made—and it is a highly individual decision despite the fact that there are relatively clear-cut patterns for FMGs trained in different nations—a new set of forces begin to act. The physician trained in the United States is subject to continuing conflicts. Ultimately this individual must decide whether to return to his or her country of medical education or stay in the United States to continue the fulltime practice of medicine.

NOTES

1. William A. Glaser, *The Migration and Return of Professionals*, New York: Bureau of Applied Social Research, Columbia, 1973, p 5.
2. Glaser's study did not include health professionals because his sponsor, The United Nations, has commissioned the World Health Organization to prepare a separate multinational study of migratory behavior of all classes of medical personnel: technicians, nurses, and physicians. The first results of this latter project are *Multinational Study of the International Migration of Physicians and Nurses: Analytical Review of the Literature*, Geneva: World Health Organization, HMD/75.7, 1975, and *Multinational Study of the International Migration of Physicians and Nurses: Country Specific Migration Statistics*, Geneva: World Health Organization HMD/76.4, 1976.
3. Examples are Pan American Health Organization, *Migration of Health Personnel and Engineers from Latin America*, Washington, D.C., 1966; S. Watanabe, "The Brain Drain from Developing to Developed Countries," *International Labour Review* (1969), *99*: 401–433; Committee on the International Migration of Talent, *The International Migration of High-level Manpower, its Impact on the Development Process*, New York: Education and World Affairs, 1970; Gregory Henderson, *The Emigration of Highly Skilled Manpower from the Developing Countries*, New York: United Nations, 1970; and United Nations Institute for Training and Research (UNITAR), *The Brain Drain from Five Developing Countries*, New York: United Nations, 1971.
4. For discussions of migration theory, see Donald Bugue, *Principles of Demography*, New York: Wiley, 1969, pp. 752–756. Also see Everett S. Lee, "A Theory of Migration," *Demography* (1966), *3*: 47–57, and Gregory Henderson, *The Emigration of Highly Skilled Manpower from the Developing Countries*, New York: United Nations Institute for Training and Research, 1970. For a critique of migration theory, see J. A. Jackson, ed., *Migration*, Cambridge: The University Press, 1969.
5. Everett C. Hughes, "Institutional Order and the Person," *American Journal of Sociology* (1937), *43*: 404–413.
6. Statistics on percentages of nations' medical graduates who migrate may be found in *World Health Statistics, Annual 1971*, Vol. III, Geneva: World Health Organization, 1975. Evidence that most physicians, at least in Argentina, consider migrating is found in Alejandro Portes, "Psicología Social de la Emigración," Buenos Aires: Instituto Torcuato Di Tella, 1973 (mimeo). Portes studied two paired samples of 60 recent graduates of Argentina medical schools—one sample had taken the ECFMG examination and the other had not—to learn about migration motivations.
7. Discussions of the structure and functioning of health care systems in capitalist countries may be found in The World Bank', *Health Sector*, Policy Paper, Washington, D.C., 1975, and John Bryant, *Health and the Developing World*, Ithaca, N.Y.: Cornell University Press, 1969.
8. The staged nature of medical careers and medical training in the United States has been described by writers such as Oswald Hall in "The Stages of a Medical Career," *American Journal of Sociology* 53 (1948), *53*: 327–336, and Howard S. Becker, Blanche Geer, Everett C. Hughes, and Anselm Strauss, *Boys in White: Student Culture in Medical School*, Chicago: University of Chicago Press, 1961.
9. Table 3.2 gives 65 measures—one for each of the 13 migration measures for each of the five career stages (these are the first five rows). Row 6 in each gives an overall measure for each of the 13 motivations. Row 7 indicates the rank order of importance for each

motivation. Table 3.3 shows, in order of importance for each of the five career stages, reasons mentioned by more than 50 percent of the sample.

10.   This is not to say that certain groups of FMGs do not feel a deep antipathy for United States culture. This is discussed in Chapters 10 and 11.

11.   Although this third motivation appears only once in Table 3.3., Table 3.2 shows that it was taken into account in between 45 and 60 percent of the decisions made in all five stages.

12.   Portes, *op. cit.*, p. 18.

13.   Portes goes on to say, however, that one should be careful not to generalize these attitudes to physicians trained in nations in which a high proportion of medical graduates migrate such as the Philippines, Taiwan, Nicaragua, Haiti, or the Dominican Republic. Nevertheless, a study carried out in the Philippines seems to indicate a similar pattern there. (See Cristina P. Parel, "A Survey of Foreign Professionals and their Employers in the Philippines," in Philippine Social Science Council, *Social Science Information*, January 1975, p. 11).

14.   Portes, *op. cit.*, pp. 31–34.

15.   As is discussed in Chapter 11, a considerable number eventually decide to stay in the United States for reasons similar to those in Portes' fifth and sixth categories.

16.   In 1971, Argentina had 620 inhabitants per physician, whereas the United States had 530. (*World Health Statistics, Annual 1971*, Vol. III, Geneva: World Health Organization, 1975).

17.   See Chapter 4 for a discussion of the United States' preferential treatment of Cuban refugees.

4

THE MECHANICS OF
MIGRATION_____

Whatever the strength of the aggregated desires of individual physicians to come to the United States, the actual inflow of physicians is controlled by important regulatory mechanisms. In the language of the stereotypical push-pull model of migration, these might be thought of as the "valves" or "faucets" of the system. In the language of social scientists, they might be called structural forces, those outside the control of the individual, exogenous in nature.

Our study focuses on a group of FMGs who have successfully hurdled a number of inhibiting mechanisms. These include, among others, (1) obtaining exit visas and posting financial bonds, where these exist, in foreign nations, (2) passing the examination administered by the United States-based Educational Commission for Foreign Medical Graduates (ECFMG), (3) acquiring a United States entry visa, and (4) finding a position in this country. In this chapter, we focus on two of these, the ECFMG examination and United States immigration policy.

For individual FMGs these two regulatory processes provide potential barriers to entry into the United States. Our findings show that successful

FMGs are those who can "play" both systems. The most important element in success appears to be *arrival* in the United States. Once here, irrespective of the type of visa or possession of an ECFMG certificate, the successful FMG has, up to now, been able to convert to the appropriate status. In these games, FMGs show considerable finesse, sophistication, and success: doctors may be among the most adroit immigrants the United States has experienced.

From our analysis of the behavior and activities of the individual FMGs, we are also in a position to comment on the operation and outcome of this nation's past and current policy to regulate two attributes of highly skilled immigrant inflow: quantity and quality. Quantity or numbers of FMGs are affected by immigration statutes and policy; quality, that is, how well trained and competent FMGs are as house officers is presumably affected by the screening examination of the ECFMG. This is extremely important because the ECFMG has been the major attempt by professional medicine to control the quality of foreign physicians in the United States, and because similar questions arise with the new Visa Qualifying Examination, a "second generation" test designed to replace the ECFMG.

Finally, the interaction of these mechanisms is examined and discussed as an overall "system of entry," which returns us full circle to the way individuals cope with the problems of arriving and remaining in the United States.

VISA CATEGORIES

Physicians come to the United States on three types of visas.[1] The permanent resident or "immigrant" visa is the one that accords a foreign national the most security once he enters this country. It is a prerequisite for naturalization and is often required by state licensing boards for licensure. It is regarded as a permanent or long-term status and permits foreign nationals to work for a living in this country. With the enactment of the Immigration Act of 1965, which abolished a long-standing system of quotas based on national origin, immigrants from the Western Hemisphere could come on this visa on a first-come, first-served basis until a general ceiling of 120,000 was reached. The ceiling for immigrants from outside the Western Hemisphere was set at 170,000, with no single country permitted to surpass a limit of 20,000.

A second visa is the exchange visitor or "J-visa," one of a larger class of nonimmigrant visas. It is numerically the most important in this category and rivals the permanent resident immigrant visa in volume.[2] It is a special status, however, created to promote educational exchange through enactment of legislation in the postwar period. Its provisions allow individuals to come to the United States for periods of training in advanced studies, including graduate medical education, until these studies are completed. At that point, the student is, in theory, expected to return home. However, through a variety of mechanisms added later, including one that permitted exchange visitors to convert to permanent resident status without having to leave the United States, the exchange visitor visa has provided thousands of FMGs the opportunity to remain here for indefinite periods of time. Visa regulations have been tightened (under Public Law 94–484) since our study was undertaken in 1974, in an attempt to make it more difficult for exchange visitors to enter the United States or to remain, but the effects of such restrictions are not yet clear. It is particularly timely, therefore, to look at exchange visitors who entered before the restrictions, to see in what ways they differ from entrants on other kinds of visa.

The third visa is actually the residual group of nonimmigrant visas such as student visas, visitor or tourist visas, and others. These, too, are temporary in nature and are usually linked with special status. In numbers, these visas play only a minor role in the immigration of alien physicians.

THE VISA GAME

What visas did the 1973–1974 cohort hold when they entered the United States? A little over one-quarter (26.3 percent) held permanent resident immigrant visas, and slightly less than two-thirds (64.2 percent) entered on exchange visitor visas. The remaining 9.5 percent entered on a variety of nonimmigrant visas. Thus, by a two-to-one margin, FMGs used the J-visa status to enter this country, reflecting in part the ease with which this visa could be obtained, as well as the relative uncertainty of their future plans to stay in the United States.

It is important to ask whether these collective choices of visa status are made with any underlying patterns. Do FMGs arrive in the United States as an undifferentiated mass of men and women who will take whatever visa status they can just to get here? The answer to this may, in part, be seen by inspection of Table 4.1. In Chapter 3 we discussed the importance of the time at which the decision was made to come to the United States and its correlation with the kinds of reasons offered for making the move. Here we see a further elaboration of this complex of factors surrounding the decision-making process: the timing of the decision is associated with the type of visa held on entry to the United States. For those FMGs deciding well out of medical school, the tendency to come on immigrant visa status is over 11 percent greater than the overall average. In contrast, FMGs deciding at earlier stages—during or right after medical school—show a greater preference not only for J-exchange visitor visas but also for other nonimmigrant visas. Moreover, the group of "late deciders" tends to cite substantially different reasons for coming to the United States.

TABLE 4.1   VISA STATUS AT ENTRY INTO THE UNITED STATES BY WHEN THE MIGRATION DECISION WAS MADE

When the migration decision was made	Visa at entry			
	Immigrant	Nonimmigrant		
	Permanent resident	Exchange visitor	Other	Total
Before medical school	14.3	61.3	24.4	100.0% (84)[a]
During medical school	23.3	68.6	8.1	100.0% (281)
One year after medical school	14.6	70.2	15.2	100.0% (122)
More than one year after medical school	37.5	56.6	5.9	100.0% (230)
Total	26.3	64.2	9.5	100.0% (667) NA = 23

[a] Percentages are weighted; *N* is unweighted.

To extend this analysis, we examined the relationship between the type of visa and the number of years of medical experience between medical school and arrival in the United States (a positive and linear relationship exists between the time at which the migration decision was made and years of experience before arrival in the United States). The finding is clear: the more years of experience a medical graduate had, the more likely it was that he or she would enter on a permanent resident visa. Despite this, even FMGs with over 4 years of medical experience find the exchange visitor visa program a major vehicle for immigration (Table 4.2).

Several implications flow from these data. First, the exchange visitor visa is the primary certificate of entry for most FMGs, regardless of stage in his or her career. The tendency for the more experienced FMGs and for those individuals deciding later in their careers to enter somewhat more frequently on permanent resident visas probably reflects an expectation that they will remain here permanently.

TABLE 4.2   VISA STATUS AT ENTRY INTO THE UNITED STATES BY YEARS OF EXPERIENCE IN MEDICINE BEFORE ARRIVAL

| | Visa at entry | | | |
| | Immigrant | Nonimmigrant | | |
Years in medicine before U.S. arrival	Permanent resident	Exchange visitor	Other	Total
None	16.7	73.9	9.4	100.0% (246)[a]
One	25.2	61.7	13.1	100.0% (214)
Two to four	31.5	63.1	5.4	100.0% (82)
Over four	43.9	51.0	5.1	100.0% (130)
Total	26.4	64.2	9.4	100.0% (672)
				NA = 18

[a] Percentages are weighted; N is unweighted.

Second, entry on exchange visitor visas is in part a function of the ease with which it can be obtained. As shown in Table 4.3, the number of individuals on permanent resident visas had increased by 32.3 percent by the time of the survey. Individuals on exchange visitor and other non-immigrant visas had declined by 26.9 percent and 5.3 percent, respectively. Perusal of immigration law demonstrates that (1) immigrant visas are, despite changes instituted in the Immigration Act of 1965, sometimes difficult to obtain, and (2) exchange visitor visa restrictions that have existed since the inception of the program, including a 5-year time limit the visa can be held, have always made it preferable to adjust to permanent resident status. In short, there is no real incentive not to adjust to an immigrant visa, if possible, unless a person has absolutely no doubt that he or she will leave this country. Current policies to limit exchange visitors to a 2-year stay make this process even more imperative.

This, then, is the first indication of what we term "visa game playing." If a country's total visa "slots" or an immigrant visa preference category is filled, the FMG's next logical step is to apply for an exchange visitor visa rather than have his name placed on a waiting list for an immigrant visa.

Often, both options were exercised by FMGs, maximizing their chances to get a more secure status here. It appears from the data that the older, more experienced FMGs worked harder at obtaining immigrant status, although it must be recognized that younger, less experienced FMGs, being at a different stage in their career development, might not have had qualms about entering on an exchange visitor visa, only to realize after arrival that it was advantageous to hold a visa allowing regular employment, even if the intent was that it would only be a temporary interlude before leaving.

TABLE 4.3   VISA STATUS AT ENTRY INTO THE UNITED STATES AND AT THE TIME OF THE SURVEY

Visa status	At U.S. entry	Survey	Percentage Difference
Permanent resident	26.4	58.6	+ 32.3
Exchange visitor	64.0	37.1	− 26.9
Other	9.6	4.3	− 5.3
Total	100.0% (672)[a]	100.0% (672)	
		NA = 18	

[a] Percentages are weighted; N is unweighted.

VISAS AND THE COUNTRY OF MEDICAL EDUCATION

Another critical variable associated with variations in visa patterns is a medical graduate's country of medical education. Table 4.4, column 1, shows, for illustrative countries, some of the variation in entry patterns. At one extreme, individuals from countries as diverse as Thailand, West Germany, and Mexico show little or no propensity to enter on permanent resident visas. At the other extreme, and a rare one at that, physicians from countries such as South Korea entered principally on permanent resident immigrant visas. (As a reminder, about one-quarter of all FMGs in our study entered with this visa.)

Further examination of Table 4.4, columns 2 and 3, shows the variability by country in the conversion from exchange visitor visas to permanent resident visas. The conversion process is in itself a significant issue that has probably provided FMGs with another avenue for staying here. The right to convert from exchange visitor to immigrant status is relatively recent, having been made possible by the enactment in 1970 of

TABLE 4.4 VISA STATUS AT ENTRY INTO THE UNITED STATES AND AT THE TIME OF THE SURVEY FOR SELECTED COUNTRIES OF MEDICAL EDUCATION

Country of medical education	Visa Status								Percentage change in individuals holding permanent resident visas
	U.S. Entry				Survey				
	PR	EV (percent)	Other	Total	PR	EV (percent)	Other	Total	
Ireland	29.3	52.7	18.0	100.0 (11)[a]	76.0	24.0	—	100.0 (11)	+ 46.7
Spain	17.3	44.7	38.0	100.0 (17)	38.0	54.9	7.1	100.0 (17)	+ 20.7
West Germany	—	77.8	22.2	100.0 (10)	66.5	33.5	—	100.0 (10)	+ 66.5
Taiwan	20.3	74.1	5.6	100.0 (62)	85.1	13.9	1.0	100.0 (62)	+ 64.8
India	25.3	71.7	3.0	100.0 (41)	71.5	28.5	—	100.0 (41)	+ 46.2
South Korea	70.2	29.8	—	100.0 (30)	95.9	4.1	—	100.0 (30)	+ 25.7
Philippines	24.3	62.9	12.8	100.0 (46)	31.5	50.0	18.5	100.0 (46)	+ 7.2
Thailand	—	100.0	—	100.0 (44)	43.3	56.7	—	100.0 (44)	+ 43.3
Iran	16.0	84.0	—	100.0 (41)	57.8	42.2	—	100.0 (41)	+ 41.8
Mexico	6.3	65.6	28.1	100.0 (26)	18.6	81.4	—	100.0 (26)	+ 12.3
Brazil	—	87.3	12.7	100.0 (20)	3.2	93.6	3.2	100.0 (20)	+ 3.2

[a] Percentages are weighted; N is unweighted.

Public Law 91–225 which abolished the requirement that an FMG on an exchange visitor visa had to leave the country for 2 years before applying for admission as an immigrant. Although the old 2-year "deportation" requirement acted as a dubious deterrent against FMGs' eventual permanent residence in the United States,[3] the abolition of this requirement eased considerably the short-term process of remaining here and enhanced the "game playing" prospects. With this loophole closing under new regulations, other ways to beat the system will undoubtedly appear.

Most of the conversion evident in Tables 4.3 and 4.4 took place within the territory of the United States. For our selected countries, conversion rates differ widely. The lowest percentages of change are for Brazil (3.2 percent) and the Philippines (7.2 percent). Countries with the highest rate of change included West Germany (66.5 percent), Taiwan (64.8 percent), Ireland (46.7 percent), India (46.2 percent). Thailand (43.3 percent), and Iran (41.8 percent). The Western European countries of West Germany and Ireland have numbers of medical graduates appreciably smaller than those of the Asian countries with high conversion rates, and one cannot exclude the possibility of randomness in the figures. The trend of most Asian nations to have the high conversion rates is important: it may be an indicator of intention to remain in the United States, a point argued elsewhere.

Nevertheless, even among Asian nations, the patterns of entry and adjustment differ from country to country. For example, Taiwanese medical graduates had perhaps the greatest success in converting from exchange visitor status to immigrant status (Figure 4.1). Thirty-eight of the original 47 had converted by the time of the survey, and an additional two medical graduates had changed from other nonimmigrant visas to immigrant status. For neighboring South Korea, relatively more individuals entered on immigrant visas to begin with, and, in addition, of the seven entering on exchange visitor visas, five had converted to permanent resident status. Other Asian nations differed markedly: Thailand had one entrant on an immigrant visa, and, by the time of the survey, only 17 of the original 44 Thai graduates had converted. The Filipino medical graduates came mostly on exchange visitor visas, and their conversion rate remained low. Indians, by contrast, had more success in visa adjustment to permanent resident status.

There is no clear pattern of entry across countries. Common sense suggests that factors inherent in each country play some role in determining which visa medical graduates will obtain, whether they will convert, and, eventually, how many will remain. For example, with respect to obtaining an immigrant visa, foreign nationals may qualify

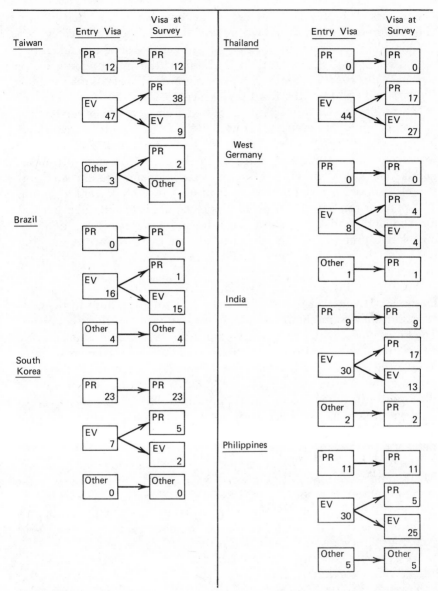

Figure 4.1 Patterns of visa and visa adjustment for selected illustrative countries of medical education.

under certain "preference" categories, or they may throw their lot into "nonpreference" categories. Two general classes of preference categories include *relative* preferences, for example, unmarried sons and daughters of United States citizens and their children (the first preference), or *occupational* preference, for example, immigrants in professions and their spouses and children (the third preference).

The proportion of immigrants admitted each year on either relative or occupational preferences varies widely from country to country. In fiscal year 1973–1974 the Philippines had a total of 19,238 men and women granted immigrant visas. Of these, 8195 (42.6 percent) immigrants obtained their visas through occupational preferences. Comparable proportions for other Asian countries are 30.8 percent for India, 21.2 percent for South Korea, 18.9 percent for Pakistan, 15.6 percent for Thailand, and 9.5 percent for Taiwan. The proportions entering on relative preferences varied much less for these countries, ranging from a high of 57.2 percent for Filipinos to a low of 40 percent for Indians.[5]

Why these countries vary so widely according to occupational preferences is unclear. It is clear that there is a rough pattern in the conversion from nonimmigrant to immigrant status among these countries. The Philippines, with 42.6 percent of all 1973–1974 immigrants entering on occupational preferences, also had one of the lowest conversion rates among the medical graduates in our sample (7.2 percent). At the other extreme, the country with one of the highest conversion rates was Taiwan (64.8 percent). It has a very low proportion of FMGs entering on occupational preferences (9.5 percent). Both countries had comparable proportions of FMGs entering on relative preferences: the Philippines, 57.2 percent and Taiwan, 59.2 percent.

One may deduce that when one path is blocked, another will be found. If, for some reason, relatively few physicians from a given country enter or are permitted to enter on one classification, they will attempt to come on some other. For example, the low conversion rate of Filipinos appears to be correlated with somewhat lower or average rates of entry on exchange visitor visas. Taiwan, with its high conversion rate, had an above average entry rate of medical graduates on exchange visitor visas. India, with a conversion rate lower than Taiwan but greater than the Philippines, had an exchange visitor visa entry rate slightly lower than Taiwan but higher than the Philippines. The proportion of FMGs entering on immigrant visas through occupational preferences was 30.8 percent, higher than Taiwan and lower than the Philippines.

This means that FMGs, if their ability to secure immigrant visas is limited or blocked, will tend to enter on exchange visitor visas as an optional course of action, and the high entry rates on exchange visitor visas appear to be connected with higher than average conversion rates. In reality, many other options exist. We describe only the most dominant of many possible patterns.

Further, in the case of graduates from countries with low numbers of FMGs entering on immigrant visas and few people converting, for example, the Philippines, those graduates have been able to stay in the United States indefinitely extending the time spent in training positions.

In the case of a country like Brazil, which is under the more restrictive Western Hemisphere immigration statutes, the "game playing" hypothesis receives even more support, and the role of the exchange visitor visa as a certificate of prolonged sojourns in the United States is seen.[6] No Brazilian medical graduate entered on an immigrant visa, and only one of 16 exchange visitors managed to convert to it by the time of the survey. Additionally, 12.7 percent of these graduates entered on other non-immigrant visas and converted to exchange visitor visas once here. Among other Latin American medical graduates, a similar pattern holds. In the case of Mexico, 28.1 percent of FMGs entered on other non-immigrant visas and by the time of the survey, all of these men and women had converted to other more conventional statuses.

A clearer understanding of what we have termed "visa game playing" may be obtained by examining some actual cases of FMGs, particularly those from Latin America. We randomly pulled from our files examples from four countries, Chile, Brazil, Venezuela, and Peru. All arrived in the United States on visitor or tourist visas; the results are revealing.

Two FMGs changed to exchange visitor visas the same month they arrived in the United States on visitor visas. Both arrived within $1\frac{1}{2}$ years of our study and both stated that study and training in the United States was the reason for changing visas (alien tourists may not work in the United States). Both want to be on a medical school faculty; both think they will "probably leave" this country, although one of them who was a first-year resident in obstetrics and gynecology bluntly stated that his United States training was "in no way" helping him to meet the medical needs of his home country, Venezuela. Each man had taken the ECFMG once in his country and succeeded in passing it.

Two other Latin American MDs held their visitor visas for an average of 1 year before converting to exchange visitor visas. One of them, from Brazil, "toured" Ann Arbor, Michigan for 11 months during which time he studied English at the University of Michigan for 4 months. Although he had passed the ECFMG several years before his arrival in the United

States, he did not do so until his seventh try. He had definitely decided to remain.

The other case, an FMG born in and a citizen of Peru, received his degree from a Spanish medical school. Although he reports that he changed 13 months after his arrival because he "started here as an intern," it is fairly clear that he intended all along to take specialist training in the United States, because he studied "postgraduate medicine" at the University of Miami during the interim. Most likely he took preparation courses for the ECFMG before passing the examination on his fourth attempt.

A blend of personal strategies within the larger framework of visa law results in much room for negotiating in the visa system. For the Latin American physicians discussed, their principal limitation was the provision in the Immigration Act of 1965 that did not permit Western Hemisphere FMGs to adjust their status from nonimmigrant to immigrant. Thus, although the rate of the adjustment of status as a percentage of total immigrants ran at 62 percent for all countries combined in 1972, the percentage of adjustments was zero for all Western Hemisphere countries, with the exception of Cuba (special legislation was passed in 1966 allowing Cuban refugees who had been in the United States for 2 years to adjust their status to immigrants). This explains why FMGs from Latin American countries, such as the Brazilians illustrated in Figure 4.1, had virtually no conversions from exchange visitor to permanent resident and why four of the 20 Brazilians entered on other nonimmigrant visas. Given the restraints of the system, the FMG seems to have been able to find some way to stay here and to manipulate the system to its limits—at least to the present.

From the structural view of visa legislation it would be erroneous to infer that FMGs come here, helter skelter, in full control of a visa program, disregarding the original intentions of the program legislation. We suggest that the period in an FMG's life at which he or she decides to come to the United States partially predicts what kind of visa will be obtained. Another factor is a country-specific composite of forces such as the general demand for certain visa categories. Yet another is the distinction made by the Immigration and Naturalization service between the Western and Eastern Hemispheres.

There are, therefore, patterns of entry of FMGs. From the point of view of the United States, with particular respect to the physician resources issue, is there any relevant pattern of entry produced by visa legislation? The answer, which has policy implications, is a tentative yes.

UNDERLYING PATTERNS OF ENTRY

We note that the later the migration decision is made, the more likely it is that an FMG holds a permanent resident visa, as well as having had more medical experience before entering the United States. For example, whereas the mean proportion of those FMGs who had not had any training posts before arrival in the United States was 36.8 percent, for the "medical school deciders" the proportion rises to almost 52 percent (51.9 percent). For FMGs making the decision a year or more out of medical school, the proportion drops to 21.3 percent.

Although this relationship may sound a bit like stating the obvious, it really is not so at all. All these physicians were in the same cohort in training, most had recently entered the United States, and thus neither group had been here longer than the other. It is not obvious why we should have found two statistically distinct groups of FMGs, one making the decision in the midst of medical education and with little medical experience, and another making the decision later and with the benefit of some years of and a wider variety of medical background.

Part of the answer to this problem is found by comparing the factors given by our respondents that encouraged migration to this country. The two most important reasons they gave are medical specialization and the level of salaries available. These two factors are "U.S. pull" factors, that is, influences emanating from the host country that exert a pull on physicians from other countries. The next five factors may be designated as "donor nation push" factors, that is, forces driving the physician from his or her own country. These include advice from professors in one's own country, a paucity of positions in one's own country, political and social problems, restrictions on practice, and military service.

To answer this question we cross tabulated these migration reasons with the time at which the decision to migrate was made. For medical school "deciders" the influence of United States pull factors is paramount. However, for physicians deciding after medical school, "donor nation" push factors take on the most important influence.

For FMGs with no previous medical experience, as well as those with one or two medical positions before in the United States, pull factors predominated; United States medical specialization led the list. For FMGs with three or more positions, the situation is entirely reversed, and "donor nation push" factors lead the list of reasons, with political and social problems most often stressed. There was a distinct decrease in the importance of medical specialization among this experienced group of FMGs.

One final attribute of these two groups was their tendency to report differential future migration plans. Overall, exactly the same proportion of FMGs reported they would leave the United States as said they would remain: 44.6 percent. Almost 11 percent (10.9 percent) were undecided. Those FMGs who made the decision to come to the United States during medical school were very close to this distribution. Medical graduates making the decision 1 or more years after graduation reported more often that they decided to remain. Medical graduates immediately out of medical school behaved more like their medical school peers, claiming 58.8 percent of the time that they would return.

The relationship holds up for the two measures of the amount of medical experience: number of positions and years spent in these positions. The farther beyond medical school the decision was made, that is, the more medical experience an FMG had, the more likely it was that he or she would report deciding to remain in the United States.

On the basis of these data, we find a distinct and unrecognized clustering of FMGs. On one hand, there is a young group of FMGs who decided to come to the United States during or directly after medical school and who tended to have little or no prior medical training experience before arriving. Additionally, they reported being attracted to the United States because of its emphasis on specialty training and better economic prospects. They tend to report that they would return to their countries more or as often as they say they would stay here. On the other hand, and in contrast, we find a somewhat older group of FMGs who decided to come to this country a year or more after medical school and who tended to have had several years of medical training in a number of different positions. They report their motivation in coming to the United States as a consequence of forces within their countries, and they have a decided opinion that they will remain permanently in this country. To a large extent, we have two opposite groups.

The existence of the two groups raises the critical issue: whether these FMGs are coming on similar or different visas. We already know from Tables 4.1 and 4.2 that entry visa is related both to the time at which the migration decision is made and to the number of years of medical experience before entering the United States. Further, when patterns of conversion are examined, it is also true that the more experienced FMGs, as well as those who make the migration decision well out of medical school, were less likely to have remained on nonimmigrant, including exchange visitor, visas.

The data support the view that—at least to some extent—United States visa policies work as apparently intended. The older, more experienced late decision makers, who leave home for reasons more related to their home countries than the attraction of the United States, appear to be coming as "true" immigrants: men and women seeking a new life and a new start in medicine. In contrast, the younger, less experienced medical graduates, who make the decision to migrate early in their medical education, are coming to the United States as "true" students or trainees, initially at least, with the intention of returning to their home countries. They come through the auspices of the exchange visitor program which, as previously noted, was originally tabbed as an educational exchange program to spread the benefits of technology in medicine.

However, the relationships are far from perfect. The possibility of converting one's visa status without leaving the United States means that many FMGs in the "trainee" group have converted and are remaining and that many FMGs in the "immigrant" group, forced to come on nonimmigrant visas, have also converted. Thus, despite the finding that in the main FMGs are arriving in the United States in an orderly, predictable manner, significant numbers of other foreign MDs are taking unusual steps in order to secure a more permanent visa status than visitor, student, and other programs permit.

More broadly, immigration policy stops functioning as a regulator of alien doctors as soon as they arrive in the United States. Although somewhat more exchange visitors initially entered into major university teaching units (see Table 4.8), suggesting a differential effect of visa status on chances of landing a top-notch training post on arrival, this edge is lost after the FMG arrives, begins adjusting visa status, and has a chance to be mobile within the United States. The important factor in considering visa status is arrival in this country. Visa "game playing," which occurs later, is one means by which FMGs secure quality graduate medical education and enlarge their future options of returning or remaining.

THE ECFMG EXAMINATION

A second major hurdle for would-be FMGs is taking and passing the examination administered by the Educational Commission for Foreign Medical Graduates (ECFMG) headquartered in Philadelphia. Certification is necessary in order to train in any AMA-approved residency program except where prohibited by state licensing laws[7]. The examination, given in test centers both within and outside the United States, contains questions derived from Parts I and II of the examination administered to American medical students by the National Board of Medical Examiners (NBME). It is in two parts: the first part tests general medical knowledge, and the second tests English language skills. Candidates must achieve a score of 75 or better (out of a total 100 points) to receive certification, and they may take the examination as many times as necessary to pass it. At the time of writing (fall, 1977), the ECFMG examination is being supplanted by a new Visa Qualifying Examination, developed by the NBME, but many of the criticisms our respondents made will apply equally to the new examination.

Much criticism has been leveled at the examination by both American medical observers and FMGs. Generally, the arguments take two forms. First, there is the feeling that the examination is too easy and allows unqualified physicians entrance into American hospitals. The proponents of this line of reasoning often underscore this by pointing to the low pass rates of FMGs on the examination.[8] Taking a somewhat different line, some have argued that the ECFMG examination serves as a poor substitute for the educational and professionalization process of American physicians, beginning during the undergraduate premedical years and culminating in the conferring of a United States medical doctor degree; this "continuum" of medical education is an essential component of the training of competent physicians, and the fact that it is not undertaken by FMGs implies a potentially inadequate preparation for practice in the United States.[9]

The second general position has been articulated mainly by FMGs who argue that the examination is taken under adverse circumstances—such as in football stadiums—which negatively affect the overall performance. Others argue that the multiple-choice format is alien to many foreign-educated physcians, and that an examination drawn from tests of U.S. medical students is inappropriate for physicians several years removed from medical graduation.

The role of examinations in admitting foreign physicians to the United States has been viewed ambivalently by government agencies. In 1975 the U.S. Department of Health, Education and Welfare began a $1.3 million program to help 350 Vietnamese refugee physicians prepare for the ECFMG examination, including stipends for travel, and housing and subsistence costs. It was hoped that these physicians would practice in underserved areas such as rural Nebraska.[10] A year earlier, there was talk, but no final action, by the National Health Service Corps, an agency of the U.S. Department of Health, Education and Welfare, on financing some of the costs of the ECFMG training program run by the Office of International Education at the University of Miami. This program has traditionally catered to Cuban refugee physicians, although a large number of other Spanish-speaking medical graduates have been trained there. (The United States government financing would have been tied to a minimum 2-year commitment from these physicians to practice in underserved areas.[11]) For practical purposes, these branches of the United

States government have regarded the ECFMG as a test for which foreign physicians can clearly be trained.

Certainly a screening examination provides no major deterrent to FMGs who are successful in other ways. Among the 1973–1974 survey cohort, nearly 70 percent of the FMGs reported passing the examination on the first attempt (Table 4.5). The majority of house staff were highly successful on the examination as measured by the number of times the examination was taken. Only 30 percent of this training group had to take the exam more than once. Comparison with the higher number of multiple takers reported by the ECFMG in its *Annual Report*, reveals that FMGs who become house officers in the United States perform much better than foreign physicians as a whole.[12] Perhaps hospital administrators and physicians in charge of recruiting house officers select foreign medical graduates who pass on the first try. In any event, most of the FMGs in approved training positions are readily qualified, by the stated criteria of the testing organization. Raising the standards or pass-rates for all physicians who take the test—many of whom never leave their own countries—will not, therefore, necessarily reduce the number of entrants to the United States.

Those medical graduates in our survey who did better than average came from Ireland and other British Commonwealth nations, Ceylon, Taiwan, South Korea, Thailand, Syria, Brazil, and non-Arab African nations. On the other hand, countries whose medical graduates fell below the average include Spain, Cuba, and Mexico. However, no distinctive national patterns emerge from the data. Individual graduates from Western Europe and English-speaking countries do both well and average; the same is true for the Far East, the mid-East, and South America.

TABLE 4.5 DISTRIBUTION OF THE NUMBER OF TIMES THE ECFMG EXAMINATION WAS TAKEN

Number of times the ECFMG was taken	FMG	USFMG
Once	69.6	67.7
Twice	21.0	22.1
Three or more	9.4	10.1
Total	100.0% (675)[a]	100.0% (39)
	NA = 1[b]	NA = 3

[a] Percentages are weighted; N is unweighted.
[b] Excludes 14 Canadians, who are exempted from the examination.

However, the gender of the respondent had some importance with respect to ECFMG pass rates. Men are more successful than women in passing the examination in foreign countries. As shown in Table 4.6, this relationship is only part of the explanation for differential pass rates, since an additional critical factor is the marital status of the female medical graduate. Single women pass the ECFMG as successfully as men. The finding that married women are appreciably poorer performers on the examination than any other group suggests that child rearing and other traditional female roles hinder the pursuit of professional credentials in medicine (although it is quite possible that married women and single women are preselected groups, the latter able to do better in any event). The causal problem cannot be answered from our data, but the correlation exists and draws into question the interpretation of a single test score as a measure of a physician's competence.

TABLE 4.6   PERCENTAGE OF FMGS WHO SAY THEY PASSED THE ECFMG EXAMINATION ON THE FIRST ATTEMPT, BY WHERE THE EXAMINATION WAS PASSED, GENDER, AND MARITAL STATUS

Where the ECFMG Was Passed	Married		Single		Total
	Men	Women	Men	Women	
	(percent)		(percent)		
United States	38.8 (62)[a]	13.5 (30)	40.3 (14)	68.1 (3)	(109)
Abroad	78.0 (394)	54.4 (40)	83.1 (103)	70.4 (26)	(563)
Total	72.9 (456)	38.1 (70)	78.0 (117)	70.1 (19)	(672) [b]
					NA = 4

[a] Percentages are weighted; N is unweighted.
[b] Excludes 14 Canadians, who are exempted from the examination.

We examine this relationship for those countries with a substantial number of FMGs in our sample found to be above, at, or below average on the distribution of times the examination was taken. In the case of Taiwan, the married women were highly successful in passing the examination on the first attempt. However, the small number of married women ($N = 2$) makes this a weak comparative case. India, which fell somewhat above the average distribution, reflected the overall pattern: married female FMGs did more poorly in the examination than any other category of Indian medical graduates. Again, the small number of single female graduates makes comparison problematic, but the pattern is nevertheless maintained. In the case of Pakistan, too, which fell very near the average distribution, female married physicians did most poorly, although male married medical graduates did more poorly than those from other countries. Single males did quite well by contrast, and the one single female passed the examination on the first try.

The overall pattern is, however, by no means uniform for all countries. Neither the country of an individual's medical education nor that person's gender and marital status follow a universal pattern for predicting performance on the ECFMG examination. Some countries have medical graduates who do well; others, who do less well. Gender and marital status appear to produce differences: usually, the married women lower the pass rates. However, where male FMGs from countries do poorly on the examination (for example, from Iran and the Philippines), the sex- and marital-linked variables decrease in importance, that is both males and females do more or less poorly.

A final critical way of assessing ECFMG examination pass rates is to analyze the relationship between the pass rates and English language skills. There was no discernable association. We measured English skills through asking our interviewers to classify the respondents' English as excellent, good, fair, or poor. Of FMGs with "excellent" English, 77.7 percent passed the ECFMG examination on the first try; of those with "good" English, 65.0 percent. "Fair" and "poor" English speakers, however, did fairly well: 60.7 percent and 69.5 percent, respectively, passed the ECFMG examination on their first attempt. What begins as a linear relationship, becomes curvilinear, and no apparent rationale is available for the result.

Nor are there clear patterns for countries in which English is the language of medical instruction. The United Kingdom, Ireland, and other British or former British holdings are all represented by medical graduates who do well on the examination, that is, pass it on the first attempt. In many schools in India, medicine is taught in English, and this is reflected in an above-average pass rate. Yet a major nation for which this does not hold true is the Philippines where, despite English language instruction, medical graduates continue to have difficulty passing the examination on the first attempt.

When country of medical education is held constant, that is, when each country is examined separately, the relationship between English language ability and the number of times the examination is taken tends to disappear or become ambiguous: thus, English appears to assume a lesser role in predicting how well the examinee will perform. This is true even for countries in which English is the language of medical instruction. We conclude that language skills are relatively unimportant as predictors of passing the ECFMG examination; certainly they are less important than knowing the country of training. As far as the individual is concerned, passing the test on the first try is the result of interacting factors. Medical school is clearly important, and it is an advantage to be single—perhaps because the career decisions of married physicians are more complex. The great strength of the ECFMG or any similar test is that it tests the individual, ignoring extraneous factors which, as we have shown, have widely varying effects.

ENTERING THE UNITED STATES WITHOUT CREDENTIALS

Some researchers have sought to characterize the problems associated with having large numbers of FMGs in the United States by pointing out the presence among them of a large body of non-ECFMG-certified FMGs.[13] We cannot estimate from our data the size of this group. However, we can affirm that nearly 16 percent of all of the 1973–1974 FMG trainees did not pass the ECFMG examination until after their arrival in this country.

This finding raises the question of what they were doing while they were uncertified. To pose the question as other researchers have done, were they engaged in medical activities for which they were unqualified, thus constituting a so-called "medical underground" of marginal clinical competence?

An answer to this question begins with the examination of the correlates of passing the examination in the United States. As shown in Table 4.7, a sizable relationship exists between taking the examination here and the number of times the examination was taken. Those FMGs taking the examination three or more times were more than three times as likely to have passed it in the United States than the overall average for FMGs. In contrast, FMGs successful on the first try were less than half as likely to have passed it in this country than the average.

This finding must be placed in context. Data presented earlier in Table 4.6 show once again the joint effect of gender and marital status. For both married and single men as well as for women taken as a group, the essential relationship between taking the examination in the United States and taking it multiple times is unchanged. However, for married women there are markedly more individuals passing it here. This is not the case for single women. Thus marital status once again emerges as a partial explanation for understanding behaviour on the ECFMG examination.

TABLE 4.7 WHERE THE ECFMG EXAMINATION WAS PASSED BY THE NUMBER OF TIMES IT WAS TAKEN

Number of times the examination was taken	Where the ECFMG was passed		
	United States	Abroad	Total
Once	7.4	92.6	100.0% (470)[a]
Twice	27.4	72.6	100.0% (132)
Three or more	52.6	47.4	100.0% (73)
Total	15.8	84.2	100.0% (675)[b]
			NA = 1

[a] Percentages are weighted; *N* is unweighted.
[b] Excludes 14 Canadians, who are exempted from the examination.

Thirty of the 110 FMGs who passed the examination in the United States were married women, a weighted proportion of 30 percent. Most of these women were here because their husbands were here. Examples include the cases of Dr. P and Dr. T, the first a native of India, the other an unusual combination of Polish birth, Scottish medical education, and New Zealand citizenship. Both entered the United States on permanent resident visas with their husbands and spent about a year as housewives. Each took the ECFMG examination (twice); the Polish-born FMG worked for 1 month as a laboratory technician. Both had working husbands, one a sanitation engineer, the other a medical resident in radiology. A revealing comment made by one respondent concerned her reason for changing medical specialties (pediatrics to pathology): the former was an "unbearable amount of work for a married woman."

Regardless of the defining characteristics of this group of FMGs who passed the ECFMG examination in the United States, they were at one time a "reserve pool" of potential physicians. The fact that they did become ECFMG certified raises once again the issue of "games playing." While biding their time, what were these men and women doing?

The roles they reported filling represent a full range of medical activities, some of which are in no way contingent on ECFMG certification, for example, research fellowships (9.2 percent). Others were doing some sort of clinical work: "hospital" positions, "students," private practice. In all likelihood, these men and women were acting as physician's aides and in other paramedical roles. Although it is clear that the line between legitimate medical activity and illegitimate and illegal assumption of physician roles can easily be transgressed, from the FMG's point of view any medical activity improves his or her chance for eventual certification. The American medical system appears to have no effective way to merge these activities in a rational manner into full physician status; thus the FMGs manage as best they can within a system that publicly impugns such practices yet privately knows that they are often vital.[14]

The prevalence of questionable medical activity must not be placed out of context with respect to this study group. Over half of these FMGs after passing the exam in the United States, reported being employed only as an intern or resident and only after having obtained proper certification. Whereas those who worked in medically related roles before ECFMG certification demonstrated an ability to "play" the system at its weak points, that is in underserved areas or understaffed hospital departments, those who did not showed great persistence in striving time and time again for their badge of admission. In either case, the groups were engaged in "games playing" in a system that willingly utilized their services and allowed them to take the examination as often as was necessary to pass it.

A final analysis demonstrates further the games playing hypothesis and highlights the "system of entry" into the United States. This analysis consists of two elements: (1) the number of times an FMG took the ECFMG examination and its correlation with his or her visa at entry into the United States and visa status at the time of the survey, and (2) the location of the ECFMG examination and its correlation with the visa variables.

Generally, FMGs who came to the country on any given visa and who had not adjusted status when we interviewed them, had taken the examination only once. In contrast, men and women who had changed visa status were more likely to have taken the examination more than once. An exception to this were FMGs converting from exchange visitor visas to immigrant visas: they passed on the first try as often as non-changers. Since this group constituted the bulk of visa changers, we can note that nonimmigrant visa status (other than exchange visitor visas) is a part of the visa system that allows considerable latitude for FMGs to work toward status as a house officer in an American hospital.

FMGs entering on non-immigrant visas who had not converted, particularly those entering on the exchange visitor program, were among the most successful ECFMG examinees. If there is among the 1973–1974 FMG house staff cohort a group of men and women who might be cause for concern it would most likely be those who did not enter on permanent resident and exchange visitor visas: that is, those who entered as dependents or tourists. They are more likely to have taken the examination a number of times before passing, probably in the United States. However, it is a very risky conclusion that this group is necessarily unqualified. Many of them, as we point out, are spouses who have followed their husbands. They are, in any event, a minority of FMGs in approved training programs.

TABLE 4.8   RELATIONSHIP OF VISA STATUS AT ENTRY INTO THE UNITED STATES BY LEVEL OF UNIVERSITY AFFILIATION OF FIRST U.S. HOSPITAL

	Level of university affiliation of first U.S. hospital			
Visa at entry	Major teaching units	Other university affiliation	Non-affiliated hospitals	Total
Permanent resident	35.7	27.1	37.2	100.0% (169)[a]
Exchange visitor	43.0	32.2	24.7	100.0% (424)
Other non-immigrant visas	44.3	17.0	38.7	100.0% (70)
Total	41.3	29.3	29.4	100.0% (663) NA = 27

[a] Percentages are weighted; N is unweighted

In a broader sense, the "system of entry" provides FMGs a number of ways to secure a training position. In Table 4.8, for example, the visa of entry plays almost no role in predicting whether he or she will obtain a full university-affiliated house officer position. In fact, the distribution of other nonimmigrant physicians—precisely those who had the least successful experiences on the ECFMG—had the greatest success in obtaining a top-flight university–affiliated post. The point is that *arrival* in the United States appears to be the critical factor. Thus the "system of entry" offers variable routes to house officer status; some avenues are widely traveled, whereas others may lack some legitimacy, but all more or less allow equal achievement.

CONCLUSIONS

Policy issues rather than theoretical constructs provide the basis for the organization of the empirical findings in this chapter. In both policy areas—immigration and medical screening—we seek to synthesize the data around the issues of regulation of quantity and quality.

We have found that immigration law and procedures do tend to differentiate and segregate "true immigrants" from "true students of medicine," and that the ECFMG examination provides some rough measure of evaluating the medical preparation of FMGs. At the same time, however, we stress the less obvious ways the original and primary purpose of different visa programs could be circumvented. We also state our concern that a screening examination may be found wanting when it comes to measuring the quality of actual medical experience beyond the medical school years. This, then, is a somewhat mixed review of two critical policy areas that almost always receive attention by analysts of the FMG phenomenon.

In our final chapter, we address some of the broad policy implications of the analysis of these two major barriers to entry into the United States. However, for our purposes here, it suffices to stress that these dual regulatory barriers provide the context within which FMGs find plenty of opportunity for individual strategies bent toward United States graduate medical education. We argue that FMGs are less the victims of forces "pushing and pulling" them from one country to the next as they are the active participants of a decision-making process based on a calculated risk that American training would benefit their careers. Part of the process in coming to this country is obtaining the necessary credentials in whatever way possible, because, as our analysis further demonstrates, entry into the United States is the first step toward successful mobility into "good" hospital positions. This is so, not in the obvious sense that one must first be here in order to work here, but rather, that once a foothold has been made, that is, once a house officer position has been secured, there commences an almost inexorable movement toward better and more prestigious positions.

NOTES

1. A comprehensive description and analysis of immigration law, visa statutes, and their effect on gross numbers of migrants with respect to physicians are available in Stephen S. Mick, "The Foreign Medical Graduate," *Scientific American* (February 1975), vol. 232, No. 2: pp. 14–21; Rosemary Stevens and Joan Vermeulen, *Foreign Trained Physicians and American Medicine*, DHEW Publication No. (NIH) 73–325, (June 1972); and Rosemary Stevens, et al., "Physician Migration Reexamined," *Science* (31 October 1975), *190*, pp. 439–442.

2. For the period 1965–1973, a total of 21,891 FMGs entered the United States on immigrant visas; however, nearly twice that number (42,037) entered on exchange visitor visas. See Table 1, Rosemary Stevens, et al., *Ibid.*, p. 440.

3. In an earlier study, the authors noted the tendency of some physicians to leave the United States and to return several years later, presumably to meet the 2-year absentee stipulation then in effect. Eighteen percent of FMGs responding to a mail questionnaire had left the United States during some portion of their career, only to return an average of 2.7 years later. See Rosemary Stevens, Louis Wolf Goodman, and Stephen S. Mick, "What Happens to Foreign-Trained Doctors Who Come to the United States," *Inquiry* (June 1974), p. 118. *XI*, No. 2:

4. Immigration and Naturalization Service, *1974 Annual Report*, Washington, D.C.: U.S. Government Printing Office, Table 8A, p. 39

5. *Ibid.*, Table 7A, p. 37.

6. The 1965 Immigration and Nationality Act placed physicians from Latin America at a disadvantage relative to their Eastern Hemisphere counterparts. There are a number of restrictions; the ones most relevant to this discussion include the absence of any preference system so that prospective immigrants simply had to wait their turn for visas along with, for example, unskilled workers. Second, the avenue to immigration of coming to the United States as a nonimmigrant and then adjusting to immigrant status was not permitted to physicians from the Western Hemisphere. Thus the few Latin American physicians in our sample who claimed to have adjusted from exchange visitor to immigrant status were either reporting erroneously or had somehow managed to circumvent the law.

7. See Rosemary Stevens and Joan Vermeulen, *op. cit.*, pp. 26–47, for a detailed discussion of the ECFMG and its examination.

8. See Aaron Lowin, *FMGs? An Evaluation of Policy-Related Research*, Minneapolis, Minnesota: Interstudy, especially Chapter 3.

9. Betty A. Lockett, "Circumventing the Continuum or How to Bypass the U.S. Medical Education System Without Really Trying," unpublished paper, (27 December 1974).

10. "U.S. to assist refugee physicians," *American Medical News* (18 August 1975), p. 1.

11. "For FMGs, a delay in 'refresher' course," *Medical World News* (10 May 1974), p. 89.

12. Readers familiar with ECFMG statistics know that in any given examination, only about 30–40 percent of all candidates achieve a passing score. Through the July 25, 1973 examination, the overall pass rate was 38.1 percent, with 38.8 percent passing that particular examination. As of that date an aggregate 56.5 percent had taken the examination for the first time, and for the July 25 examination specifically, 50.2 percent were first-time candidates. Finally, the cumulative numbers of people scoring 75 percent or better over the years was 119,802 out of 315,885 examinations administered, yielding an overall cumulative pass rate of 67.8 percent. Thus our study group did substantially better than the bulk of FMGs. (See the *Annual Report 1973*, Philadelphia: Educational Council for Foreign Medical Graduates, Tables 1A and 2A, pp. 10–11.

The apparent discrepancy between our data and published ECFMG statistics is a product of several methodological issues inherent in the research design of our study. First, since the study is cross sectional and composed of a rough cohort of interns and residents, it cannot nor was it expected to represent a specific group of ECFMG examination candidates. FMGs in our sample passed the examination over a wide span of years, the earliest being in 1960, with the bulk falling between 1969 and 1972 (58.5 percent) and the latest year being 1973. Thus our sample is representative of no single cohort of candidates.

Second, it must be remembered that our data are derived from the successful FMGs, those who have entered and were currently in AMA-approved house staff positions. As such, we probably over-represent by some unknown factor FMGs who pass on the first try. The fact that in any given examination sitting many more FMGs fail is quite consistent with our findings, since these latter FMGs would not appear in the sample.

A third, and related point, is arithmetical. We do not include those FMGs who consistently fail year after year because, as mentioned, they would not have been found in approved training programs. Thus, in a sense, our base or denominator of FMGs is smaller than it would ordinarily have been were we to have drawn our sample from a list of names of physicians sitting for the examination all over the world.

These methodological considerations are important for several reasons; the first is to counter the argument that the FMGs in our sample were erroneously reporting information regarding the ECFMG. Although a certain amount of response error is expected in any survey, the reasons just outlined are, in our judgment, more than adequate as explanations for the distribution of responses obtained.

13.   See especially R. J. Weiss, J. C. Kleinman, V. C. Brandt, J. J. Feldman, and A. C. McGuinness, "Foreign Medical Graduates and the Medical Underground," *New England Journal of Medicine* (30 June 1974), vol. 290, No. 25; pp. 1408–1413, and R. J. Weiss, J. C. Kleinman, V. C. Brandt, and D. S. Felsenthal, "The Effect of Importing Physicians—return to a Pre-Flexnerian Standard," *New England Journal of Medicine* (27 June 1974), Vol. 290, No. 26: pp. 1453–1458.

14.   For an argument that FMGs are used in critical shortage areas, see A. Goldblatt, L. W. Goodman, S. S. Mick, and R. Stevens, "Licensure, Competence, and Manpower Distribution," *New England Journal of Medicine* (16 January 1975), Vol. 292, No. 3: pp. 137–141.

5

RECRUITMENT AND EXPECTATIONS_____

INTRODUCTION

The foreign medical graduate who has decided to come to the United States and has passed the ECFMG examination has all but one of the prerequisites for an American graduate education: the final element is obtaining a hospital position. Finding a hospital is perhaps the most difficult aspect of migration for the individual FMG. It is also, as a process, perhaps the most interesting. Few physicians come to the United States under organized matching programs or even under government or university sponsorship. Each individual must do the best he or she can with whatever information is available to find a job in an internship or residency—in one of 1700 American hospitals, each of which makes its own appointments.[1]

In finding a position, however, FMGs reveal the same ingenuity and a willingness to explore all possible channels that distinguish the visa and examination systems. A Filipino physician with 12 years of professional experience heard about his first American hospital from an employee in a travel agency who had traveled in the United States and remarked that this hospital (a community hospital in Ohio) had many foreign interns and residents. An Ecuadorian physician discussed hospitals with an American physician attached to the Peace Corps. An Indian physician writes to physician friends in the United States for possible openings where they are working. A Romanian physician learned of his first American hospital through the staff at U.S. Information Services (USIS). An Argentinian physician came directly from a hospital run by the Seventh Day Adventists in Argentina to one run by the same group in the United States. A Norwegian physician, already in the United States, was helped to find a job by the American university where her husband worked. The examples are numerous, but the motif is simple: Entry to the American hospital system and thus by definition to American cultural life and to the professional system of American medicine depends on individual communications and coping mechanisms.

Since the granting of a United States visa is usually conditioned on a job opportunity, the FMG must make his or her job arrangements from afar through a battery of letters. There are exceptions, notably for those entering the United States on temporary (visitor) visas, women physicians who come in as dependents, and others entering as tourists or able to gain jobs in the United States, nonmedical or medical, while looking around for graduate positions or completing requirements for the ECFMG. However, these are options for the minority. Of the 732 FMGs and USFMGs in our study group, only 72 reported that they spent their first 3 or more months in the United States in activities other than training positions. The great majority of FMGs seek jobs and are hired sight unseen.

This chapter describes how foreign physicians based in cities as distant from the United States as Manila, Seoul, Addis Ababa, or Bangkok get themselves recruited (or recruit themselves) to American hospitals. How a physician lights on the name of a particular residency program in a given hospital, in a specific state, has long been something of a mystery. What information is available, and what is used? How far does the institution chosen through the particular method of recruitment meet the individual's expectations?

These are critical questions with respect to the individual FMG career, for migration marks a radical career shift from the professional/educational systems of one country to another. If the individual is uninformed about the United States, he or she may move inadvertently from a prestigious position in the home country to one of low prestige in the United States. If so, future career decisions may be affected. The physician may become disillusioned, "turned-off," or, conversely, more eager than he or she would be otherwise to "make it" in the United States system. Either attitude (or both, held simultaneously) may change the FMG's career plans with respect to further training and ultimate practice location; most obviously, whether the physician returns home or remains in the United States.

In sociological terms the individual may move from a position of "status consistency" in the home country to one of "status inconsistency" in the United States, that is, from a position of generally high prestige and satisfaction to one of role conflict and marginality: high prestige as a physician, but low prestige by virtue of a particular training setting, as well as by being a foreigner or "stranger."[2]

Some disorientation and difficulty in adjustment may be experienced by all FMGs on entry to the United States—for they have taken up their roots in a familiar system and are entering one that is unfamiliar. Knowing *what to expect* in the United States may alleviate the problem considerably. Knowing *how to choose* a hospital makes possible a careful weighing of priorities. For example, a physician offered a job in a medium-sized community hospital with a minimal university connection when he or she would prefer a position in a large hospital that is an integral part of a medical school might decide (1) to reject the job offer in favor of remaining in a university training setting in the home country, (2) to reject the job offer in the hope of landing a better American offer, or (3) to accept the offer knowing that it is not ideal, on the grounds that once in the United States it will be easier to find the optimal position. Each of these choices requires, however, a firm grasp of information about the American hospital system.

Our pilot studies suggested that the decision to come to the United States, a very important decision in terms of both career and personal goals, is made with a dearth of real information about what graduate medical education in the United States is like.[3] The study findings confirm this conclusion. The foreign graduate has the general impression that American education is good and that it will meet his or her needs for specialized training; however, the range of opportunities and programs and the chances of being accepted into one program rather than another are questions outside the physician's competence, since he or she has little knowledge of the American system and in some cases overconfident assumptions and unrealistic expectations.

The type and extent of information available to FMGs about the United States job market and specific training opportunities, although largely neglected in the literature, are important to examine from several perspectives. From the point of view of the American hospital system, what the FMG knows about the hospital may seem unimportant, even

irrelevant. In terms of hiring, the onus is on the hospital to justify its
. choices on the basis of whatever information it has about its applicants.
Each hospital seeks a house staff of proven excellence to fill its available
positions. Each thus competes to attract the best new graduates of American schools, graduates (USMG or FMG) working in other American
hospitals who are willing to transfer to a better, more advanced position,
and the "cream" of potential migrants applying from outside the United
States.

Letters and applications from foreign physicians flow into the offices of
administrators, directors of medical education, and chiefs of service in
American hospitals, sometimes by the hundreds, every year. The hospital makes its choices of new house staff (who usually begin work on July
1 of each year) as best it can, on the basis of its personal knowledge of
candidates, their training and experience, and personal recommendations. Applicants who can appear for an interview, who come from
world-renowned schools, and/or who come highly recommended by
known individuals have the advantage in this process. Unknowns must
trust their luck or judgment in finding an available vacancy.

From an organizational point of view, this selection process may be
quite rational. Indeed, it can be argued that both hospitals and FMGs may
be benefited. At least some hospitals attract good candidates who might
not have applied to them if they had known more about the training
offered, and such candidates are not disappointed by being rejected by
more prestigious hospitals. From the individual point of view, however,
the process is characteristically irrational, haphazard, and informal.
Grapevines help in providing information, as they have for innumerable
other groups of immigrants. The "Green Book," the American Medical
Association's *Directory of Approved Internships and Residencies*, used as a
primary source of information by one-third of our FMGs and as a
secondary source by at least one-fourth, provides considerable information. Nevertheless, the vagueness persists. The individual FMG may
not be able to maximize his or her opportunities by entering the most
appropriate training hospital, because the FMG cannot usually tell from
available information where that is, nor where there may be a suitable
vacancy. In the long run, American hospitals cannot benefit by being
staffed by disappointed physicians.

From other perspectives, too, knowledge of the information and
recruitment process is essential. In terms of understanding the behavior
of physicians as migrants, who are potentially but not necessarily permanent immigrants to the United States, we must know how each man-
ages his specific process of entry to the American sociocultural system.

One possible mechanism, for example, is the process of "chain migration" such as that described by Lochore in looking at migration from Europe to New Zealand: a pioneer group arrives and becomes settled, sometimes accidentally, after originally intending to return home; the first group encourages others to join them, and eventually the immigrants form stable settlements with their own native institutions.[4] Translated to FMGs in the United States, one might assume a recruitment process targeted on jobs in specific hospitals, speading to surrounding areas. In some cases the process may be a function of individual recommendation (for example, a highly regarded FMG intern or resident in an American hospital vouches for a friend); in some, deliberate hiring policy by the institution. Thus one Connecticut hospital seeks graduates of Turkish schools; a Long Island hospital seeks graduates from Sri Lanka (Ceylon).

Even if the numbers are small, the resulting chain or cluster effect is undoubtedly important in the migration of doctors, both in terms of long-term assimilation into American culture and as a means of access for new arrivals. There were, for example, 40 Thai FMGs in Buffalo, New York in 1973, half of whom were interns and residents. This cluster of fellow nationals, together with Thais in other fields in the same city (there is a published *Directory* of Thais in Buffalo), can provide information as well as concrete assistance to physicians in Thailand who are seeking to come to the United States.[5] Thus one would expect a snowballing effect, and this we see. Although some FMGs return home after completion of training, some from each cohort remain, expanding and reinforcing the local network.

However, although local networks or clusters of fellow nationals in the same professional field provide a natural entry point for those physicians who know someone in such a group, they may also limit the choice of training programs available to the individual FMG by providing definite geographic scopes. Given the fact, for example, that two-thirds of all Thai physicians in the United States in the early 1970s were located (in descending order) in the states of New York, Illinois, Pennsylvania, Michigan, and Maryland,[6] one would expect these states to exert more attraction than others to new job seekers from Thailand, at least for those whose primary access was through local (U.S.) reference groups. Similar comments hold for other nationals, although some groups are more "spread out" than others. (Colombian physicians, for example, although found in greatest numbers in New York, Illinois, Ohio, Rhode Island, and Washington, D.C., were also relatively strong in Connecticut, Pennsylvania, Virginia, Michigan, and Massachusetts, the combined total for all these states including approximately two-thirds of the group.) In short, what may be advantageous for an *immigrant* in terms of ready cultural assimilation is not necessarily the best opportunity for the migrant *student* whose primary goal is specialized training. Given the choice, an individual FMG might prefer optimal training irrespective of its location in the United States over a less than optimal opportunity in a city with strong ethnic ties and friendship networks.

Irrespective of such informal networks as a source of information about the American health care system, all groups expose themselves to the tensions inherent in the physician's dual role as potential immigrant and international student. Migrant doctors who enter the United States to join fellow nationals may carry essentially conflicting perceptions in belonging to two quite different communities—an ethnic community of immigrants on one hand, and an international medical community on the other. However, the migrant doctor who relies wholly on his or her position in the international medical community may not fully appreciate the cultural gulf to be bridged in moving from the professional system of one country to that of another.

Besides friends, the most important channel of information for recruitment into American hospitals is the "Green Book," published every year by the American Medical Association. However, a directory, however detailed its information, cannot prepare the foreigner for the complex patterns of prestige, behavior, speech, and role expectations that distinguish any sociocultural system. The American medical graduate knows instinctively, or has learned through the normal socialization process of 4 years in an American medical school, those hospitals which are "good" graduate training positions, in which specialties, and those regarded as "not so good." The foreigner without an inside track lacks this vital information, and may not realize that he or she lacks it.

In choosing to migrate, the FMG finds himself in transition between well-defined professional systems. Already launched on a career, the FMG abandons the familiar professional milieu, the medical profession of his own country, and the intimate knowledge gained of the workings of that system. A profession usually brings with it certainty; the FMG must now learn to cope with uncertainty. There is at once a breakdown of previous professional ties and a lack of ready assimilation into American medicine. American medical graduates with whom FMGs compete for jobs are already 4 years down the track. From being an insider in a familiar system, the FMG becomes a "stranger" in an alien system. For the first time in his or her career, the FMG may be forced to make decisions on the basis of inadequate information.

RECRUITMENT NETWORKS

For American medical graduates, entry to a first-year graduate position as an intern or resident is a natural progression in an ongoing process of professionalization. After 4 years of medical school, the USMG moves to 4 or more years of graduate education (the length depends on the specialty). Table 5.1 shows that USMGs rely heavily on their professional contacts and knowledge of the American system in finding their first internship or residency: 57 percent of the USMGs found their first training position through their own medical schools, through a clerkship in a particular hospital during their medical education, or through other professional sources. In short, the process of recruitment into first graduate positions for USMGs is predominantly through their insider's role in the professional system, substantially buttressed by the help of friends (typically others in training) in the United States. As a result, the USMG relies on directories and other formal sources to a minimal extent, although he or she may use a directory as a secondary source of information.

The process of recruitment for FMGs has greater variety, but it is distinguished by its lack of reliance on professional networks, either in the United States or in the home country. FMGs rely far more heavily than USMGs on personal connections and directories in finding their first training position: 76 percent of the FMGs found their first job through these channels, compared to 32 percent of the USMGs. Few FMGs were able to draw on professional resources in their own countries in finding a job in the United States; few could benefit from professional networks in this country.

American medical schools were the primary source of information about the hospital at which the FMG was subsequently employed for only one FMG out of our total sample of 690 (an estimated 0.2 percent of all FMGs). Generally, the American professional system was hostile or indifferent to recruiting FMGs. For FMGs the process is one of self-selection.

These findings undoubtedly reflect the house staff market system. Hospitals select USMGs first, then FMGs known to them, then other FMGs. There were, on the average, more FMG applicants for jobs than there were jobs available. Thus hospitals were not motivated to recruit FMGs deliberately. (Less than 1 percent of FMGs in our study group were recruited via hospital solicitation and 3 percent by advertisement). United States medical schools felt an obligation to place their own graduates in suitable positions and provided a ready source of general information for medical students. No such obligation or access existed for the majority of FMGs.

TABLE 5.1   HOW DID YOU FIRST HEAR ABOUT YOUR FIRST HOSPITAL OF
TRAINING IN THE UNITED STATES?

Primary source of information	FMG (percent)	USMG (percent)	USFMG (percent)
Personal connections	40.4	25.3	29.3
Friends in U.S.	22.2	20.2	28.1
Friends in CME[a]	7.7	NA	1.2
Family	6.0	2.8	—
Knew person at hospital	4.5	2.3	—
Formal sources	35.7	6.7	10.5
Directories	31.7	6.7	9.3
Medical journals	3.3	—	1.2
US/UN agencies	0.7	—	—
Professional networks, foreign	10.7	—	12.5
CME medical school	6.5	—	8.1
Persons in CME who had been to U.S.	4.2	—	4.4
Professional networks, U.S.A.	8.8	56.5	21.2
Intern/resident matching program	6.0	2.8	1.2
Well-known hospital/person	1.8	8.1	8.8
Hospital solicitation	0.8	5.2	1.2
U.S. medical school	0.2	30.1	4.4
Worked at hospital during medical school	—	10.3	5.6
Previous U.S. exposure	1.1	7.4	21.9
Other	3.3	4.4	4.4
Total	100.0 (681)[b]	100.0 (130)	100.0 (40)
	NA = 9	NA = 3	NA = 2

[a] Country of Medical Education.
[b] Percentages are weighted; N is unweighted.

Advice from the FMG's own professional milieu, including professors
and deans in the country of education, appears also to have been of little
assistance. Tables 5.1 and 5.2 indicate quite plainly that professional
sources in the home country are of little practical value in job seeking;
hence the latter's reliance on friends and directories. Although 40 percent
of the FMGs said they were influenced a "great deal" or "fair amount" by
teachers in their country of medical education in their decision to come to

TABLE 5.2   RATING OF INFORMATION USED BY FMGS IN SEEKING A U.S. HOSPITAL POSITION

Source of information	Reported by FMG as Helping				
	A great deal	A fair amount	A small amount	Not at all	Total
AMA Directory of Approved Internships and Residencies (Green Book)	50.3	16.8	7.4	25.6	100.0% (689)[a]
Friends who had been in the U.S.	34.2	23.4	16.4	26.1	100.0% (688)
National Internship and Residency Matching Program	12.5	2.4	3.3	81.9	100.0% (688)
Educational Commission for Foreign Medical Graduates (ECFMG)	8.7	20.4	18.0	52.9	100.0% (689)
Professors/deans at CME[b] medical school	7.7	12.4	21.2	58.7	100.0% (689)
Advertisements in U.S. medical journals	7.1	13.1	16.8	63.0	100.0% (688)
U.S. government offices (like USIS or consulate)	2.3	4.4	8.6	84.8	100.0% (689)

[a] Percentages are weighted; N is unweighted.
[b] Country of Medical Education.

the United States (Chapter 3), this advice appears largely hortatory. Only 20 percent of the FMGs found their teachers equally helpful in seeking an American hospital job, and 7 percent used them as the primary source of information about the hospital in which they actually found a position.

FMGs also received little help from American examining and governmental agencies. Help from the ECFMG, when it did exist, appeared to consist largely of directory assistance.

Advertisements in American journals were used by a few FMGs, although they were reportedly of some help to about one out of three (Table 5.2), perhaps by indicating the kind of information FMGs should seek in determining the relevance of a specific position. Our findings that 7 percent of FMGs found that advertisements helped them a "great deal," but only 3 percent learned of their first job from this source, suggests that the primary role of advertisements is educational or informational rather than as a direct employment procedure.

Advertisements in journals such as the *Journal of the American Medical Association*, which has a section "Interns and Residents Wanted," do not directly solicit FMGs. Some restrict applications to USMGs or experienced FMGs already in the United States by such requirements as a 1-year American internship, or the holding of a license to practice in the state. Others include statements such as "nondiscrimination in employment" or "equal opportunity employer," which may encourage FMGs as well as women and minority USMGs. One may hypothesize that the FMG who applies to an advertisement unsuccessfully will learn from the process and will know how to apply to other institutions, perhaps directly. More generally, the advertisements provide information that hospitals feel is important in their solicitations and may not be apparent from the Green Book. For example, a note by a New York City hospital that it is in a "good neighborhood" may alert the FMG to the fact that many American hospitals are in inner-city areas in which living conditions may be less than ideal. Information about hospital affiliation with universities may also instruct the FMG about the variations in American teaching situations: statements in advertisements that "full-time staff hold faculty appointments," "full educational program with university teachers," or "active academic program"[7] suggest, by their very inclusion, that all hospitals are not so blessed. Finally, information on varying salaries and fringe benefits (housing, meals, laundry, and insurance) may also provide useful background information to the FMG with little practical knowledge of the American system.

In terms of actually finding a job, however, the great majority of FMGs relied primarily on their friends, the Green Book, or both in combination. Table 5.2 shows that two-thirds of all FMGs said they were helped a "great deal" or "fair amount" by the Directory of Approved Internships and Residencies, and half were helped a "great deal" or "fair amount" by friends who had been in the United States.

FMGs who rely on the Green Book tend to apply to a number of hospitals, selected by area of the United States, by having heard of the hospital or by knowing of others who had gone to these places. Those FMGs relying on friends may choose to apply only to hospitals at which their friends are situated or may have jobs actually lined up for them. Although there are many other patterns of recruitment, it is striking how little FMGs are able to rely on professional networks such as medical schools or associations here and abroad. The results of this process are distinctive patterns of recruitment for FMGs compared to those for USMGs entering their first graduate educational position.

FORMAL SOURCES OF INFORMATION

The Green Book lists every hospital offering approved training programs in the United States by state, location, hospital size, specialty of training, number of positions offered, length of training, and salary. The directory also notes the administrative control of the hospital (i.e., whether it is a nonprofit corporation, Veterans Administration hospital, state hospital, etc.); whether the hospital is affiliated with a medical school and to what extent, how many of the house staff were foreign and how many non-foreign during the previous year, and the hospital's necropsy rate (percentage of patients who died in hospital on whom autopsies are performed), a presumed rough indicator of the institution's research emphasis. The Green Book thus provides considerable information not only about the location and size of the institution, but about its nature and status, at least to those familiar with the American system.

However, for those not familiar with the system, the detail of the Green Book is both bewildering and insufficient. Comments by FMGs in our hospital case studies emphasize that no advice was offered as to what was meant when it was said that a hospital has 400 beds or was a "community hospital." Information is provided, but the FMG lacks the criteria for interpretation.

In some ways, the Green Book may make the selection process more difficult. For example, although 90 percent of the training hospitals were affiliated with university medical schools in 1974, affiliation can range from the true "university" situation of a university hospital unit to a relatively loose affiliation agreement between a community hospital in one town or city and a medical school in another. In the latter, department chiefs may hold honorary university appointments and/or university faculty members may visit the hospital for teaching, but the hospital may offer a quite different teaching milieu from the university unit expected by many FMGs entering an "affiliated" hospital in the United States.

The American Medical Association classifies the hospitals affiliated with the universities into "major teaching units" (the hospital is a major unit in the medical school's M.D. teaching program), hospitals with "limited affiliation" (used for undergraduate teaching to a limited extent), and hospitals affiliated "for graduate training only." These categories speak for themselves in giving the highest status to hospitals most closely linked with undergraduate medical education, in which the USMG has an automatic entree. We use the categories throughout this book as indicators of levels of affiliation. However, there are wide differences within these categories: a "major teaching unit," for example, may include both a university unit staffed primarily by full-time faculty and

USMGs and run on strong departmental lines, and a community hospital run by private attending physicians, whose house staff is made up predominantly of FMGs. The USMG making a choice from within the status system is able to distinguish between the two. The FMG, poring over the Green Book in a medical library in a distant city, does the best he or she can given the information available. Our findings suggest that FMGs expect American graduate education to be uniformly excellent, based on the patterns of university medical schools, whereas USMGs know that there are wide variations.

Reliance on the directory also encourages FMGs to make numerous applications to American institutions; the FMG casts his or her net as wide as possible (Table 5.3). Although FMGs and USMGs tend to make single applications at rather similar rates, the average number of applications made by FMGs is much higher.

About one-fifth of both FMGs (23 percent) and USMGs (19 percent) were hired by the only hospital to which they applied, usually because they were assured of the position in advance. FMGs typically received such an assurance from family or friends or from the hospital's Director of

TABLE 5.3   NUMBER OF HOSPITALS APPLIED TO BY FMGS BY SELECTED SOURCE OF INFORMATION ABOUT FIRST U.S. JOB

Primary source of information	One	2–4	5 or more	Total
Family	51.5	34.5	14.0	100.0% (45)[a]
CME Medical School	39.4	31.2	29.4	100.0% (40)
Knew person at hospital	35.0	17.3	47.7	100.0% (34)
Friends in U.S.	32.0	23.1	44.9	100.0% (146)
Persons in CME who had been to U.S.	31.7	4.0	64.2	100.0% (25)
Friends in CME	17.7	22.9	59.5	100.0% (52)
National Internship and Residency Matching Program	6.7	7.5	85.8	100.0% (22)
Directories	6.4	15.4	78.3	100.0% (212)
All Sources[b]	22.8	22.2	55.0	100.0% (677) NA = 13

[a] Percentages are weighted; N is unweighted.
[b] Includes sources other than those selected above; for complete list, see Table 5.1

Medical Education (DME). USMGs were usually hired in advance by the DME or by faculty in an American medical school.[8]

Almost all USMGs who made multiple applications applied to fewer than nine hospitals: 52 percent applied to two, three, or four hospitals, and another 39 percent to between five and nine institutions, leaving 8 percent who applied to 10 or more hospitals. FMGs who applied to more than one hospital took a more scattershot approach: 29 percent applied to two, three, or four institutions, 25 percent to between five and nine, and 46 percent applied to 10 hospitals or more. Of our total sample of 690 FMGs, 118 applied to 20 hospitals or more in the hope of landing their first job.

The interview schedules ring with remarks such as these:

I applied everywhere—from the Green Book. (A male Indian FMG who applied to 98 hospitals, eventually gaining an appointment as an intern at a nonaffiliated hospital in the Northeastern United States.)

I looked through the books that have all the listings (A male FMG from Ecuador who came to the United States without the ECFMG certificate and took a job as a house physician in a Florida hospital before finding a rotating internship at a small county hospital.)

I applied to many hospitals and I got a contract from City. (A female Pakistani FMG).

I sent letters to hospitals and this hospital was the first to answer. (A male Honduran citizen, graduate of a medical school in Spain.)

I just wrote them through the Directory of Approved Residencies. (A male FMG from Eire.)

I came here without a job and then looked for one—Medical directory—green pages. (A male FMG from India who, having located his choices, then made use of the telephone and the Yellow Pages.)

Generally, FMGs who take the ECFMG examination in the United States apply to fewer hospitals than those taking the ECFMG abroad and use the Green Book less: 70 percent of the FMGs who passed the ECFMG abroad said that the Green Book helped them in their hospital search a "fair amount" or a "great extent", compared to 53 percent of those who passed it here.

These findings suggest either that FMGs already in the United States have better information and professional contacts open to them in the process of job selection than those applying from other countries, or tie their applications to a particular area or city. We conclude that at least some of those who enter the United States without the ECFMG certificate may have an advantage over their peers in the American job market rather than, as is sometimes supposed, a disadvantage because they are initially unqualified for American graduate education.[9] This is particularly apposite for FMGs who take work in hospitals in nontraining positions for which the certificate is not necessary, as a "house physician" or "house surgeon" or technologist. Such physicians have the opportunity to soak up the peculiar culture of the American hospital or the hospital system from a relatively neutral position. When they enter the training system, they know what it is like and how they will be treated.

Knowing what it is like is also an important prerequisite for effective use of the job-matching program widely used by American graduates, the National Intern and Resident Matching Program (NIRMP): 92 percent of the USMGs in our study said they used the matching program. As indicated in Table 5.2, the great majority of FMGs said the NIRMP was of no help to them in their search for an American hospital position.

The usefulness of the matching program is undoubtedly diminished for FMGs seeking their first job because the plan requires applicants to list their hospitals of preference—this presumes some foreknowledge of which hospitals will accept them. Ideally, physicians visit each hospital, are interviewed by hospital staff, and learn about the training program on a first-hand basis. The applicant then lists hospitals by preference, the hospital rates its applicants, and the NIRMP matches the applicant and hospital according to the two rank order lists. Such a system works well for American medical students, allowing them the chance to see hospitals and a standardized process of selection: all appointments under NIRMP are announced on a single date. Most FMGs have neither the opportunity to visit hospitals nor adequate information to make a selection.

Moreover, the NIRMP appears to present difficulties even to FMGs who are already in the United States. The scheduling of the ECFMG examination is such that it is impossible for an applicant to take that examination (passage of which is a prerequisite for NIRMP) and receive the score in time to enter the matching program in the same year. Those FMGs who enter the United States without the ECFMG certificate but with the intention of gaining it as rapidly as possible are thus almost bound to seek jobs independently; otherwise they will be jobless for several months.[10] Finally, those who enter the United States and hear of excellent training programs may apply to them through the matching program but may be rejected by all their selections.

Dr. A. provides an example of this "Catch–22" situation. This Nicaraguan citizen, who took his medical education in Brazil, came to the United

States in 1971 to take the 5-month preparation course for the ECFMG examination in Miami. After passing the examination, he applied for internships through the matching program at hospitals initially recommended to him by his professors in Brazil, including Johns Hopkins and the University of Michigan. He was soon to find out, however, "that these places are not going to hire you." Somewhat bitter at having lost a year by relying on his superiors (Dr. A. had meanwhile returned to Nicaragua), he took informal advice from colleagues who had been to the United States and applied to 12 more modest American hospitals directly; the result was an internship at a community hospital in Louisiana, predominantly staffed by FMGs.

INFORMAL PATTERNS OF RECRUITMENT

Dr. A's story shows the interweaving of the various recruitment networks and the importance of information from colleagues and friends as a direct line to specific training institutions. Friends in the United States were cited as the primary source of information about their first American job by 22 percent of all FMGs (Table 5.1), friends in the country of medical education by another 8 percent, members of the family by 6 percent, and connections at the employing hospital by another 5 percent; 40 percent of all FMGs found their first American job through this informal network of family and friends. As indicated in Table 5.2, many others also referred to such connections as part of the process of job selection. Informal patterns of recruitment and selection are thus the single most important vehicle for FMGs in overcoming the systemic biases of the American system against the ignorance and lack of status of outsiders.

Of our total sample of 690 FMGs, 64 applied to one hospital because they had been assured by friends that a job was there or because they had family in the area; another 47 said they had a "special interest" in this one hospital, a term that may include personal connections. (USMGs, in contrast, rarely rely on such personal networks.)

Thus an FMG from Ceylon, interviewed in a hospital in Chicago, chose this hospital because "my brother worked here." A female physician from Cuba said of her choice of a hospital in Miami: "We went directly there because my family was there and also we have a friend who is a doctor who worked [here]." Another Cuban, trained in Spain, chose Orlando, Florida, because "I knew they needed trained personnel in surgery." An FMG from Costa Rica chose Atlanta, Georgia, for a similar reason. A Jordanian citizen who had graduated from medical school in Germany chose a nonaffiliated hospital in Ohio for his first position in a city selected because his three Jordanian brothers-in-law had settled there: the hospital itself he selected from the Green Book.

Such examples not only illustrate the reliance of FMGs on kin and friendship networks, but also describe the way in which "chain migration" or clustering takes place. In some cases the process can be seen in development. For example, the Indian FMG in our sample who applied to 98 hospitals selected from the Green Book was able to provide a basis for subsequent migration. His sister, also a physician, has come to join him at the same institution, and they have set up house together.

Familial clusterings are by no means unusual and indeed may have been influential in the FMG's decision to come to the United States. Thus a Singapore physician came to the United States because "all the family is out here." This physician not only had family in San Francisco, where he settled, but cousins at Cornell and Johns Hopkins. An Iranian FMG joined the staff of a New Jersey hospital because his aunt, a registered nurse in that hospital, told him of a "good possibility" there. Another Iranian was influenced in his choice of a hospital in Florida by his cousin in private practice: "She is in Ob-Gyn. When she visited us in Iran, she told me they have a very good department here."

Friends provide a similar supporting role. A Pakistani physician joined a friend working at a Connecticut hospital. A Filipino woman physician found out from her friends in Baltimore, "that they had an opening"; a second joined two nurse friends at a hospital in Chicago; a third, in the United States as a dependent, heard of a job opening while having her second baby at a New Jersey hospital from a friend on the staff there. A Mexican physician remarked: "It was an accident, I was at the University of Miami [taking courses for the ECFMG] and met a friend who was instrumental in getting me the application to the hospital and they accepted me. Originally I expected to go elsewhere." An Iranian physician joined a friend, "My wife's friend actually," in Cleveland.

These grapevines are not only useful as points of contact with the American system, they are undoubtedly an advantage in the job market. The hospital can rely on a known person to vouch for the character of an unknown; the FMG can join his or her peers. Table 5.3 indicates that half of the FMGs who relied primarily on information from their family, and a third of those who relied on the advice of friends in the United States or who knew someone at the hospital or someone who had been in the United States, negotiated with only one American hospital—the one that offered them a job.

Friends and family are most useful in discovering job availability, but not necessarily in locating the most appropriate training locations. A distinction must be drawn between access to the United States, specifically to the hospital system, the primary role of friendship networks, and matching training opportunities to individual needs. Typically, the migrant enters the United States (as have other immigrants) as an employee, taking jobs that might not otherwise be filled in locations already served by immigrants. Access to the job market is the key to the successful assimilation of immigrants, and one expects new migrants to join the market at a relatively low level. Such positions are not necessarily the best training positions for international exchange students who expect to return to their own nations, who may have no desire to be assimilated into American life (quite the reverse), and who come to the United States to experience the best in specialized techniques.

Reliance by FMGs on friends and directories for information about a first American position fosters the first process (immigration), not the second (international exchange). Thus a Brazilian exchange visitor selected 15 hospitals from the Green Book and was appointed to one that had no university affiliation. A Malaysian-Chinese graduate of a medical school in Taiwan also entered as an exchange visitor to a nonaffiliated hospital, lined up by a doctor friend. An Indian physician selected a church hospital in Illinois with a total house staff of two, because he had heard of it through friends from his medical school who had also interned there. We hypothesize that such processes actually encourage FMGs to *perceive themselves as immigrants*, who will wish to climb the status ladder in America, rather than as international exchange students.

FMGs for whom advice was most nearly matched with appropriate training opportunities were probably those with a direct line of contact between their own medical schools and specific hospitals. Over one-third of the FMGs who heard of their first hospital via their own professional medical school networks were accepted to the one hospital to which they applied. However, these FMGs represent a small minority of all migrant physicians. Generally, FMGs appear to accept the first job made available to them, either by direct introduction or a letter of acceptance.

EXPECTATIONS OF THE AMERICAN SYSTEM

We suggest that the FMG holds a series of conflicting attitudes and roles in coming to the American hospital system. The decision to come to the United States puts many FMGs in a double-bind situation in which there are disadvantages as well as advantages (Chapter 3). A second series of conflicts arises in the clash between "culture-free" and "culture-specific" aspects of medicine. FMGs as a group tend to think of themselves as internationally mobile scientists, with skills that can be applied anywhere in the world.[11] Entry to an American hospital, in contrast, jolts the FMG to recognition of his or her status as an alien or outsider. Finally, the channels of information about American hospitals available to FMGs set up tension between the physician as an exchange student and the physician as a United States immigrant.

The insecurities arising from these conflicts are inevitably exaggerated by a lack of concrete—very basic—information about American hospital life (Table 5.4). The size of the hospital poses little problem: the number of beds is clearly stated in the Green Book. FMGs are also relatively well

TABLE 5.4   ADEQUACY OF INFORMATION ABOUT FIRST U.S. POSITION IN THE LIGHT OF EXPERIENCE

As it turned out, once you began working at (first U.S. hospital), did you feel you had been adequately informed:	Percentage answering "Yes" to each question		
	FMG	USMG	USFMG
About the hospital's size?	95.4[a]	95.5	100.0
About the hospital's location?	87.0	100.0	100.0
Whether or not the hospital had an affiliation with a university medical school?	76.3	97.7	97.6
Those entering			
Major teaching units	83.4	98.4	100.0
Limited affiliation	75.7	90.4	100.0
Graduate training only	80.7	100.0	77.9
Nonaffiliated units	68.0	100.0	93.1
About the working conditions in general?	74.1	88.1	97.6
About the duties of your position?	61.8	83.6	82.4
About the quality of the hospital's teaching program?	57.9	86.4	84.8
Those entering			
Major teaching units	65.9	87.1	81.8
Limited affiliation	54.6	86.0	100.0
Graduate training only	52.7	100.0	77.9
Nonaffiliated units	49.0	84.3	93.1
About the social and economic characteristics of patients?	50.9	97.7	98.8
Percent base (N)	(690)[a]	(133)	(42)

[a] Percentages are weighted, N is unweighted.

informed about the hospital's location, because the hospital's address also appears clearly in the Green Book. However, the first note of the "strangeness" of the American experience appears in this question with respect to the 13 percent of FMGs (94 members of our study group) who felt they were inadequately informed about some aspects of the location of American hospitals, including the fact that many large hospitals are in poverty areas of major cities. One-third of these FMGs elaborated by citing "bad neighborhood"; one-third gave no explanation, and one-third blamed themselves for not asking about the neighborhood or gave assorted reasons, including five FMGs in our group who had trouble finding the hospital on arrival.

Almost one-fourth of the FMGs said they were inadequately informed about the hospital's affiliation with a university medical school. Of these ($N = 122$), 44 percent said they were sent false or misleading information by the hospital (for example, that X hospital is affiliated with Y medical school when that means a very loose affiliation rather than university teaching in the hospital), 25 percent said they found the hospital was not affiliated after they got there and felt that they should have been told; 3 percent found affiliation more limited than expected. A lucky 10 percent made a positive discovery: the hospital was affiliated more closely than they expected. The remaining 18 percent cited miscellaneous reasons or proffered no explanation.

Lack of information was marked for the 208 FMGs in our study group who entered nonaffiliated hospitals; almost one-third said they were inadequately informed about affiliation when making their initial hospital selection. It seems clear that many FMGs come to the United States with little notion of the importance of university affiliation to their training.

The resulting awakening can cause bitterness, as a few examples illustrate:

> The AMA said [there would be] a great deal of affiliation with a university medical school but there was not as much as they said. (A Japanese exchange visitor, looking forward to returning to Japan, in a hospital predominantly staffed with FMGs, affiliated with a new, still developing American medical school.)

> It said [it was affiliated] somewhere in the hospital paper, but it had no university affiliation. Legally it was, but in practice it didn't exist. (A New Zealand physician trained in Britain.)

> I should have been told the truth. I was disappointed. I was told they were affiliated with [University] but instead the only affiliation they ever had. . .was when their residents went [there] for lectures. The whole thing was very disappointing. . . (A Filipino physician.)

. . .It was not affiliated and there is no full time teaching staff or approved medical residency. (A Pakistani physician entering a program approved for internships only.)

The truth—everything they said was wrong—they are lying about such affiliation. (An Iranian physician.)

Our conclusion is not that American hospitals deliberately distort information about the degree of university affiliation, but that the term "university affiliation" as used in the American hospital system leads physicians trained in other systems to erroneous assumptions. In many countries a university hospital is one staffed by fulltime university faculty and used intensively for the teaching of medical students. Other hospitals are not referred to as university affiliated even if the staff includes some parttime medical school faculty; not so in the United States. The custom of American hospitals of including a note of their affiliation with a stated university on their letterhead and in their brochures may well give FMGs the impression that the hospital is a primary source of teaching for the university and that they will be taught by university staff, whereas, in fact, outside the university unit proper, interns and residents are taught by fulltime community hospital staff, some of whom have courtesy university appointments, and by private practitioners.

These are distinctions in the social organization of medicine—in medicine's culture-specific attributes—and can be attributed to lack of perception of the American system as much as to lack of information. Perception is closely related to expectations. One of the few publications written for FMGs makes this point explicitly by listing the many ways in which American medicine is different from what the FMG may have previously experienced or labeled as "good" in his or her own system.

Among the distinctions: American medical education is research oriented, teaching about the unusual or the unknown, whereas most schools elsewhere teach about common conditions. Most physicians in the United States are specialists, not general practioners. Hospitals vary enormously in type and nature. The practice of medicine in America is unique with regard to legal matters (malpractice claims) that may arise between doctor and patient, including the importance of the medical record as the basis for a lawsuit, factors that may shock FMGs from other nations. In the hospital, the FMG may be faced with large case loads, long hours, a faster pace, and language difficulties. Added to these are broader social distinctions, including the attitude to death (FMGs are warned not to appear unfeeling), and the narrower gap between men and women—

the nursing staff must be treated as equals.[12] The American hospital is full of the unexpected.

Such considerations may well explain our findings that 26 percent of FMGs felt inadequately informed about general working conditions in American hospitals, 38 percent about the duties of his or her new position, and 40 percent about the quality of the hospital's teaching program (Table 5.4). By far the most frequent comment on house staff duties by FMGs was that they had more work, more patients, or more responsibility than they expected. Comments about working conditions concentrated on the fact that much of the work was routine, at least with respect to their previous expectations.

Some physicians, used to the more authoritative role of physicians in many societies, were surprised to find that they had to wheel patients themselves or take prescriptions to the lab if they wanted speedy service. An Indian FMG in a large city hospital remarked "everything must be done yourself." Some found, in the words of another Indian physician, that they had no responsibility for decision making in the actual medical care of patients: "The history and physicals of patients is the major responsibility for residents." A Cuban woman physician remarked, "Our culture is different and we had different work assignments. We didn't have to do any IV's, inserting catheters in men—in our country we didn't do that, usually the nurse did it, but here we have to do these things." Such duties are not necessarily any different for FMGs than the USMGs in similar situations. The difference is that USMGs, having done clerkships in American hospitals, are aware of what to expect.

Complaints about the quality of teaching ($N = 280$) included comments about little or poor teaching and ambiguous or nonexistent information sent to FMGs; a few said that the hospital was a private hospital and that they were not aware of the implications of this, that is that the house staff worked for private attending physicians, or that the hospital had no residency program and that they were unaware of the importance of this, since much teaching of juniors is done by residents. Only 3 percent of the respondents remarked that, although they were uninformed about teaching quality, their discovery was a happy one: teaching was better than expected. Again, such discoveries may require considerable personal adjustments.

As a final illustration of "culture shock," half of all FMGs said they had been inadequately informed about the social and economic characteristics of American patients (Table 5.4). Some FMGs were surprised to find themselves in largely private hospitals catering to middle-class Americans. A general criticism of this milieu as a first post was that house staff had relatively little responsibility (compared with a university hospital, for example), because the private attending physicians were often unwilling to delegate responsibility.

Others expected to find white, middle-class patients and were faced with patients from urban ghettos in large city institutions. Some FMGs may never have had to deal directly with poverty before; others expected all Americans to be relatively affluent and well educated. An Iranian physician in Baltimore complained, "The patients are almost all Black; for the first few months I could not understand them." A Lebanese citizen, trained in the United Arab Republic, says, "I didn't know there were so many Puerto Ricans, Blacks, welfare patients." An Icelandic physician found that "it was and still is difficult for me to adjust to the ethnic group (Puerto Rican) because for me it is completely foreign to my own." A Filipino said, "I should have been told about which class they belonged to—they are such a low class of people, all of them." A Brazilian said, "They are poorer than I expected and less educated."

Although many of those who said they were uninformed about the social and economic characteristics of American patients added that, in fact, such lack of knowledge made no difference to their own experiences, the strangeness of entry to the American hospital cannot be gainsaid. FMGs arrive knowing relatively little about the nature of, and variations in, the American hospital patient population, the organization of the hospital system, or the complicated systems by which American patients pay for medical care, usually through private health insurance, Medicare, or Medicaid.

Perhaps foreigners can never be adequately informed about the complexities of the American hospital system; knowledge may only come from working in it. However, the lack of basic information experienced by many FMGs suggests areas in which some difficulties could be ameliorated or avoided. An Iranian FMG remarked that if he had been told what kind of patient population there was at his hospital, he could have been more helpful. Introductions to the American sociocultural medical system through formal courses or other forms of orientation might also have helped the Filipino who "didn't expect to find the patient who couldn't pay put in a separate place. . . I just didn't understand it"; the British physician who said, "I come from a socialized medicine area and was shocked at the number of people here who have inadequate health insurance"; or the Pakistani who assumed, to the contrary, that America had no health insurance: "I feel I would have liked to know that there was an extensive health insurance program so I could have ordered things sooner." A Taiwanese graduate said bluntly, "The hospital should give instruction about U.S. health programs, such as Blue Cross, Medicare, and such."

CONCLUSION

Some FMGs, coming to the United States with vague expectations of specialized training, are disillusioned and condemnatory of the sociocultural aspects of American medicine, notably, the lack of a national health service, the prevalence of malpractice claims, and general attitudes to poverty populations. However, the series of adjustments FMGs experience on entering the United States may well have a cumulative effect on all FMGs. Culture changes themselves pose difficulties to many: "The food and the climate and the customs were strange." For some, housing posed enormous problems. Orientation programs, when they existed, were frequently frail vehicles to remedy the FMG's lack of information. Previous ignorance of American hospital patients, house staff duties, working conditions, and hospital affiliation is thus compounded.

We conclude that FMGs lack essential information about the American system that might affect their hospital selection, perhaps even the decision to come. As far as selection and recruitment is concerned, FMGs are matched to hospitals on pragmatic lines, relating primarily to job availability. Information programs, developed by United States Government agencies, by hospitals or by professional associations, could go a long way to easing the process of transition. Orientation programs which include analysis of the American medical system, health insurance and other organizational aspects of medicine, could help further to develop realistic responses to the American experience.

The conflicts in the FMG's roles and status described in this chapter indicate, however, that questions of recruitment and expectations are by no means simple questions of adequate or inadequate information. Both the FMGs themselves and the American hospitals that advise them appear to consider "medicine" as a readily transferable international entity, yet studies of the sociology of undergraduate medical education emphasized long ago that medicine is by no means solely the mastery of common techniques. An important part of medical education is how to cope—to behave—when faced with uncertainty: uncertainty deriving from limitations in the state of knowledge, from the individual's imperfect mastery of that knowledge, and from inconsistent or ambivalent information.[13] Behavior is always culture specific, not readily transferable across international lines. A physician works in a specific sociocultural environment. His or her role is conditioned by social expectations, professional traditions and the operation of a particular medical care system.

After migrating, the FMG must readjust his or her professional responses and learned modes of behavior and become reeducated— resocialized—in a foreign system. Such processes, already complex, are made more so by the fact that FMGs must rely largely on their own initiative in seeking their first American position.

NOTES

1. In 1973–1974, 66,000 internships and residencies were offered in 1711 American hospitals. Although almost 90 percent of these hospitals were by then affiliated with a university medical school, selections are usually done by staff in the individual hospitals, often specific specialty departments for appointments in those areas. The system applying to our sample is described in *Directory of Approved Residencies*, Chicago: AMA, 1974 (appears annually).

2. See for example Leonard Broom, "Social Differentiation and Stratification," in *Sociology Today, Problems and Prospects* Robert K. Merton et.al. (Eds.), Harper and Row: Vol. II, New York, 1965, 429–41.

3. Stephen Smith Mick and Eileen Hoffman, *Preliminary Report on the Hospital Case Studies*, New Haven: Yale University (mimeographed), 1972. Gary Dean Sax, *Foreign Medical Graduates in Yale-Affiliated Community Hospitals*, an essay presented to the Department of Epidemiology and Public Health, Yale University, in candidacy for the degree of Master of Public Health, 1973.

4. R. A. Lochore, *From Europe to New Zealand*, Wellington, 1951. For a later discussion, see Charles Price, "The Study of Assimilation," in Jackson (Ed.) *Migration, op cit.*, pp. 181–237.

5. See Myron D. Fottler and Thanin Thanapisitikul, "Some Correlates of Residence Preference among Foreign Medical Graduates: A Case Study of Thai Medical Graduates in Buffalo," *Medical Care* (1974), 12: 778–87.

6. J. N. Haug and B.C. Martin, *Foreign Medical Graduates in the United States, 1970*, Chicago: Center for Health Service Research and Development, AMA, 1971, pp. 216–17, 249.

7. Examples are from the *Journal of the American Medical Association*, October 21, 1974, pp. 504–05.

8. For FMGs who applied to one American hospital ($N = 172$), "Did someone assure you of the position in advance?" Yes, 55.4 percent; No, 44.6 percent. "If yes, Who?": Family connections, 40.7 percent, U.S. Director of Medical Education, 37.1 percent; Supervisor in CME, 13.4 percent, other, 8.9 percent. "Why did you apply to only one hospital?": Friends knew job was there or family lived in area, 33.6 percent; special interest in the hospital, 27.1 percent; R was accepted right away, 22.2 percent, other 17.1 percent. For USMGs who applied to one American hospital ($N = 27$). "Did someone assure you of position in advance?" Yes, 59.6 percent. "Who?" U.S. Director of Medical Education, 32.3 percent; medical school supervisor, 26.3 percent; family connections, 15.2 percent; other, 26.3 percent.

9. See, for example, Robert J. Weiss, "The Effect of Importing Physicians—Return to a pre-Flexnerian Standard", *New England Journal of Medicine* (1974), 290: 1453–58.

10. We did not ask our FMG respondents directly whether they used the NIRMP, only how far it helped FMGs in their search for an American hospital position: 93.0 percent of FMGs who took their ECFMG in the United States said the NIRMP helped them "not at all," compared to 79.6 percent of those taking it abroad: an average of 81.9 percent for both groups (see table 5.2).

11. "In general, medicine is a science which can be practiced anywhere in the world regardless of social and cultural differences." FMGs agree strongly (71.9 percent), agree somewhat (15.2 percent), disagree strongly or somewhat (12.8 percent).

12. Yvan J. Silva, *Career Development for Foreign Medical Graduates in the United States*, Springfield, Illinois, Charles C. Thomas, 1973.

13. See Renée C. Fox, "Training for Uncertainty," in Robert K. Merton, George G. Reader, and Patricia Kendall (eds.), *The Student-Physician*, Harvard University Press, Cambridge, 1957, pp. 207–41.

6

PATTERNS OF ENTRY TO THE U.S. HEALTH CARE SYSTEM_____

INTRODUCTION

Patterns of selection and recruitment have an obvious effect on the distribution of FMGs in the U.S. training system. The influence of friends and chain migration encourages FMGs to join others, concentrating foreign physicians in particular hospitals, cities, and states. Reliance on the Green Book to find a hospital also encourages entry into specific states, because the foreign physician may note at a glance that FMGs are in the majority of positions in virtually all training hospitals in some states (New Jersey is a prime example), whereas in others (e.g., California) the reverse is evident.[1] In the absence of other assistance, reason would suggest to the FMG that applications to the former rather than to the latter states are more likely to be successful. Why apply, for example, to the University of Colorado Affiliated Hospitals, with a house staff of 465, but only 13 FMGs? Would not the Brooklyn–Cumberland Center in New York City seem a more likely prospect, with its house staff of 163, of whom 157 were FMGs in 1973?[2] Assuming that FMGs exercise judgment on the basis of all available knowledge, the recruitment process encourages entry to specific hospitals and certain states.

In fact, the process of self-selection and the demand of American hospitals for residents work interdependently. Each process encourages the biases of the other. The selection process for FMGs is built on the assumption that jobs are usually available in certain areas and institutions because they have not been filled by USMGs. At the same time, the availability of a relatively large supply of FMGs allows "favored" institutions and states such as California to take the great majority of their house staff from U.S. medical schools, leaving few openings for foreign physicians; institutions that are relatively less attractive to USMGs are unable to fill their available posts and are willing to offer jobs to foreign physicians. The effect of this market system, geared as it is to the selection of USMGs, has led to skewed distributions of USMGs in terms of available training positions and thus, in progression, to skewed distributions of FMGs. For whatever reason, as this chapter shows, FMGs are distributed in their first American positions in ways that are quite different from the initial distributions of USMGs. Although these patterns may be the product of wide disparities in training opportunities in the American system as a whole, FMGs tend to begin their U.S. training in different states, in hospitals with a lesser degree of university affiliation than is available for USMGs, with fewer training opportunities, and to join house staffs that are filled with other FMGs.

This is the first nationwide study to examine the entry patterns of FMGs into the American health care system. Annual figures collected and tabulated by the American Medical Association show only where *all* FMGs in house staff positions are located in any given year; they give a static snapshot. Thus it has been possible to show, for example, that FMGs are found disproportionately in hospitals without university affiliation, in smaller hospitals than USMGs, and in the Northeast, Mid-Atlantic, and East North-Central States,[3] but we have not known whether this is because the "entry system" for FMGs has steered new arrivals in these directions or whether FMGs tend to gravitate toward certain positions after their first American job has been completed.

Knowledge about entry patterns is important from three distinctive points of view: first, with respect to the impact of American educational and immigration policies on the flow of new entrants; second, to the organizational role played by American hospitals in assimilating new entrants; and third, to the FMG's American career. If the number of entering FMGs is to be cut back drastically by changes in the immigration laws (as new legislation suggests),[4] it becomes important to evaluate the effects this might have on the pattern of entry of FMGs who continue to come to the United States. Will the number be reduced, but the distribution patterns remain the same, with FMGs continuing to enter similar hospitals and states? To look at this, we must know whether all American hospitals receive new FMGs at similar rates, or whether there are identifiable types of hospitals that act as portals of entry to the system.

Different questions arise from examining the impact of the hospital system on the careers and perceptions of individual FMGs. In entering graduate medical education—the period of internship and residency—the physician commits himself (herself) to a vaguely defined apprenticeship in a complex and structured institution. Professionally, the hospital becomes his home; he has to learn the household rules. Indeed, success in learning depends, in large part, on successful integration of the resident in the hospital social system and on acceptance by members of that system: by patients, nurses, other members of the house staff, chiefs of service, and attending physicians. In turn, the resident is molded by the expectations inherent in the hospital, and such expectations may vary according to the nature and structure of each institution. The first graduate educational position plays, in short, an important role in socializing the young physician into the nuances of the American medical profession. Since this is certainly true for new American graduates, it is reasonable to suppose that the first American training hospital is also of particular importance in the socialization of alien physicians.

That there are distinctive expectations and definitions of the house staff role in different American training hospitals has been demonstrated in the literature.[5] Different hospitals produce different role models for house staff to follow at a critical stage in their career. Where the FMG goes first for American training may have a profound effect on his or her definition of the "ideal" American physician, attitude to American hospital life, expectations of training, and future career.

FIRST AMERICAN TRAINING POSITION

Graduate educational positions for physicians fall into three basic types: internships, residencies, and research positions.[6] The internship, originally designed as a general first year of graduate education, is in the process of being phased out. However, our findings show that the great majority (94 percent) of the USMGs in training in 1974 had completed or were in the process of completing an internship; their normal pattern of graduate education was a 1-year internship followed by a specialist residency of from 3 to 5 years. Three-fourths of the USMGs entered internships in hospitals designated as major teaching units, that is, with the closest degree of affiliation with a university medical school.

This pattern provides a paradigm against which FMG entry positions can be measured. However, because of the substantial prior training and experience of FMGs as a group, one would expect many FMGs to enter the American system above the basic internship level.

TABLE 6.1 TYPE OF FIRST U.S. HOSPITAL POSITION

	FMG	USMG	USFMG
Internship	78.3	94.1	73.3
Residency	18.0	5.3	26.8
Research position	3.7	0.6	0.0
	100.0% (690)[a]	100.0% (133)	100.0% (42)

[a] Percentages are weighted; *N* is unweighted.

Table 6.1 indicates that FMGs were, indeed, more likely than USMGs to enter American graduate positions at the residency level, although, in fact, less than one in five FMGs actually did so; in addition, a small minority (4 percent) entered research positions. Thus, 78 percent of the FMGs began their American training as interns, compared with 94 percent of the USMGs.

When the positions are considered in terms of type of position and hospital affiliation, wider differences in entry patterns emerge. Almost three-fourths of the USMGs began their graduate careers in internships in major teaching units; however, little more than one-fourth of the FMGs entered the American system via this pathway.

The overall differences by type of affiliation are striking. Thus 41 percent of the FMGs began their American training in a hospital with a major university affiliation, 29 percent in other affiliated units, and 29 percent entered the system as an intern or resident in a hospital with *no* university affiliation. Comparable figures for USMGs were 78 percent, 14 percent and 8 percent. In short, USMGs almost always entered training at hospitals with at least some medical school affiliation, whereas almost one-third of the FMGs began their American training in positions that had no university teaching supervision.

A number of explanations can be advanced for these patterns. One is that FMGs choose specialties that fall with relatively great frequency outside the affiliated units. Our findings show, however, that approximately 60 percent of both USMGs and FMGs began their American careers without a specialty (Table 6.2), that is, in general positions, typically in rotating internships; the preferred location for USMGs entering such positions was in hospitals with a major university affiliation. Specialty alone cannot explain the differences.

TABLE 6.2   SPECIALTY OF FIRST U.S. POSITION[a]

	FMG	USMG	USFMG
General training (no specialty)	58.2	65.7	63.2
Surgical specialties	13.0	5.0	8.2
Medical specialties	12.1	19.1	7.7
Hospital-based specialties (anesthesiology, pathology, radiology)	6.0	2.9	8.3
Psychiatry	2.3	3.4	1.2
Obstetrics/gynecology	1.6	0.5	5.3
Pediatrics	1.6	2.9	.0
General/family practice	0.8	.0	1.2
Other	5.5	0.5	4.8
Total	100.0% (686)[b]	100.0% (133)	100.0% (42)
	NA = 4		

[a] Figures include specialty of first U.S. position of any kind, including those FMGs whose first U.S. job was not an approved graduate training position ($N = 72$). The "other" category includes FMGs whose first job was nonmedical ($N = 33$), as well as those in other medical specialties.
[b] Percentages are weighted; N is unweighted.

Moreover, the differences in entry patterns hold for individual specialties. Although our figures for specialty groups are small, the results are striking: the USMG begins his training in a major teaching unit, irrespective of specialty; the FMG begins outside such units. FMGs who enter training at the first-year (internship) level are much more likely than USMGs to begin training outside major teaching units. Only those who entered pediatric and obstetric internships in our study were the exceptions to this general rule; three-fourths of the FMGs entering pediatrics internships took positions in major teaching units, together with half of those entering internships in obstetrics. In all other cases, a minority of

FMG interns entered major teaching units, compared to the vast majority of USMGs.

Generally, FMGs entering the American system as residents were more likely than other FMGs to enter major teaching units. Half of the FMGs entering residencies in primary care (general practice or family medicine, internal medicine, and pediatrics) began their American training in major teaching units. Residents in psychiatry were least likely to enter major teaching units, whereas FMGs entering residencies in the hospital-based fields of anesthesiology, radiology, and pathology were the most likely of all groups to begin their training in major teaching units, with more than 80 percent entering such units. Even here, however, the rate for USMGs exceeded that of FMGs; all the USMGs in the hospital-based specialties began their training in major teaching units.

The relatively small proportion of FMGs entering major teaching units undoubtedly reflects employment realities. FMGs compete with USMGs for the jobs in major teaching units, but compete largely with each other for jobs in other types of hospitals. FMGs appointed to residencies at first position may be more carefully screened by employing hospitals than other FMGs; that is, FMGs entering the American system as residents may be outstanding candidates and thus more likely to be appointed to major teaching units than to other hospitals. In addition, or alternatively, such FMGs may have better access than other FMGs to the American professional system, enabling them to find both a residency and a prestigious entering position; but such entrants are in the minority. For most FMGs the entry channel is the internship. The differential patterns of entry reflect these processes; FMGs begin graduate training outside major teaching units irrespective of their chosen specialty.

Two other facets of specialty interest should be noted. First, despite the fact that the primary reason for FMG interest in the United States is the desire for more medical specialization (Chapter 3), FMGs actually tend to begin training in nonspecialized training positions. One possible explanation of this is that all American training positions may seem "specialized" to the FMG seeking to enter the United States: the question may thus be one of semantics rather than substance. It is also likely, however, that the patterns reflect practical elements, including the requirement by American state licensing boards of a year of internship, similar requirements by specialty boards, and last (but not least) the availability of general rather than specialist internships at the time most of our sample was job-hunting.

This conclusion is strengthened by a second aspect of specialist entry evident in our study findings. There is no relationship between the strength of the FMG's desire to come to the United States for specialization—that is, whether the physician regards "more medical special-ization in the United States" as influencing him a great deal, to some extent, or not at all in the decision to migrate—and the chance of a first job in a major teaching unit, presumably the most specialized type of pro-gram. Of the 268 FMGs who said that they were influenced "a great deal" by medical specialization in coming to the United States, 44.2 percent began their American training in major teaching units, 28.0 percent went to other affiliated units, and 27.9 percent to nonaffiliated hospitals. These proportions are virtually the same as those for all FMGs.

On the other hand, there is a relationship between entering hospitals and the FMG's sources of information about the American hospital sys-tem. Notably, FMGs who were accepted into major teaching units for the first hospital position relied more often on professional contacts in the United States and on friends in seeking their first American hospital than did FMGs entering nonaffiliated hospitals.[7] Those entering nonaffiliated hospitals, in contrast, were heavily dependent on the help of directories. Almost half of the FMGs whose first job was in a nonaffiliated unit relied on formal sources of information, compared to little over one-fourth of those entering major teaching units. Those entering nonaffiliated hos-pitals also relied less frequently on friends in the United States, although they relied more frequently on their family, and friends in the CME. It appears, then, that those entering the major teaching units are those with the most highly developed contacts within the American training system. Those who go to nonaffiliated units do so either because they are unin-formed about other possibilities or because they join family members already in a specific location (the classic pattern of immigration).

Taken together, the findings in this section support our previous con-clusions that FMGs choose their first position by job availability rather than by the potential for training; that is, FMGs enter positions in non-affiliated hospitals and in hospitals with limited affiliation because they are offered such positions, rather than because of unique training advan-tages by specialty.

ENTERING AFFILIATED AND NON-AFFILIATED HOSPITALS

If specialty is not a factor in the entry of FMGs to major teaching units, what is? In the next sections, three other variables are explored: the respondent's academic background as revealed in the respondent's place in class during medical school, the country of medical education and race, and the respondent's visa status.

Academic Background

The academic background of physicians is important in determining whether there is, as generally supposed, a ranking process in graduate medical education, with the best graduates entering the most prestigious training situations. Harrison observed from data on house staff collected in the late 1950s that both USMGs and FMGs in affiliated hospitals were drawn disproportionately from the top quarter of their medical school class.[8] Our findings show some relationship between class standing and first hospital affiliation, although this is clearly only one of several potential causative factors in the distributional patterns by hospital affiliation. The results are shown in Table 6.3.

TABLE 6.3   ACADEMIC BACKGROUND OF RESPONDENTS AND ENTRY TO AFFILIATED AND NONAFFILIATED HOSPITALS

	FMG	USMG	USFMG
Respondents in upper third of class	76.0	47.7	68.8
Entered major teaching units	34.0	39.1	46.4
Entered other affiliated units	23.0	4.8	14.5
Entered nonaffiliated hospitals	19.0	3.8	8.0
Respondents not in upper third of class	23.9	52.4	31.2
Entered major teaching units	7.2	39.0	5.1
Entered other affiliated units	6.2	9.1	13.0
Entered nonaffiliated hospitals	10.5	4.3	13.0
	100.0% (690)[a]	100.0% (133)	100.0% (42)

[a] Percentages are weighted; *N* is unweighted.

Respondents in our study were asked to rank themselves according to whether they were in the top, middle, or lower third of their class. The results, self-perceived, must be taken with some qualification, since there is undoubtedly some inflation of position, if only from wishful thinking. Thus half of the USMGs ranked themselves in the top third of their class, a mathematical impossibility; so did most of the USFMGs and three fourths of the FMGs, and virtually no one in any group admitted to being in the lowest segment. Within the two basic levels of response—top third and middle third—there were, however, suggestive patterns of entry to major teaching units. Thus 45 percent of the FMGs who said they were in the top third of their medical school class entered American training in major teaching units, compared to 30 percent of those with lesser credentials. Comparable figures for USMGs were 82 percent and 70 percent.

However, these patterns must be viewed in the context of how the various groups were actually distributed. The USMGs entered major teaching hospitals whether they were in the top third of their class or not. For USMGs, place in class is not a major determining factor in initial placement in a major teaching unit, although it may well affect the particular hospital or program entered. For FMGs, class standing appears to have an effect on some individuals but not on others.

There seem to be two ranking processes at work. As a group, USMGs have a far better chance of entering the most prestigious training positions than USFMGs, and USFMGs in turn have a higher chance than FMGs. FMGs say they are drawn from the top of their class more often than do the other groups. Class standing has some influence within each group, but it is not an overriding factor in initial distribution to type of hospital; almost two-thirds of the FMGs in the nonaffiliated hospitals said they had graduated in the top third of their class. However, it remains true that the USMG in the top third of his class has the greatest likelihood of entering a university teaching unit; the FMG from the lowest third of the class has by far the *least* chance of entering a major university program. From the beginning of training, therefore, there is some differential selection of interns and residents appointed to different types of hospitals.

Another variable, initial success in the ECFMG examination, was also tested as a predictor of entry by FMGs to affiliated positions. No relationship was found. Although 73.4 percent of the FMGs entering major teaching units said they passed the ECFMG on the first attempt, compared to 69.8 percent of those entering the nonaffiliated hospitals, this difference was too small to be significant. If such measures do represent a level of competence, there is no evidence here that competence is a major predictor of entry by FMGs to different categories of hospital.

Country of Medical Education and Race

FMGs are, however, selected differentially into different categories of hospitals by their country and/or region of medical education. Interestingly, these patterns appear to have little to do with the decision to come to the United States in terms of the range of options available to FMGs with respect to their country of medical education (discussed in Chapter 3). Rather, FMGs from countries most like the United States enter major teaching units at the highest rates. Physicians entering the United States from the predominantly white countries of the British

Commonwealth, including Canada, are much more likely to enter major teaching units and far less likely to go to unaffiliated hospitals than FMGs from other country groups. FMGs from Asian schools have the least likelihood of entering major teaching programs. Two-thirds of the graduates from British Commonwealth countries (excluding countries in Asia) entered American training in major teaching units, compared to little more than one-third of the graduates from schools in Asia and the Far East.

However, there are differences among countries in the different groups. Notably, physicians graduating from schools in Ceylon and Japan go into the various types of training program at a rate not too different from that of physicians entering from schools in Eastern Europe, that is, about half enter major teaching units. These patterns are different from those of, say, India and the Philippines, where about one-third of the graduates enter major teaching units, one-third other affiliated programs, and one-third nonaffiliated institutions.

Differences within other broad groups emphasize that the country of medical education, as well as region, affects where FMGs enter the American training system. For example, Brazilian graduates have a relatively high rate of entry to major teaching units (55.0 percent), whereas the rate for Colombian graduates is low (11.8 percent); graduates from Spain show higher rates (38.1 percent) than graduates from West German schools (12.5 percent). Such findings emphasize the heterogeneity not only of motivations, but also of informational networks, of different members of the FMG population within broad interregional population categories.

In all country groups, however, FMGs enter training in major teaching units at a lower rate than USMGs. Graduates from the British Commonwealth (excluding Asia) and Eire and from Eastern Europe have, however, a higher chance of entering major teaching units than the American graduates of foreign medical schools.

The combination of country and regional differences results in differential distributions of FMGs by broad racial characteristics. Although race itself may not be a determining factor in hospital appointments, the initial distributions produce different racial distributions in the house staff entering affiliated and unaffiliated hospitals. Most positions in major teaching units are filled by USMGs, and most USMGs are white (95 percent of our respondents); thus the staffs of these units are predominantly white. All the USFMGs in our group were white; half of these were in major teaching units. Unaffiliated units rely, on the other hand, largely on FMGs, who are, in turn, predominantly Indo-Asian.

Within the FMG population, entry patterns are also associated with racial characteristics. Black FMGs in our sample (most trained in European schools) had the highest chance of gaining a first position in a major teaching unit and the lowest rate of entry into unaffiliated institutions. Those coded by our interviewers as "Orientals" had the least chance of entering major teaching units and the highest rate of entering unaffiliated programs. These differences must be borne in mind in interpreting other aspects of the house staff data, since to some degree race may be a proxy for cultural differences, which may, in turn, affect the relative ease of assimilation of FMGs into the American professional system.

Visa Status

Since patterns by country of medical education may be the result of the extraneous pressures of visa status, we also looked at visa status as a final background factor that might affect the differential selection of FMGs into the American training system. As noted in chapter 4, exchange visitors enter major units at a somewhat higher rate than permanent residents; conversely, relatively more permanent residents are in unaffiliated hospitals than the exchange visitors. To some extent, therefore, visa appears to be a determining factor in the type of hospital of entry, but the differences are by no means as great as might be expected. Although two-thirds of all the FMGs appointed to first positions at major teaching units arrived in the United States as exchange visitors, so did well over half of those who began their American training at unaffiliated institutions. As with the other characteristics examined in this section, visa provides only a limited and partial explanation for differential patterns of entry.

Conclusions

We conclude from this study of background factors that FMGs have a greater chance of beginning their American training in a major teaching unit if they are of high academic standing, come from a white British Commonwealth country or are Black and/or are on an exchange visitor visa than others in these various categories, but that none of these factors explain the differential patterns of entry. Rather, the patterns appear to be the result of a complex series of interactions between the employing hospitals and individual FMGs.

FMGs from different regions are probably selected by American teaching hospitals according to perceived levels of success by the employing hospitals; this perception may in part be an assessment of known levels of medical education in various countries, in part a cultural perception.

Thus hospitals choose USMGs first. As a second line come graduates from White British Commonwealth countries and Eastern Europe, together with Black graduates and USFMGs. This group can be regarded as culturally similar to USMGs. Third are countries that may be known by employers to have high medical educational standards: graduates of schools in Ceylon, Japan, South Africa, schools in the Near East, Central America, Western Europe, and South America. Other regions of the world form the final cadre. The large pool of graduates from the Far East, in particular, provides a major source of entrants for the nonaffiliated programs. There is no reason to conclude from our findings that this latter group varies in technical competence from any other group of FMGs.

These patterns of employer preference are layered over the selection processes of individual FMGs. Selection into a particular hospital is thus part luck, part a matter of knowledge on the part of FMGs, part contacts, and part a series of background attributes considered by specific employing institutions.

CHARACTERISTICS OF FIRST HOSPITAL OF TRAINING

The discussion so far has centered on FMG patterns of entry to American training in relation to broad categories of medical school affiliation, on the grounds that FMGs who enter training in the United States would presumably wish to enter programs with the greatest degree of university affiliation. However, there are other noticeable differences in the hospitals entered for training by USMGs and FMGs.

Our findings bear out the common observation that FMGs are more likely to enter training than USMGs in the smaller community hospitals. One-fourth of all FMGs (25.2 percent) entered training in nongovernmental, nonprofit hospitals (including church hospitals) that were not affiliated with medical schools, a much higher proportion than for USMGs (7.2 percent) and somewhat higher proportion than for USFMGs (19.9 percent). These patterns account in large part for the overall tendency of FMGs to enter nonprofit hospitals at a greater rate than USMGs. Three-fourths (75.3 percent) of the USMGs entered training in such hospitals, compared to half (47.9 percent) of the USMGs.[9]

FMGs were also likely to enter the smaller hospitals. Half of the FMGs began their American training in nonprofit hospitals with fewer than 500 beds, compared to less than one-third of the entering USMGs. Generally, USMGs gravitated to the larger institutions with major university affiliation, irrespective of whether these were nonprofit, federal, or state or local government institutions, whereas FMGs were more likely to be recruited by smaller hospitals with a lesser degree of affiliation.

Our findings do not bear out the hypothesis that FMGs disproportionately enter local government (city or county) hospitals; quite the reverse. USMGs were more likely than FMGs to begin training in such hospitals. However, there are differences when the data are analyzed further. Virtually all the USMGs (97.4 percent) who enter local government hospitals choose positions in hospitals with a major affiliation with university medical schools: hospitals like Boston City Hospital, for example, which provides teaching services for Harvard, Boston University, and Tufts. In contrast, little more than half of the FMGs; (56.7 percent) who entered local government hospitals began in major teaching units. The remainder were concentrated in local government hospitals with a limited affiliation (22.4 percent) and in nonaffiliated units (20.8 percent).

State hospitals showed an exaggerated version of a similar trend. All the USMGs who entered training in state hospitals entered hospitals with a major university affiliation. Although the great majority of FMGs who entered state hospitals also chose major teaching units (83.0 percent). others entered hospitals with limited affiliation (6.7 percent) and no affiliation (10.2 percent). Thus university affiliation appears to be the dominant characteristic of hospital of training, rather than the hospital's administration—i.e. whether it is run by a nonprofit corporation, church or non-church-affiliated, or by federal, or state, or local government.

In all categories of hospitals, USMGs entered major teaching units more frequently than FMGs. The least striking difference was, interestingly, in hospitals under church auspices, largely because relatively few USMGs were in church hospitals with a major university affiliation. There appeared to be no overriding religious reasons for the choice of a church hospital by different groups of FMGs. More than one-third of the Filipinos (35.6 percent) and Colombians (41.2 percent) entered church hospitals, but so did a similar proportion of graduates from the United Arab Republic (42.9 percent); FMGs from Argentina (11.1 percent) and Spain (23.8 percent) went to church hospitals comparatively rarely. These patterns probably reflect the clustering effect of different groups of FMGs in different institutions rather than any religious motivations.

Apart from differences by hospital affiliation and control, FMGs were, as noted, differently distributed from USMGs by size of hospital. Since size and complexity of acute general hospitals are related, this suggests that FMGs disproportionately entered *the least complex training situations.*

Such a situation, of great importance in evaluating the relative training of USMGs and FMGs, deserves fuller scrutiny through a more precise definition of "complexity." One aspect of complexity is the degree to which a hospital is specialized, and one indicator of specialization is the number of residency training programs offered, that is, the number of major specialties up to a maximum of 20 in which approved training is given. The number of residency programs thus gives a useful indicator of training milieu by hospital complexity.[10] We analyzed our data on an FMG's first American hospital according to this indicator.

If the number of residency programs and hospital specialization are indeed related, FMGs were much less likely than USMGs to enter complex training settings: 40.7 percent of FMGs entered training in hospitals with less than five residency programs compared to only 6.6 percent of the USMGs. These patterns persist when the size of the hospital and the number of residency programs are run together. Thus half (49.9 percent) of the FMGs entered training in hospitals with less than 500 beds and fewer than 10 residency programs, compared to one-fourth (23.2 percent) of the USMGs. At the other end the scale, only one out of seven FMGs (14.0 percent) entered hospitals that had 700 beds or more and 15 or more residency programs, compared to one out of four of the USMGs (26.4 percent).

Generally, the distribution of house staff by size and complexity of hospital follows the pattern of entry to major teaching units: indeed, all three variables are related. Distributional patterns for United Kingdom graduates, for example, were similar to those of USMGs. FMGs who had become American citizens by the time of the study also followed the USMG patterns of distribution. For many countries, however, the pattern of entry is predominantly to hospitals with a relatively low degree of specialization. Only 32 percent of the USMGs entered training in hospitals with nine or fewer residency programs, compared to 80 percent or more of the graduates from South Korea, Cuba, West Germany, India, Colombia, and the Philippines.

The implications of differential distributions by hospital complexity raise potentially important questions of appropriate training locale for USMGs and FMGs. As with other specialty measures there appears to be no direct relationship between the FMG's desire for a particular level of specialization and the actual hospital of entry. Thus the FMGs most strongly motivated by specialization as a factor in coming to the United States began their American training in no more specialized hospitals than did other FMGs. Half of all FMGs said that specialization influenced them to come a "great deal" or "fair amount" and began their American training in hospitals with nine or fewer residency programs, the least complex training institutions. These findings suggest, again, that coming to the United States is the salient factor for FMGs in seeking training, rather than coming to world-renowned specialized training centers: FMGs, entering hospitals because of job availability, obtain the least sought-after training positions. The resulting patterns of entry to the hospital system are thus quite different for USMGs and FMGs.

Besides differences in the level of affiliation, size, and hospital complexity, the initial training locale of FMGs differs in two other qualitative respects from the training locale of USMGs. FMGs tend to enter hospitals in which FMGs form the majority of trainees; USMGs tend to train with other USMGs. The great majority of USMGs begin their graduate medical education in hospitals in which a majority of the house staff are USMGs and USFMGs. A much smaller proportion of USFMGs and a small minority of FMGs begin at such hospitals. Almost one-third of the FMGs began their American training experience at hospitals in which the entire house staff was composed of FMGs; more than two-thirds began training at hospitals in which FMGs represent more than three-fourths of all trainees.

These differences in the social and professional milieu of the first American training hospital are joined by differences in the research emphasis of the various training institutions. Hospital necropsy rates (the percentage of patients dying at a given hospital on whom postmortem examinations are performed) provide an indicator of research interests. Necropsy rates are used by the American medical profession's residency review committees in evaluating residency programs for approval, since the basic medical sciences may be strengthened in most fields from studying applied gross and microscopic anatomy from necropsy as well as surgical specimens. The "Essentials" for approving residencies note: "It is expected that hospitals assuming responsibility for residency training will maintain a high autopsy rate."[11]

FMGs and USMGs enter hospitals with widely different necropsy rates; 12 percent of the FMGs were in hospitals in which the necropsy rate was 51 percent or over, compared to 41 percent of the USMGs. Necropsy rates, like hospital complexity, are related to the hospital's level of affiliation; thus the lower rates for FMGs reflect in large part the concentration of FMGs outside the major teaching units.[12]

The various factors taken together, show major differences in the educational setting of American hospitals entered by USMGs and FMGs for training. USMGs tend to train with other USMGs in major teaching units, whereas FMGs train with FMGs in other affiliated and non-affiliated hospitals. Indicators of the complexity and research emphasis of the hospitals suggest that USMGs generally go to the most developed training programs and FMGs to the least. Thus there are differences in

TABLE 6.4 DISTRIBUTION OF FMGS, USMGS, AND USFMGS BY PROPORTION OF FMGS AND LEVEL OF AFFILIATION, FIRST U.S. HOSPITAL OF TRAINING

	FMG	USMG	USFMG
Major teaching unit			
With 0–25% FMGs	7.8	51.6	10.8
With 25–50% FMGs	7.9	16.9	15.1
With 50–100% FMGs	27.0	10.5	30.9
Hospital with other university affiliation			
With 0–25% FMGs	1.6	12.8	6.5
With 25–50% FMGs	1.3	0.6	1.4
With 50–100% FMGs	27.5	0.6	19.4
Hospital with no university affiliation			
With 0–25% FMGs	0.2	0.6	0
With 25–50% FMGs	0.5	1.3	5.0
With 50–100%	26.3	5.1	10.7
Total	100.0% (621)[a]	100.0% (121)	100.0% (37)
	NA = 69	NA = 12	NA = 5

[a] Percentages are weighted; *N* is unweighted.

both the cultural and the scientific milieu of training.

Among the categories of university affiliation, too, there are levels of distinction between the two groups. FMGs and USMGs are distributed distinctively within each category of affiliation (Table 6.4). Most FMGs whose first hospital was a major teaching unit entered training situations in which the house staff was predominantly composed of FMGs. Only 16 percent of all FMGs began training in hospitals that were major teaching units predominantly staffed by USMGs, presumably the most desired training location. The comparable figure for USMGs was 69 percent; in addition, USMGs were much more likely than FMGs to enter other affiliated hospitals in which FMGs were in the minority. FMGs, in contrast, were concentrated in situations at all levels of affiliation in which house staff was composed mostly of FMGs. Almost one-fifth of all FMGs entered nonaffiliated hospitals for their first American position in which the house staff was composed 100 percent of FMGs.

Differential entry of USMGs and FMGs into affiliated and nonaffiliated hospitals and into relatively more or less complex training situations suggests qualitative differences in the professional environment and the initial training received by USMGs as a group and by FMGs. If one assumes that USMGs and FMGs form a single pool of entrants to graduate training in the American system, there is an allocative process whereby USMGs enter the most complex major teaching units and other affiliated hospitals, where they are taught with other American graduates. If no FMGs were admitted to the United States, this allocation would result in large numbers of internship and residency posts standing vacant, particularly in hospitals with no or relatively little university affiliation.

ENTRY INTO DIFFERENT U.S. STATES

Geographical differences provide a further dimension to such considerations. The differential selection of FMGs into some American states and not others can be clearly demonstrated (Table 6.5). Over 60 percent of the FMGs entered training in hospitals in New York, Illinois, Michigan, and Pennsylvania. In contrast, only 37 percent of the USMGs took a first job in these states. The USFMGs present a third pattern, with a highly concentrated entry into New York and New Jersey.

Virtually none of the FMGs entered California, where few internships and residencies are available. One out of six USMGs began their graduate training in California, but less than one out of 100 FMGs. The nationality patterns of entrants to California are also different from those of entrants to other states. Virtually all the FMGs who began training in California were graduates of schools in Canada, Argentina, Brazil, and countries in Eastern Europe.

Idiosyncracies in entry patterns by country of medical education can be shown in virtually every state, the result, no doubt, of chain migration. Illinois and Michigan provide a case in point. Both draw heavily on the FMG population and lightly on USMGs, but they select FMGs in quite different arrays. Illinois, which draws two-thirds of its new FMGs from countries in Asia, provided an apparent mecca for the Taiwanese. One-third of all Taiwan graduates in our study began at hospitals in Illinois. Graduates from Taiwan represented about one out of eight of all FMG entrants to the United States, but one-fourth of the FMGs entering Illinois.

In contrast, Michigan also drew half of its FMGs from countries in Asia, but few (less than 5 percent) came from schools in Taiwan. On the other hand, Michigan was a relatively popular state of entry for South Koreans,

TABLE 6.5 ENTRY OF USMGS, FMGS, AND USFMGS INTO FIRST HOSPITAL POSITION IN SELECTED U.S. STATES

States ranked by number of house staff on duty	Percentage of all house staff[a] (national figures)	Percentage of graduates in our study who began training in selected states		
		FMG	USMG	USFMG
New York	16.5	25.0	20.0	37.9
California	10.6	0.9	17.1	0
Pennsylvania	6.4	9.8	9.7	2.4
Illinois	5.9	14.8	4.6	8.3
Ohio	5.3	5.8	3.2	8.3
Massachusetts	5.0	3.9	5.7	0
Michigan	4.5	10.9	2.2	0
Texas	4.3	0.6	2.7	2.4
Maryland	3.4	3.6	3.4	4.1
New Jersey	2.8	5.7	0.5	14.8
Minnesota	2.5	0.5	0.5	0
Missouri	2.4	1.8	0.5	0
12 largest states	69.6	83.3	70.1	78.2
All other states	30.4	16.7	29.9	21.8
Total	100.0 (58,777)	100.0 (690)[b]	100.0 (133)	100.0 (42)

[a] As of December 1973, from Educational Number, *Journal of the American Medical Association.* Figures include house staff in all years of training.
  One other relatively large "importing" state for FMGs, excluded from this table, was Connecticut: 5.1% of the FMGs began their U.S. training in that state.
[b] For sample data, percentages are weighted; N is unweighted.

Thais, and Indians. One-fourth of the South Koreans began their American training in Michigan.

In Connecticut and Pennsylvania, in contrast, less than half of the FMGs were drawn from Asia. Connecticut drew a relatively strong contingent of FMGs from medical schools in the Near and Middle East and Central America. New Jersey drew more than half of its FMGs from countries in Asia and the remainder chiefly from the Middle East and Western and Eastern Europe. At the same time, New Jersey attracted no FMGs from South America, Canada, Britain, Eire, or the British Commonwealth.

New York draws strongly on all countries, but here, too, there are wide differences in its attractiveness to different groups. One-fourth of all our FMGs began American graduate training in New York. However, the state appeared unusually attractive to Taiwanese and Pakistan/Bangladesh graduates and relatively attractive to graduates from Thailand, Argentina, and Brazil (but not other countries in South America) and Central American countries, excluding Mexico and Cuba. In contrast, relatively few (one out of ten) of the graduates from the Philippines, Iran, or South Korea entered New York for their first American position.

Country-specific figures must be interpreted carefully, because they are based on relatively small numbers in each cell. However, different patterns of migration are suggested according to the respondent's country of medical education. Thus outside New York, Thai graduates entered the United States system at greater than average rates into Illinois, Connecticut, Michigan, Maryland, and Missouri. Argentinian FMGs went disproportionately to Michigan and Pennsylvania, but at less than average rates to Illinois and Connecticut, whereas none of our group entered either New Jersey or Ohio. Brazilian graduates favored New York, California, and Connecticut.

These figures suggest "pockets of welcome" for FMGs from different countries in different states. One area or hospital becomes a focus for graduates from Sri Lanka, another for graduates from Turkey or the Philippines. For example, 27 percent of the Argentinians but only 3 percent of the Brazilian FMGs entered Michigan and Illinois, whereas 66 percent of the graduates from Pakistan entered New York and Illinois, compared to 45 percent of the Indian graduates.

These conclusions are reinforced by the absence of major geographical entry patterns for FMGs from specific continents. South and Central Americans, for example, do not appear to concentrate in the American south, nor Europeans on the East Coast nor Asians on the West. Indeed, FMGs from countries in the same world region enter training in quite different American states. American states are, in short, drawing their new graduate physicians both from a different basic cadre (USMGS and FMGs) and from different countries within the body of FMGs.

Other general observations arise from the data. Because of the skewed entry patterns of FMGs into different American states, the exchange visitor program is also concentrated in particular states. One-half of all FMGs entering training as exchange visitors begin training in New York (22.3 percent of exchange visitors), Illinois (18.0 percent), and Michigan (12.5 percent). These entry patterns are similar in terms of distribution by state of entry to those of FMGs on permanent resident visas.

California, although providing a major source of training for USMGs, offers little to FMGs who come to the United States as exchange visitors. The underlying reason, again, is that entry patterns are determined in large part by the American domestic market for interns and residents.

CONCLUSIONS

The conclusions that FMGs fulfill a residual role in the American employment market and that job availability is the single most important element in the initial placement of FMGs have emerged throughout this discussion. FMGs from some countries fare better in entering the American marketplace than others. United Kingdom graduates, in particular, are likely to enter major teaching units, to be trained with USMGs, to be in more scientifically oriented training situations, and to enter the most complex institutions. None of the United Kingdom entrants entered first hospitals in which the necropsy rate was less than 40 percent, and a minority entered hospitals with less than 10 specialties approved for residencies. FMGs from other countries entered distinctively different situations. The great majority of FMGs from Taiwan, Cuba, Iran, Spain, and Thailand, for example, entered hospitals with low necropsy rates and few residency training programs. At least one-third of the graduates from Taiwan, Cuba, West Germany, Iran, South Korea, Peru, Thailand, and the Philippines began training in hospitals that were totally (100 percent) staffed by FMGs.

When the various factors are considered together, broad country patterns emerge. If the percentage of FMGs in the first training hospital, the necropsy rate, and the number of residency programs are taken together as a "package" of attributes indicating the hospital's prestige in the American system, its scientific emphasis, and its degree of specialization, FMGs from different countries can be ranked on a continuum. Those from countries like the United Kingdom show patterns of entry similar to USMGs: they go to hospitals with the fewest FMGs, the greatest scientific emphasis, and the greatest degree of specialization. Next on the continuum come FMGs from countries such as Brazil, Colombia, the United Arab Republic, and Argentina. In a third group are graduates from countries such as India, Spain, Peru, and Thailand; in the fourth are Taiwan, West Germany, South Korea, the Philippines, and Iran. The fifth and last group in our study comprised the Cuban refugees who entered the least prestigious and scientifically oriented training situations.

Although there are clearly many interlocking reasons to explain these patterns, generally the selection process of American hospitals seems to accept FMGs who are culturally most like USMGs into the prestigious, scientific teaching situations, whereas hospitals with the least university affiliation and the least opportunities for a research-oriented curriculum act as residual portals of entry for other FMGs. From the beginning of American training, the average FMG is in a different cultural, professional, and educational milieu from the average USMG.

In addition, within the FMG population, opportunities vary according to the physician's country of medical education. These opportunities are not directly related to the range of options available to physicians in deciding to come to the United States in the first place[13]—a not surprising finding given the recruitment process, and the lack of information available to FMGs in choosing their first American hospital positions.

The geographical clustering of FMG entrants in certain states is primarily a function of job availability: some states have more positions available to FMGs than others. Variations within countries can be explained by chain migration. However, the relative proportion of FMGs and USMGs entering graduate training in individual states has potentially important policy implications.

Our figures for states must be viewed cautiously, but they are suggestive. Taking the states with 15 or more respondents in our study, FMGs represented less than 10 percent of the new entrants to graduate medical education in Alabama, California, Colorado, Kentucky, and Oklahoma. It may be remarked about these states that any reduction in the entering supply of FMGs would be of little importance to the total supply of new physician entrants. In states such as Illinois, with an estimated 60 percent entering FMGs, Connecticut, Michigan, and New Jersey, with more than 70 percent entering FMGs, any large reduction could, in contrast, be of immense importance to the staffing of hospitals by interns and residents. Since some states draw heavily on FMGs from certain countries, changes in government policy in those countries or in United States visa policy will have an additional impact in selected states.

A review of the first hospital positions of FMGs and USMGs raises important questions of American educational and manpower policies. With respect to changes in the supply of FMGs in the future, it is essential to recognize that FMGs enter the United States in a few major "FMG states," with distinctive patterns of entry for graduates from different countries. With respect to the recruiting institutions—the gateway to American graduate education—FMGs enter the United States in training settings that are not only professionally and organizationally different from those entered by the great majority of USMGs, but that provide few American role models on the house staff to guide FMGs, as they struggle to understand an alien system.

NOTES

1. In California in 1973–1974, 86 percent of the residencies offered were filled by American graduates; in New York the proportion was 46 percent; in New Jersey, 22 percent. *Directory of Approved Internships and Residencies 1974–75*, Table 10.

2. *Ibid.*, pp. 46, 71.
3. *Ibid.*
4. Public Law 94–484, *Health Professions Educational Assistance Act of 1976* includes provisions for tightening up exchange visitor procedures and examination requirements, which promise to reduce the number of entrants considerably.
5. For example, Mumford's study of interns in two types of hospitals, a university center and a community hospital, found not only different patterns of interactions and communication in the two places, but also variations in the sources of rewards and punishments and differences in the objective situations the intern most often must meet; university hospital interns saw themselves as a "proud company," those working in a community hospital put more stress on their milieu as a "friendly place." *Interns: From Students to Physicians*, p. 150 and passim.
6. In 1973–1974, the academic year in which our study was administered, there were 11,031 physicians in internship positions in the United States, of whom 3425 were foreign graduates, together with 49,078 residents (including 14,923 foreign graduates) and 9324 other graduate trainees (of whom 3499 were foreign graduates). Of the total of 69,433 physicians represented in these categories, therefore, approximately 16 percent were interns, 71 percent were residents, and 13 percent were in other types of training, including research and teaching positions. Figures for "foreign graduates" exclude Canadians. Anne E. Crowley, Ed. "Medical Education in the United States 1973–74," Journal of the American Medical Association Supplement (1975), *231*, Tables 14 and 24.
7. FMGs entering major teaching units ($N = 260$) ascribed their primary source of information to personal networks (40.1 percent), formal sources (27.1 percent), professional networks USA (16.3 percent), professional networks CME (11.8 percent), other (4.7 percent). Those entering nonaffiliated hospitals ($N = 206$) noted formal sources (45.9 percent), personal networks (30.2 percent), professional networks CME (18.3 percent), professional networks USA (2.1 percent), other (3.4 percent).
8. Barbara Harrison, *Foreign Doctors in American Hospitals*, pp. 31, 437.
9. For the overall distribution of first hospital administrative characteristics, see Table 7.3.
10. On the validity of using the number of residency programs as a proxy for complexity, see Wolf Heydebrand, *Hospital Bureaucracy—A Comparative Study of Organizations*, Dunellen, New York, 1973. Of our total study group of 690 FMGs, 72 (10.4 percent) entered hospitals that according to the "Green Book," offered no approved residency positions; that is they either offered free-standing internships only or were not approved for graduate medical education. Comparable figures for USMGs were 9 (7.3 percent) and for USFMGs 5 (13.5 percent). These respondents are excluded from the data on complexity.
11. Essentials, 1969–1970, p. 310.
12. Of all our respondents (USMG, USFMG, and FMG) who began their American graduate training in major teaching units, 69.3 percent were in hospitals with a reported necropsy rate of at least 40 percent; comparable rates for those entering hospitals with limited affiliation were 53.0 percent and for those entering nonaffiliated hospitals, 29.2 percent.
13. When the variables for 100 percent FMGs on the house staff, a low necropsy rate (less than 40 percent), and least complex training settings (less than 10 residency programs) are run together, the ranking from low to high on selected countries is United Kingdom, Brazil, United Arab Republic, Argentina, Colombia, Spain, India, Peru, Thailand, West Germany, Taiwan, South Korea, Philippines, Iran, Cuba.

7

MOBILITY WITHIN THE
AMERICAN SYSTEM _____

The discussion thus far has suggested that the FMG enters the American graduate educational system in a pattern of stratification in which USMGs are generally in positions of the highest prestige and FMGs are in lesser positions. However, the FMG's efforts to cope in an alien professional system do not suddenly stop once he or she has become a member of that system. Entry patterns do not necessarily imply a continuing disadvantage. FMGs who can cope—or who can learn to cope—with the nuances and prestige rankings of the American system may move quickly from a disappointing job to a better one, maximizing their opportunities by a series of moves from position to position. This chapter argues that FMGs as a group do indeed demonstrate some degree of "upward mobility" in the American system, suggestive of successful coping mechanisms.

However, such adjustments fall short of full assimilation of FMGs into the American health care system. FMGs carry a continuing stigma of the stranger in an alien professional world. Those FMGs who begin their American careers in a less than optimal program may also be identified with that experience in their search for more prestigious positions. All else being equal, the physician who begins in a small, nonaffiliated program is likely to be disadvantaged in seeking a second American job in competition with FMGs who entered major teaching units, as well as with USMGs. Thus although the first American job may be a springboard to other opportunities, the type of first position may mold or predetermine subsequent training opportunities. In short, the first American job may be critical as a vehicle for entry, but it provides, too, an initial labeling process for FMGs that may influence their future careers in the United States.

Such concepts are neither mutually exclusive nor sufficient to describe adequately the complex personal processes that determine the individual career. Illustrations of the decisions taken by individual FMGs are given here to illuminate the range of experiences in the careers of FMGs once they are in the United States. The purpose of this chapter is not, however, to define new stages within the stages of the medical career, but to investigate mobility from the point of view of the role of the FMG in the American system.

Almost all the literature on FMGs has assumed that FMGs are static recipients of American graduate education. Notably, the relative concentration of FMGs in nonaffiliated hospitals has been viewed as if the FMGs in such hospitals were there for the whole of their American careers. In this model such FMGs form a distinctive cadre of physicians who may perhaps have received a less rigorous education than USMGs, who receive an education in the United States that is regarded within the medical profession as inferior to training in other locations. FMGs in such hospitals can therefore be regarded as doubly disadvantaged, and there are quick shifts from here to conclusions about "quality." However, there has been no evidence till now that FMGs in nonaffiliated hospitals do in fact remain there for their American careers. Some FMGs who begin in such positions, as we show here, move to the most prestigious training programs in the United States.

This chapter presents an exploratory analysis of the mobility of FMGs in the United States, measured by comparisons between their hospital of entry and the hospital of training at the time the survey was administered. The underlying questions have both social and organizational implications: If FMGs remain where they begin, those who begin in the least desirable positions may be regarded as disadvantaged in the American system. If they are mobile, they may represent a relatively successful process of socialization. Other questions are of immediate political interest. If FMGs tend to remain in their position of entry, changes made in recruitment by such hospitals have merely parochial implications. If, on the other hand, FMGs begin in one milieu and move to others, changes made in the entering hospitals will have repercussions throughout the American system.

BASIC PATTERNS

Ideally, a study of mobility would begin with one entering cohort of house staff and follow them up, prospectively, as they move from position to position over a specific period of years. The format of our survey, administered to a group of house staff in training in 1974, means that career decisions by FMGs after their arrival in the United States can only be viewed retrospectively. The data show where an individual was in 1974 and what were his or her previous positions. One can thus work backwards and hypothesize about the pattern of individual career decisions from the point of entry to the American system. However, it should be remembered, first, that our respondents entered the American system at different times; second, that other FMGs may have entered the system with many of our respondents but left before the study was administered. Thus the figures may not give a complete picture of all FMGs entering the United States, but they are complete in showing the relationship between the current job held by a representative group of house staff in 1974 and their original positions of entry to the American system. It is on this basis that our arguments are presented.

The majority of our respondents were in their second or subsequent training positions at the time of the survey. Approximately 30 percent of the USMGs and FMGs were in their first American jobs in 1974, 60 percent in their second or third posts, with the remaining 10 percent in their fourth or later training positions. The distributions for USMGs and FMGs were quite similar. We found few "career trainees," that is, physicians who graduate from training position to training position beyond a normal period of completion of training. Seven of the FMGs in our sample of 690 were in sixth, seventh, or eighth American positions, compared to one of the 133 USMGs.

The average length of training of FMGs and USMGs is also broadly similar. The average FMG in our study group was in month 32 of American graduate education, compared to the 28th month for the average USMG. Thus in terms of the time frame for comparing the mobility of FMGs and USMGs in the United States, we may be reasonably confident that each group is similarly distributed. Although FMGs have, on average, a much longer professional history than USMGs because of previous foreign experience, in terms of their role in the American graduate system they are at similar stages of their careers.

If these patterns stood alone, one might assume that the careers of USMGs and FMGs would be broadly similar, allowing for the greater tendency of FMGs to enter directly into residencies and to take research positions.[1] Table 7.1 indicates that FMGs are, however, much more likely than USMGs to move away from the initial hospital of training and more likely to move from state to state. Approximately 60 percent of the FMGs were working, at the time of interview, at a hospital that was not their hospital of entry: more than 30 percent had moved to a hospital in a different state. Some members of each group were particularly mobile: 20 percent of the FMGs and 11 percent of the USMGs had received training at three or more American hospitals, and a handful in each category were in the fifth training hospital at the time of survey.

TABLE 7.1 INTERHOSPITAL MOBILITY, FIRST AND CURRENT HOSPITALS

	FMG	USMG	USFMG
Same hospital	40.9	60.9	49.7
Same state/			
different hospital	26.4	20.3	23.7
Different states	32.7	18.8	26.6
	100.0 (690)[a]	100.0 (133)	100.0 (42)

[a] Percentages are weighted; N is unweighted.

We argue that the greater interhospital mobility of FMGs can be explained in terms of their lower initial placement level, in part because of a lower initial level of information: FMGs learn about the American system while in their first job and, where possible, better their position for their second post on the basis of better contacts and information. USMGs are initially better informed and have better access to the system; thus they are able to enter the appropriate hospital immediately. Moreover, having entered a high status institution as an intern, the USMG may also have the opportunity of remaining in that hospital for residency training, whereas the FMG, entering a lower status hospital or one not ideal for his needs, is much more likely to move on. In some cases, too, hospitals may appoint FMGs who have been hired sight-unseen for a 1-year period, with the expectation that the contract will not be renewed. Mobility is then mandatory.

Whatever the reason, there appears to be a considerable shifting of locations during the graduate educational period, although most trainees remain in the same state, if not in the same institution. For both USMGs and FMGs, such shifts appear, generally, to represent adjustments from a less desirable to a more desirable position, as seen from an individual point of view. In seeking the next training opportunity, the physician looks first at other hospitals in the same state and then to hospitals farther afield.

EXAMPLES OF HOSPITAL MOBILITY

Individual case histories illustrate the kinds of decisions made as FMGs move through their individual careers. The following examples have been selected not because they are necessarily representative of all FMGs, but to emphasize the importance of individual career decisions and to provide a context in which the statistical data can be better understood.

Dr. A provides a good example of the adjustments that may be made by FMGs who come to the United States with relatively little information and with few friends or acquaintances in the system. Dr. A graduated from medical school in Iran in 1966, did military service and worked in that country until 1972; he passed the ECFMG examination in 1969. Dr. A came to the United States in 1972 as an exchange visitor with the intention (which remains) of returning to Iran, where he intends to establish a new hospital with a group of colleagues. His first American post was an internship in a nonaffiliated community hospital in Connecticut that was entirely staffed with FMGs. This was one of 40 hospitals selected from the "Green Book" which, together with advertisements from American medical journals, appears to have been his only source of information.

Dr. A said that he was initially hampered in the United States by his lack of fluency in English, which caused difficulties in communication, particularly with professional staff. However, 2 years in his first position provided a basic training in English, and he was able to move on. The process of mobility had begun. For his second post he moved to a residency in obstetrics at another nonaffiliated hospital in New York State, and he was there when interviewed in 1974. His choice of specialty was a long-time career intention. Dr. A's evaluation of his experiences so far are mixed. He rates his present mix of patients only "fair," and he does not agree that United States programs are the best in the world. These comments may reflect the fact that, although Dr. A has moved within the American system to his chosen specialty, the training for which he came has so far been acquired without the help of friends within the system and

has been outside university-affiliated units. Dr. A is only partially socialized into the American system and remains on the periphery of graduate
education.

Dr. B, a graduate from Ecuador, has been much more successful. Dr.
B., resident in anesthesiology in a major university teaching unit when
interviewed in 1974, originally entered the United States in 1969 without
the ECFMG certificate and spent his first 3 years in an assistantship
position at a hospital in Florida. His second American post, his first in an
approved graduate educational position, was as a rotating intern in
another Florida institution, a small county hospital. However, this proved unsatisfactory to Dr. B in several respects, notably, he reports, in
terms of long working hours, and after 1 year he moved to his present
residency program in a major university.

Dr. B's career thus moved him within a few years from a position
outside the normal professional system (as an "assistant"), to a training
position at the center of professional prestige (a major teaching unit),
although in a relatively nonprestigious specialty (anesthesiology). If his
original American job was assumed to be appropriate to his skills, Dr. B
might be regarded as a member of the medical "underground," a physician working in a noncredentialled position because of his inability to
pass the ECFMG examination. In fact, Dr. B appears to have used this job
as a springboard into the American system, and he was not apparently
stigmatized in his subsequent career by beginning outside the professional structure. Dr. B expects to remain for practice in the United
States.

Dr C's career progression is rather similar.[2] Dr. C is a Filipino graduate
with considerable experience in the Philippines who began his American
career as a "surgical assistant" in a nonteaching hospital in Wisconsin in
1970. For his second post he moved to another Wisconsin hospital as an
intern, having passed the ECFMG examination. From this base Dr. C
progressed to a residency in general surgery at a Veterans' Hospital in
California, in a program with a limited university affiliation. The basic
pattern of his American career, like that of Dr. B, is transfer from one
hospital to another in the same state and then a move to a different state,
each move representing a gain in status. Whether Dr. C will move again,
perhaps to a major teaching unit, remains to be seen.

Dr. D's career shows a similar "upward" progression, although he
started and ended at different places. Dr. D graduated from medical
school in India in 1964 and came to the United States in 1966. He entered a
rotating internship in a small children's hospital in Illinois to which he
was introduced by friends from medical school who had also interned
there. After a year he moved to a large Veterans' Hospital in Illinois,

where he stayed for the bulk of his American training, completing a 4-year residency in general surgery and a 1-year residency in thoracic and cardiovascular surgery. Taking his specialization a step further, this was followed by 2 months of pediatric cardiac surgery in a children's hospital. In 1973 Dr. D moved from Illinois to Arizona, to a position as clinical fellow and cardiovascular surgeon in a hospital with major university affiliation.

Dr. D's career, moving as it did from a rotating internship to a highly specialized university program, can be seen as a classic story of the successful immigrant. Dr. D has become socialized as an American physician. Like many of his American peers, his future location will be "somewhere warm . . . definitely not Chicago." Wherever it is, Dr. D has every intention of remaining in the United States.

Many FMGs cope far less successfully. For example Dr. E, a Brazilian graduate and exchange visitor, entered an internship in a thousand-bed, university-affiliated city hospital in the Eastern United States in 1972. He did not enjoy this experience, chiefly because he felt adrift in an alien system. No one taught him the routine of work; he had no orientation program; he was disappointed by the lack of elective rotations; the patients were poorer and less educated than he expected; and English was a problem to a "moderate extent." Instead of adjusting to these conditions, Dr. E moved to a residency in a Veterans' Administration hospital in Louisiana where again he dealt with low-income patients. He is reportedly bitter about his American experience and plans to return to private practice in Brazil.

The individual nature of these reactions must be stressed. The lack of initial guidance in the American system is relatively commonplace and does not necessarily lead to alienation. For example, Dr. F's initial response to his first position was very similar to that of Dr. E, but he eventually adjusted to the system. Dr. F, an Indian, joined the staff of a large university-affiliated county hospital in Chicago in 1971. He too said he had insufficient information about his duties, the job, training programs, and working conditions; after 5 months, Dr. F. moved to a residency in a small nonaffiliated hospital in upstate New York. After 1 year there, however, Dr. F returned to his first location, gaining in the process a university fellowship in a medical subspecialty. Meanwhile, his views of the hospital have changed, and he reports that he is enjoying his position, the excellence of the training experience, the confidence of the staff, and the gratitude of patients: "I am serving a population I think would be neglected and I feel that those patients I see would probably not get the quality and quantity of care I deliver [if I were not there]."

The individual nature of these responses precludes any easy classification. For some, successful adjustment may encourage the FMG to remain here for his career; alternately, the wish to remain may ameliorate the process of socialization. However, satisfaction with the system is not necessarily a predeterminant of the desire to remain, because this decision is, as we show in Chapter 11, based on a complex of considerations. In the individual career histories we see a spectrum of experiences, from those who adjust readily and quickly to the American system to those who are frustrated by certain of its aspects and those who are alienated from it.

For example, Dr. G, a Malaysian who moved from an entry position in a nonaffiliated hospital in Ohio to a residency in pathology in a major university hospital in Indiana, reports that he is "disgusted at the treatment of foreign doctors in Indiana," largely because of his problems with licensing arrangements for FMGs in that state. Dr. H, a graduate of Ceylon, who had been a government medical officer in charge of a rural hospital, began his American career at a community hospital with limited university affiliation, where he had a few adjustment problems, but moved after 9 months to a first-year residency in psychiatry at a major university unit in Chicago. From there he moved to a world-renowned psychiatric training program as a second-year resident; he is now considering community mental health work in Oregon or Maine.

Dr. I from Iran, began at a hospital with limited affiliation in New Jersey, staffed almost entirely with FMGs. He too was given little initial instruction or orientation, but he adjusted and moved for his second position to a residency in a large city hospital with a major university affiliation in Washington, D.C. He then moved to a nationally renowned teaching hospital as a resident, then as a research fellow, and plans to go back to Iran to teach. Dr. I's experiences are thus very different from those of our first example, Dr. A, who also plans to return to Iran.

These examples illustrate the potential for mobility through the American system as seen in the careers of selected FMGs. Although it is a potential that remains unfulfilled for many FMGs, these examples point to characteristics of career progression in the United States that can be measured in analyzing the statistical data. These characteristics include mobility among hospitals with different levels of university affiliation, mobility from state to state, and differential mobility by specialty, country, sex, and race.

MOBILITY BY TYPE OF HOSPITAL

Table 7.2 shows the movement of FMGs, USMGs, and USFMGs among categories of hospitals, taking their first and current hospitals as the point of reference. The table provides a yardstick for the degree of mobility between categories of hospitals, measured in this instance by the level of university affiliation. It thus tackles the question of whether a first position in a particular category, for example, in a nonaffiliated hospital, predetermines future positions in this or other categories.

TABLE 7.2   MOBILITY OF USMGS, USFMGS, AND FMGS BETWEEN FIRST AND CURRENT HOSPITAL

	All respondents[a]			Those who changed hospitals[b]		
	FMG	USMG	USFMG	FMG	USMG	USFMG
Indicators of stability						
First and current hospitals are:						
major teaching units	36.3	75.6	48.6	25.3	64.8	30.5
other affiliated units	14.5	11.9	7.6	8.2	3.5	0
nonaffiliated units	15.9	1.1	13.9	9.6	0	9.7
Subtotal	66.7	88.6	70.1	43.1	68.3	40.2
Indicators of upward mobility						
Moved into major teaching unit						
from other affiliated unit	13.0	1.1	12.5	22.1	3.2	25.0
Moved into major teaching unit						
from unaffiliated unit	8.5	5.6	6.3	14.6	15.5	12.5
Moved into other affiliated unit						
from unaffiliated unit	5.2	0	0	8.9	0	0
Subtotal	26.7	6.7	18.8	45.6	18.7	37.5
Indicators of downward mobility						
Moved from major teaching unit						
to other affiliated unit	2.4	3.0	1.4	4.1	8.3	2.8
Moved from major teaching unit						
to unaffiliated unit	2.6	0.6	4.9	4.5	1.6	9.7
Moved from other affiliated						
to unaffiliated unit	1.5	1.2	4.9	2.5	3.2	9.7
Subtotal	6.5	4.8	11.2	11.1	13.1	22.2
Total	100.0%[c]	100.0%	100.0%	100.0%	100.0%	100.0%
N	(690)[c]	(133)	(42)	(389)	(52)	(20)

[a] Includes respondents who were in first hospital (i.e., had not changed hospitals) at time of study
[b] Excludes respondents who were in first hospital (i.e., had not changed hospitals) at time of study.
[c] Percentages are weighted; N is unweighted.

The table shows that the great majority of USMGs (88.6 percent) were in the same category of hospital as their hospital of entry to the graduate educational system when interviewed. Most USMGs begin their graduate education in a major teaching unit and either stay in the same hospital for subsequent training or move to another major teaching unit. Thus, although there was indeed mobility by USMGs from one hospital to another, the moves were nearly always lateral, from one major teaching unit to another. Those USMGs who moved among the categories of affiliation were also most likely to move into major teaching units.

The majority of FMGs (66.7 percent) also remained in the same category for training, but the patterns were rather different, since the initial distribution of FMGs was quite distinct. Like USMGs, the FMGs (and USFMGs) who began their training in major teaching units tended to remain in the same category for further training. Only 5 percent of all FMGs began their American training in a major teaching unit and had moved to another category of affiliation by the time of survey; the comparable figure for USMGs was 4 percent.

Having begun at a major teaching unit, the chances of staying in this category appear to be quite favorable. Of the FMGs who began training in such units, 88 percent were still in such units at the time of survey, together with 96 percent of the USMGs and 89 percent of the USFMGs. The limitations of the mobility data should be recognized in drawing general inferences. Nevertheless, it would appear that an initial position in a major teaching unit is a strong predictor of the location of the physician's subsequent training.

It should be remembered, however, that although most USMGs began training in major teaching units, this was true of only a minority of FMGs (41.3 percent). An essential question to be raised is how many FMGs who began in other units were successful in moving into major teaching units, that is, how far the case histories of "upward mobility" characterize a general process.

Table 7.2 (column 1) shows that a relatively large minority of all FMGs (21.5 percent) began their American training outside major teaching units but had moved into such units by the time of survey. Another group (5.2 percent) moved from nonaffiliated programs to programs with limited university affiliation. In summary, therefore, whereas 33.3 percent of all FMGs had moved from one category to another, 26.7 percent had moved "upwards" in the ranking system.

The last three columns of Table 7.2 show the mobility patterns for those who had made a hospital change by 1974: a total of 389 out of our 690 FMG respondents. Here the process of upward mobility is shown more clearly. Almost one-half of those who had moved from one hospital to another had "bettered" their position in terms of university affiliation. Most others had switched hospitals within the same affiliation category. Relatively few had moved to hospitals with a lesser degree of affiliation than the hospital of entry. Only 7 percent of those who moved had begun their American experience in an affiliated hospital and moved to an unaffiliated unit by the time of survey.

Part of this "mobility" may be an artificial reflection of the fact that during the period of training of our respondents, a large number of hospitals that were originally unaffiliated developed affiliation agreements with universities. The shifts from the nonaffiliated category to the category of limited affiliation may thus reflect, at least in part, a change of status of the hospitals rather than a complete change of venue of FMGs. However, even if part of the shift can be explained this way, it remains true that during their training the potential for university contact was generally increased for FMG respondents.

It should be emphasized, moreover, that FMGs who were in their first American position at the time of survey ($N = 190$) were distributed in nonaffiliated hospitals at rates similar to the first position rates for other FMG respondents. There appeared, in short, to have been little actual change in the number of FMGs entering different types of affiliated units.[3] These findings strongly suggest that for a substantial group of FMGs the nonaffiliated programs act both as a portal of entry to the United States and provide a "base camp" in which the FMG can acclimate to and be assimilated by the American system. Hospitals with limited affiliation may also serve a similar function for FMGs who later move to major teaching units.

We conclude, that FMGs as a group experience more interhospital mobility than USMGs and that this mobility tends to be in the direction of the affiliation patterns of USMGs, that is, toward training in major teaching units. Some FMGs may find that their needs are best served in particular programs with a lesser degree of affiliation, as illustrated in the case histories of FMGs who moved away from first positions in the major teaching units of large public general hospitals to less demanding situations. Generally, however, the trend is toward the major teaching unit, with few who begin there moving out, whether FMG or USMG.

FMGs in major teaching units also seem to be somewhat more satisfied with their progress than FMGs in other types of units. When asked to compare "this year's training" with "last year's," almost 60 percent of the FMGs in major teaching units said "this year's training" was better than the previous year, and another 30 percent rated it "about the same." The least contented groups of FMGs were, interestingly, those in the second category of affiliation, in hospitals affiliated for "limited use teaching." Less than 40 percent of these FMGs rated their training as better than the previous year, whereas another 40 percent considered it about the same.

These differences may reflect a tacit and unfavorable comparison by FMGs in hospitals with such limited affiliation to hospitals with major university programs: a "so near and yet so far" basis of evaluation. It may be hypothesized tentatively that FMGs in hospitals with the second level of affiliation are more likely to be dissatisfied because they aspire to position in major teaching units; thus the figures may reflect the more general processes of interhospital mobility. FMGs in hospitals affiliated "for graduate training only" or without affiliation may be more content with their situation, perhaps because they do not make direct comparisons with major teaching units. Alternatively, they may be more recent arrivals who are still adjusting to the American system or who may expect to move to major teaching units without a period in a hospital with the second level of affiliation. Whether these hypotheses can be substantiated, the conclusion remains that a substantial proportion of FMGs who begin their training in nonaffiliated hospitals or hospitals with limited affiliation stay there for only a limited period.

THE INTRODUCTORY ROLE OF THE NONAFFILIATED HOSPITAL

These findings have substantial implications for both the individual careers of FMGs and the role of unaffiliated hospitals in introducing FMGs to the American system. The definite movement of FMGs out of the nonaffiliated hospitals can be readily demonstrated by looking at those who had changed hospitals: 44 percent of those originally in nonaffiliated programs had moved to major teaching units by the time of survey; 27 percent more had moved into limited-use teaching units; 29 percent remained in nonaffiliated units. In contrast, all USMG "changers" who started in nonaffiliated units had moved into major teaching units.

Although the predominant movement is "up," a second interesting organizational finding is the extent of downward movement of FMGs in contrast to that of USMGs. For example, slightly over 25 percent of the FMGs who began in major teaching units and had changed hospitals, had moved away from such units by the time of survey. In contrast, only 13 percent of the USMGs experienced similar movement. These findings indicate that FMGs who initially begin in nonaffiliated hospitals do move up and out over time, although a substantial number do not move at all. Additionally, over time, some FMGs leave the affiliated hospitals and enter nonaffiliated ones.

Presumably others who were in the early stages of their American careers at the time of survey will also move to other categories of affiliation before completing their training. Thus the final mobility patterns may show a greater tendency to move out of unaffiliated units and generally to "play the system."

From the organizational point of view, the nonaffiliated hospital appears to play a distinctive role in introducing FMGs to the American health care system. To some extent, these hospitals may protect the major teaching units by taking responsibility for teaching new recruits: the university selects those with some familiarity with American hospital life and with demonstrated skills. A second function of the nonaffiliated hospital is the screening or sifting of new recruits; thus those able to move upwards can do so.

To some degree, the performance of nonaffiliated hospitals may also have a "cooling out" function, a term Burton Clark adopted from Erving Goffman.[4] This is the process of lowering and/or redirecting FMG aspirations away from certain desirable aspects of American medical practice: lucrative specialties, university teaching, and specialty board certification. Our findings do show an association between the type of hospital affiliation and the choice of career: FMGs in major teaching units are much more likely to consider university teaching, whereas those in nonaffiliated hospitals look to private practice or fulltime hospital staff positions.[5] This association may well be determined by the type of hospital of training. One may hypothesize that hospitals inculcate values that influence house staff in certain directions, that they offer instruction that leads towards these paths, and that the quality of the instruction that is available is likely to be lower in nonaffiliated units relative to the levels necessary for successful achievement. If so, the nonaffiliated program prepares the way for what Clark calls "structured failure."

Other observations arise from the data. If our description of "upward mobility" is correct, those American hospitals with a primary role as portals of entry have a continuing turnover of FMGs and the continuing burden of introducing new groups to the American system. It follows that although some hospitals have "FMG problems," they may not necessarily have a problem because they have too many FMGs, but because they have too many people who have just arrived from abroad and need a special type of teaching.

The new physicians may be competent physicians in a familiar milieu, but they may lack "cultural competence," the ability to deal with the American system. Hospitals that experience a constant influx of entrants—perhaps one-third of the total house staff each year—have a special role in assimilating and socializing FMGs as American physicians. At the same time, the more prestigious hospitals, notably the major teaching units, are able to recruit FMGs who are not only more experienced in American medicine but are also more experienced in America.

From another point of view, we may conclude that the differential array of FMGs among different types of hospital affiliation reflects, to some extent, differential experience as FMGs move in their careers among different categories of affiliation. The "better" hospitals attract FMGs who are the most thoroughly assimilated into the United States. These may not always be those FMGs who have come to the United States for advanced training to take back to foreign countries. Rather, the patterns reflect the sum of individual coping mechanisms. Those who can cope best, do best in their experiences within the American system.

MOBILITY AND OTHER HOSPITAL CHARACTERISTICS

Shifts among categories of affiliation are important not only in themselves, but also because they are associated with other characteristics of American training. Tables 7.3 and 7.4 show, in summary form, the mobility of FMGs by a series of hospital administrative attributes and socioprofessional characteristics. Generally, FMGs moved to larger hospitals during their American careers. There also appears to have been some movement away from church hospitals. Thus 23 percent of the FMGs began training at church hospitals, but only 15 percent were in such hospitals in 1974. Concurrently, there were some apparent shifts into state and federal institutions.

Changes in the cultural and scientific milieu of training can be observed as FMGs move in the American system. Only one-fifth of the FMGs entered American training in hospitals in which the majority of the house staff were USMGs, yet in 1974 one-third of the FMGs were in such locations. The research emphasis (indicated by the hospital necropsy rates) showed less change, but again there was a shift in similar direction: 12 percent of the FMGs began in hospitals with a necropsy rate of at least 51 percent compared to 18 percent of the FMGs in 1974. These changes indicate a general process of mobility toward larger, more complex hospitals, with fewer FMGs. In each respect, as with the type of hospital affiliation, the shifts suggest a gradual assimilation of FMGs into the patterns of training of USMGs—although, as the figures show, this process is limited, partial, and by no means complete.

USMGs, providing the benchmark for comparison, show relatively little mobility as measured by these variables. Beginning in the most university-oriented, largest, and most complex institutions, they remain there in patterns similar to those at entry to the system, but slightly enhanced in each respect. Again, we may conclude that FMGs are both mobile in the American system and that, beginning in relatively modest training situations, they show a greater degree of change than USMGs once their first American position is completed.

TABLE 7.3 FIRST AND CURRENT HOSPITALS—ADMINISTRATIVE CHARACTERISTICS

	First hospitals (Percents)			Current hospitals (Percents)			Percent difference (Percents)		
	FMG	USMG	USFMG	FMG	USMG	USFMG	FMG	USMG	USFMG
Affiliation									
Major teaching unit	41.3	78.3	54.1	58.0	82.0	66.2	+16.7	+3.7	+12.1
Limited affiliation	29.3	13.9	26.1	22.2	14.7	12.5	− 7.1	+0.8	−13.6
Nonaffiliated	29.4	7.8	19.9	19.8	3.3	21.3	− 9.6	−4.5	+ 1.4
	100.0	100.0	100.0	100.0	100.0	100.0			
Admistrative control									
Nonprofit, nonchurch	52.0	36.2	53.4	46.7	35.2	48.1	− 5.3	−1.0	− 5.3
Church	23.3	11.7	18.3	14.9	12.5	14.4	− 8.4	+0.8	− 3.9
City-country	17.8	21.5	14.8	19.0	20.0	9.3	+ 1.2	−1.5	− 5.5
State	3.8	12.4	2.7	8.8	12.3	8.1	+ 5.0	−0.1	+ 5.4
Federal and Miscellaneous	3.3	18.1	10.7	10.7	19.8	20.0	+ 7.4	+1.7	+ 9.3
	100.0	100.0	100.0	100.0	100.0	100.0			
Size (number of beds)									
0–400 beds	39.3	23.8	24.0	28.3	20.7	22.8	−11.0	−3.1	− 1.2
401–600 beds	32.0	29.7	28.0	26.9	28.4	22.7	− 5.1	−1.3	− 5.3
601 beds and over	28.7	46.5	48.0	44.8	50.9	54.5	+16.1	+4.4	+ 6.5
	100.0	100.0	100.0	100.0	100.0	100.0			

a Percentages are weighted.
b Totals may not add to 100.0%, due to rounding.

TABLE 7.4 FIRST AND CURRENT HOSPITALS—SOCIOPROFESSIONAL CHARACTERISTICS

	First hospitals (Percents)			Current hospitals (Percents)			Percent difference (Percents)		
	FMG	USMG	USFMG	FMG	USMG	USFMG	FMG	USMG	USFMG
Number of residency programs									
1–4	40.7	6.6	9.3	22.0	7.4	14.4	−18.7	+0.8	+ 5.1
5–9	28.0	25.7	38.9	30.4	19.2	20.6	+ 2.4	−6.5	−18.3
10–14	10.9	15.3	25.9	15.0	17.3	22.5	+ 4.1	+2.0	− 3.4
15 and over	20.4	52.4	25.9	32.6	56.1	42.5	+12.2	+3.7	+16.6
	100.0	100.0	100.0	100.0	100.0	100.0			
Percentage of FMGs on house staff									
0–25	9.5	65.0	17.3	14.2	71.8	17.5	+ 4.7	+6.8	+ 0.2
26–50	9.6	18.8	21.6	18.7	14.5	31.9	+ 9.1	−4.3	+10.3
51–99	50.5	12.4	59.7	53.7	13.1	40.6	+ 3.2	+0.7	−19.1
100	30.5	3.8	1.4	13.4	0.6	10.0	−17.1	−3.2	+ 8.6
	100.0	100.0	100.0	100.0	100.0	100.0			
Necropsy percentage									
0–25	10.2	4.4	11.4	8.6	3.6	8.0	− 1.6	−0.8	− 3.4
26–50	78.1	54.5	66.6	73.6	51.2	68.6	− 4.5	−3.3	+ 2.0
51–100	11.7	41.1	22.0	17.8	45.2	23.4	+ 6.1	+4.1	+ 1.4
	100.0	100.0	100.0	100.0	100.0	100.0			

[a] Percentages are weighted.
[b] Totals may not add to 100.0%, due to rounding.

149

Organizationally, we see that FMGs are assimilated into the American system through institutions that are foci for training FMGs. Although there may be some practical advantages in entering an American hospital in the company of other foreigners, all of whom are asking similar questions, it can be hypothesized that this experience reinforces the identification of the FMG as an alien or "stranger" from the very beginning of his stay in the United States.

The tables also show quite clearly that despite interhospital mobility, there remain considerable variations between FMGs and USMGs with respect to their continuing (current) training situations. Although both groups gravitate toward hospitals of similar size, the average FMG is far more likely than the average USMG to train outside a major teaching unit, in the least complex and least scientifically oriented hospitals, and in the company of other FMGs. The majority of FMGs were training in major teaching units in 1974, but less than one-half were in hospitals with 10 or more residency programs, only one-third in programs staffed predominantly with USMGs, and only one-sixth in hospitals with relatively high necropsy rates.

GEOGRAPHICAL MOBILITY

These findings suggest differences in the quality of education experienced by FMGs and USMGs. However, before any firm conclusion can be drawn, we must examine whether the distribution of FMGs may be explained, in part, by geographical restrictions, perhaps self-imposed, that are implicit in the FMG's state of entry. We know, for example, from Table 7.1 that although 60 percent of the FMGs changed hospitals between their first and current American post, almost one-half of these individuals shifted to another hospital in the same state. To some extent, therefore, the state of entry predetermines the subsequent career patterns of FMGs in the United States.

Location and mobility patterns by state are given in Table 7.5. Among the states that were the largest employers of house staff in 1973, New York, California, Massachusetts, Michigan, and Texas gained slightly in the number of FMGs within our group between first and current American jobs. Pennsylvania, Ohio, Maryland, New Jersey, Minnesota, and Missouri were "loser" states; fewer FMGs were located in these states in 1974 than had entered training in those states, whereas Illinois had the same proportion of entrants as of current trainees. There is more geographical diffusion of FMGs after their first position; however, there is also a continuing concentration of FMGs in certain states. More

TABLE 7.5 LOCATION OF TRAINING OF RESPONDENTS IN 1974, SELECTED STATES

State ranked by number of house staff on duty, December 1973	Percentage distribution of respondents by state in 1974			Percent difference compared to first hospital distributions[a]		
	FMG	USMG	USFMG	FMG	USMG	USFMG
New York	27.3	15.5	40.9	+2.3	−4.5	+3.0
California	1.9	19.5	4.1	+1.0	+2.4	+4.1
Pennsylvania	7.7	8.5	6.5	−2.1	−1.2	+4.1
Illinois	14.8	3.5	8.3	0	−1.1	0
Ohio	3.7	4.8	4.1	−2.1	+1.6	−4.2
Massachusetts	4.8	7.0	4.1	+0.9	+1.3	+4.1
Michigan	13.5	1.7	0	+2.6	−0.5	0
Texas	0.9	1.6	2.4	+0.3	−1.1	0
Maryland	2.8	4.6	0	−0.8	+1.2	−4.1
New Jersey	4.3	1.1	13.0	−1.4	+0.6	−1.8
Minnesota	0.6	1.6	0	+0.1	+1.1	0
Missouri	1.6	1.6	0	−0.2	+1.1	0
Twelve largest states	83.9	71.0	83.4	+0.6	+0.9	+5.2
All other states	16.1	29.0	16.6	−0.6	−0.9	+5.2
Total	100.0 (690)	100.0 (133)	100.0 (42)			

[a] For first hospital distributions, see Table 6.5.
[b] Percentages are weighted.

than one-half of the FMGs were located in New York, Illinois, and Michigan.

Such observations give a useful picture organizationally but provide only a partial picture of mobility of individual FMGs. Those FMGs in Illinois in 1974 are not necessarily the same physicians who entered Illinois initially. One FMG may start in Illinois and move to Michigan, whereas another starts in Michigan and moves to Illinois. The numerical result is the same as if both had remained in their entry state, but the patterns have different implications.

Studies of the geographical patterns of FMGs from selected countries indicate that there is in fact considerable mobility among a few states. There appears to be a veritable shuttling of personnel among the states located on the northeastern seaboard and westward to the Great Lakes: from Massachusetts to Washington, D.C., back to Illinois and Michigan. Few FMGs, however mobile, appear to break away from these geographical limitations. Presumably, this is the major market for FMG jobs.

Examples drawn from the countries of medical education with the greatest number of survey respondents give the characteristic flavor of geographical mobility. There were, for example, 47 Filipino graduates in our sample. By the time of survey, 31 had moved from their first hospital of training, of whom 13 had moved to other hospitals in the same initial state: one had moved to another hospital in Connecticut, two in Illinois, three in Maryland, one in Michigan, two in New Jersey, one in New York, one in Ohio, and two in Pennsylvania. The 18 Filipino graduates who have moved out of state revealed a mixed bag of experiences. Two moved to Ohio, one from an entering position in Georgia, one from Pennsylvania. Of the others who began in Pennysylvania, one moved to Illinois, one to Maryland, and one to New Jersey, thus continuing in high FMG states. Similarly, two FMGs who began in New Jersey moved to New York, whereas two who began in New York moved to Pennyslvania; one who began in Ohio moved to New York, and another who began in Illinois moved to Michigan.

Only seven of the total group of 47 Filipino FMGs moved outside the so-called "FMG states" or began outside such states, although Filipinos appeared more mobile than most country groups. One Filipino moved from California to Oregon, another from Wisconsin to California; one moved into Texas (from Connecticut), one to Arizona (from Illinois), one to Indiana and one to Iowa (both from New York), and one to Tennessee (from Wisconsin). In short, most FMGs from the Philippines tended to move to another hospital in the same state or to remain within the relatively small group of FMG states.

To a greater or lesser extent such patterns hold for other country groups. Of the 44 FMGs from Thailand, 26 had moved, including 14 who had moved to other hospitals in the same states: Illinois, Maryland, Michigan, Missouri, New Jersey, and New York. The 12 who shifted states showed few surprises. Five moved into New York from Colorado, Connecticut, Illinois, Michigan, and Missouri. One moved from Illinois to Michigan; one from Maryland to Missouri; one from Rhode Island to Maryland. The four who moved outside the major FMG states included three with apparent contacts in Tennessee—one moved from Tennessee to Alabama, one from New York to Tennessee, and one from Michigan to Tennessee—whereas one moved from Pennsylvania to Oregon.

The Pakistani graduates in our sample were more mobile as a group: 29 of the 31 Pakistani FMGs had changed hospitals by the time of interview, and 19 had moved different states. But again mobility tended to be within the major FMG states: into Ohio, Connecticut, New York, New Jersey, Michigan, Maryland, Missouri, and Pennsylvania, from these and neighboring states. Only five Pakistani graduates who began there moved away from the Eastcoast–Great Lakes complex: two to Texas (one from Illinois, one from New York), one to Colorado (from New York), one to Virginia (also from New York), and one to South Carolina (from Michigan).

The Taiwanese group in our sample ($N = 62$) showed a similar clustering effect. Although 17 moved out of their state of entry (and 18 others moved within their first state), the moves tended to be within a small number of states. Four Taiwanese FMGs moved out of Illinois, for example, but they moved to Michigan, Missouri, New York, and Pennsylvania. Six moved out of New York, but three went to Pennsylvania, one to Connecticut, and one to Washington, D.C.; only one "broke ranks" and entered training in Alabama. Pennsylvania appears to have had a particular attraction. Six Taiwanese moved into Pennsylvania from other states, whereas only one moved out of the state.

Some Indian and Iranian graduates were relatively adventurous. Three Indians (out of 41) moved into Arizona and Tennessee, whereas four Iranians (out of 43) went to Florida and Louisiana from the Northeastern–Great Lakes complex. However, none moved to California, the nation's second largest training state. These patterns, based as they are on retrospective data, must be interpreted cautiously. Nevertheless, we feel reasonably confident in concluding that when FMGs begin the process of upward mobility they tend either not to move very far geographically or to move to states in which there is already a substantial group of FMGs. For some, family and friendship networks continue to be important; FMGs join friends in other locations. Others may be motivated by the availability of jobs for FMGs in these states. Some hospitals may rely on interviews that require a personal appearance—easier to organize in contiguous areas. The combined effect is to perpetuate the per-dominance of FMGs in certain locations.

We have shown that FMGs are more mobile than USMGs in terms of changing hospitals and states and that mobility tends to be in an "upward" direction, toward hospitals with greater university affiliation and specialization. However, the shifts take place in merry-go-round fashion within a limited number of states. States such as New York, Illinois, Michigan, and New Jersey continue to attract a relatively large proportion of FMGs compared to the relative distribution of USMGs. States such as California attract a relatively small proportion of FMGs.

If one could show that the type, nature, and quality of house staff training varied systematically by state of training program, these findings would be of considerable interest in helping to explain other features of the FMG experience. Studies of the actual training offered in each state or by degree of university affiliation, types of program, specialty dis-tributions, and other variables, have, however, not yet been done. We cannot say whether, for example, the nature of training in California is the same, better, or worse than that offered in New York or even whether the experiences are different. Lacking evidence on this point, we can draw no causal inferences about the importance of the state of training inde-pendent of other variables. As far as the states are concerned, we observe that a few states are heavily involved in educating new entrants; that the "cream" of this process may then move to other states; but that, gen-erally, those states with a major recruitment function benefit most from FMGs who are already assimilated into American culture. To some extent there is a self-perpetuating FMG system.[6]

DIFFERENTIAL FMG HOSPITAL MOBILITY

As a final theme, we examine whether the broad patterns of mobility we have observed hold equally for all groups of FMGs. Since there were differences in the entry patterns of FMGs into the American hospital system by country of medical education and other variables, different groups may have different mobility experiences within the United States. Thus initally disadvantaged FMGs may "catch up" with others by adjust-ing their position after arrival. Alternately, those who begin with advan-tages may continue to be advantaged in the American system.

Our findings show that FMGs who are most like Americans move quickly upward in the prestige system from initially "disadvantaged" positions. For example, only one-half of the graduates of Eire began their American training in major teaching units, but the great majority of the remainder had moved to such units by 1974. Thus at the time of study 94 percent of the Irish graduates were in major teaching units.

Other country groups with relatively high adjustment rates in terms of hospital affiliation include West Germany, Syria, Colombia, and the United Arab Republic. Cuba, an unusual case in that none of the Cuban FMGs in our sample began in major teaching units, also showed considerable "upward mobility," with 41 percent of graduates in major teaching units by 1974.

The West Germans in our group, few of whom entered major teaching units (probably because of initial lack of information), were particularly "upwardly mobile." Three-fourths (75.1 percent) had switched hospital categories between their first and current hospitals, all toward hospitals with a great degree of university affiliation: 58.5 percent had moved into major teaching units from other types of hospital, whereas 16.6 percent had moved out of first hospitals that had no affiliation into hospitals with a limited university affiliation.

FMGs who might be expected to experience most cultural differences between their countries and the United States were least likely to "play the system" or, conversely, to be offered university jobs. Japanese and Thai physicians illustrate the point. Japanese physicians entered the United States in positions in major teaching units at a rate similar to graduates from Mexico and Peru, and considerably above that of India. However, there was no noticable movement of Japanese FMGs into major teaching units. Thus in 1974 only 43 percent of the Japanese FMGs were training in major teaching units, compared to an average of 58 percent for all FMGs. In contrast, 73 percent of the FMGs from Peru were in such units, 62 percent of the Indians, and 57 percent of the FMGs from Mexico.

Graduates from Thailand entered the United States in major teaching units at rates similar to graduates from the UAR and Spain, and above those of Taiwan. Mobility patterns for Thai graduates were, however, different from those of the others. Thus at the time of survey 45 percent of the Thai FMGs were training in major teaching units, together with 54 percent of Taiwanese FMGs, 61 percent of the FMGs from Spain, and 72 percent of the UAR graduates.

To some extent these variations may reflect an unwillingness to move at all—for example, out of an area with strong family and ethnic ties. However, such reasoning reinforces our conclusion that cultural affinity is an important aspect of "making it" in the American graduate educational system. Whether it should be is another question.

Mobility should not, however, be overstressed. For many FMGs, the nature of the first hospital determines the nature of subsequent American hospital training; inertia appears throughout the system, and generally those countries with a relatively large initial intake of FMGs into non-affiliated units tended to have a relatively large proportion in such units for continuing training. Graduates of Taiwan are a case in point: 36 percent of the Taiwanese FMGs began their American training in nonaffiliated hospitals, 22 percent remained in this type of hospital, and they were joined by others who had begun in different levels of affiliation, to make a current proportion of 34 percent. Graduates of Colombia, South Korea, and Cuba showed varying patterns, but in each case the results were similar: a relatively large proportion of FMGs from these countries entered training in nonaffiliated hospitals, and a relatively large proportion remained there in 1974. In short, there are simultaneous patterns of "upward mobility" for some and "stasis" for others. Some groups move rapidly, such as the West Germans or the Irish, and other groups tend to remain in their category of entry. In each group there are individuals who are mobile, and others who are not.

The resulting patterns are in part a function of entry patterns, part of relative mobility. If the complexity of hospitals is taken as an index of a suitable location for specialized training, Irish graduates assimilate most successfully, followed by Eastern Europeans and Canadians. Least assimilated on this scale are graduates from Ceylon, Philippines, India, and Thailand. One-third of all FMGs were training in hospitals with 13 or more residency training programs in 1974. However, more than two thirds of the FMGs from Eire were in such units, together with at least one-half of the graduates from Eastern European and Canadian schools. In contrast, less than one-fifth of the graduates from Thailand, the Philippines, and Ceylon were in such programs in 1974.

One-third of all FMGs were in relatively noncomplex units (one to six residency programs). Over one-half of the Philippines and Taiwanese graduates were in such programs, together with almost half of the graduates from Ceylon and South Korea. In contrast, FMGs from Thailand, India, and Pakistan were clustered in such units at less than the average rate, as were graduates of Canada, Eire, Eastern Europe, and the United Kingdom.

Because of the variation among individuals, these patterns are difficult to assess. One Filipino graduate may enter and remain in a major teaching unit, as did 26 percent of the FMGs from the Philippines; another may enter and remain in a nonaffiliated unit, as did 29 percent; another may move in an "upward" direction. Since Filipinos are less mobile in the American system than, for example, Indian FMGs, the choice of first hospital appears to be particularly important for this group. We suggest that choice of first hospital is largely accidental: there is no overriding qualitative sorting among categories of hospital. Yet if certain groups of FMGs are relatively concentrated in less prestigious hospitals, assumptions may be drawn that these are the less "qualified" FMGs, and if training and experience are different in these hospitals, such assumptions may be borne out by the American experience.

CONCLUSIONS

We cannot conclude from our data that FMGs who entered and remained in major teaching units are distinguishable from their countrymen who entered and remained in nonaffiliated units; for example, that a South Korean in a university unit is more likely to be "university material" than his counterpart in a nonaffiliated unit, or that the Pakistani or Indian FMGs, the majority of whom were in major teaching units in 1974, were—on entry to the American system—better prepared than or qualitatively different in other respects from Filipino graduates, who were less mobile in terms of hospital prestige.

Some general conclusions can, however, be drawn from our data. First, it is clear that FMGs as a group not only enter less prestigious positions than USMGs, but remain, on average, in less prestigious positions even after several years of training. The location of the first hospital appears to be a predictive element in the FMG's career. However, within the FMG group there is further stratification. Women appear less upwardly mobile than men, Orientals than Whites or Indians. Generally, those most like Americans gravitate to training settings similar to those of USMGs. Although our study did not measure the competence or quality of FMGs, it is doubtful that these patterns reflect technical competence. More probably, they reflect *cultural competence*, the ability to "make it" as American physicians.

One consequence of this phenomenon is that FMGs who wish to be most fully assimilated into American graduate education must assimilate most fully as Americans: they must, in fact, *become* American physicians, in role, outlook, work, and attitudes. The lack of special exchange programs—the "sink or swim" nature of the American experience—may serve to socialize the FMG to such a point that he or she becomes de facto an American immigrant. It follows that FMGs constantly compare their performances to those of USMGs, instead of those of other countrymen or their native country's needs.

At the same time, the American health care system works in such a way as to stigmatize FMGs by not assimilating them fully into American graduate education; indeed, by ensuring that FMGs have quite different training experiences. This duality haunts the FMGs as they make their way in the American system.

Mobility itself is largely an individual characteristic. Some FMGs, like other immigrants before them, assimilate readily to the system. Others appear baffled by its complexities. Some members of defined groups—from individual countries, for example—appear to "rise" through the system, irrespective of their portal of entry, whereas others appear trapped by their initial selection. These terms are not intended to be pejorative: some nonaffiliated hospitals or "FMG states" may offer better programs than university units or states catering largely to USMGs. The general processes are, however, toward programs that are most like those of USMGs. Given the choice, FMGs, like their USMG peers, choose to be educated with USMGs rather than in a mix of FMGs from a variety of countries, and to be in major teaching units and complex, research-oriented institutions.

These movements are at odds with apparent assumptions that FMGs are static recipients of American benevolence, that is, that "good" FMGs go to "good" hospitals, whereas "poor" ones go to others, and there they stay: in short, that there is no games playing by FMGs in the American system. Our findings show that, if little else, FMGs develop their own coping mechanisms, It is possible, if unusual, to begin as an intern in a small, nonaffiliated hospital and move by steps to a fellowship in a major university: the classic idealized career of the successful immigrant.

Generally, however, the first hospital of training is a critical determinant of the FMG's subsequent American career. The FMG learns that there is a system of stratification in the system, in which FMGs are expected to take lower positions and that "success," including acceptance as a highly competent professional, is related to the ability to present oneself as American.

NOTES

1. As might be expected, virtually all the interns we interviewed began their American training in internship positions: indeed, these respondents were typically in their first American positions. Others who entered the system as interns had moved into a residency or research position by 1974. Although FMGs had a greater likelihood of entering the American system directly into residencies, whereas the typical pattern for USMGs was to begin as an intern, the job shifts for each group are quite similar, reflecting a predominant pattern of movement from internships to residencies. For those of our respondents who did an internship, the average length of training was 12 months for both USMGs and FMGs, with a slightly longer period (16 months) for USFMGs.

    FMGs appear, however, somewhat more likely than the other groups to enter a research position at some point in their American careers, although research jobs do not seem an important avenue into approved internship and residency training: only 2 percent of the FMGs came to the United States for research jobs and moved later to an internship or residency. However, reverse movement is evident. Most of the 77 FMGs who were in research positions in 1974 began their American careers as interns or residents.

These patterns may be the result of labeling difficulties: there is not always a clear-cut distinction between a "residency," supposedly training for clinical practice, and a "research position," which may also involve clinical work, but the figures are worth noting as a feature of American training as a whole. Our findings indicate that, at a minimum, 10 percent of USMGs hold a defined position in research as part of their graduate education, as do 16 percent of the FMGs and 14 percent of the USFMGs. Since these figures refer to only two types of American post, the current position and the position of entry, they probably understate the complete pattern: an additional number of respondents may have held research posts between their first American position and their position at the time of survey.

2. It should be noted, however, that beginning an American house staff career as an "assistant" is unusual. Our findings show that 91.1 percent of the FMGs begin work in the United States as interns, residents, or in research/postdoctoral positions, whereas another 1.6 percent originally entered the United States as medical students: an example is a graduate from West Germany who took a clinical clerkship in an American institution as part of his medical school experience. Only 2.7 percent of the FMGs began their American careers in hospital positions that were not approved graduate positions. The remainder held other jobs or gave responses that were inappropriately coded (including nonpaying work such as "house spouse" or "studying for the ECFMG").

3. First position of all FMGs ($N = 657$): major teaching unit, 41.3 percent; other affiliated, 29.3 percent; nonaffiliated, 29.4 percent. First position of FMGs who were in their first American training position in 1974 ($N = 190$): major teaching unit, 43.7 percent; other affiliated 23.7 percent; nonaffiliated, 32.5 percent.

4. Burton R. Clark, *The Open-Door College: A Case Study*, McGraw-Hill, New York, 1960

5. See Chapter 9.

6. Some states have, moreover, experienced an increase in reliance on FMGs: Illinois is a case in point. The percentage of FMGs in internships in Illinois rose from 47 percent in 1967–1968 to 65 percent in 1972–1973, whereas the percentage in residencies rose from 45 to 53 percent. Most were situated in Chicago and its immediate environment. Since physicians in private practice were moving to the suburbs in the same period, one can see a shift in the type of care offered to the population in the inner city, as well as in the training environment of young physicians and in the impact of the American professional culture on entering FMGs. See Kong Meng Tan, "Foreign Trained Physicians in Illinois," *Illinois Medical Journal 144* (December 1973); Donald Dewey, *Where the Doctors Have Gone: The Changing Distribution of Private Practice Physicians in the Chicago Metropolitan Area, 1950–1970*, Illinois Regional Medical Program, 1973.

8

HOUSE STAFF
RESPONSIBILITIES_____

INTRODUCTION

Curiously, many hospitals in the United States have become international training centres almost by default. Not all of these are large, public metropolitan hospitals. Community hospitals in relatively affluent areas have also become cosmopolitan centers for specialty training. A house staff may be composed entirely or predominantly of foreign physicians who are, in turn, taught by American private practitioners. The question arises: What is it that these foreign physicians actually do? What role do they play in the hospital, and what value do they have to the community's practitioners?

Such questions have been largely unexamined, yet they are intrinsic to any study of the trade-offs involved in graduate education. An intern or resident learns by working. In rating any house staff position, the FMG or USMG must balance out in his mind the amount and type of work the hospital wishes done and the value of the experience in terms of training.

An analysis of the role of the FMG in the U.S. health care system is complicated in three respects. First, there has been remarkably little information about the roles, responsibilities, and contributions of house staff as a whole, whether USMG, USMFG, or FMG. Second, even where information has been available, there have been problems of interpretation.[1] Finally, a number of stereotypes have developed that shroud the facts in additional mist. It appears to be generally believed that house staff are exploited, that unaffiliated hospitals are particularly guilty in this respect, and that FMGs are exploited in particular. House staff work is alleged to include much work inappropriate to the status of physicians. House staff were also regarded, until very recently, as essential for the staffing of outpatient departments and emergency rooms. Hospitals appeared as villains, willing to attract the relatively low-paid intern or resident for service needs rather than for the young physician's education.

Standing in stark contrast to these views are other stereotypes. The internship, it has been argued, is necessarily a long and arduous experience, since it stands as a "baptism by fire," a "rite of passage" into the mysteries of the medical profession.[2] More mundanely, it teaches the acolyte to react appropriately to stress, particularly in the middle of the night. Outpatient and emergency experience are especially important, because here the house officer has the greatest responsibility and the least supervision. FMGs are allegedly less "competent" than USMGs and are given less exacting tasks to do.

There may be some truth in all these claims. However, stereotypes are dangerous because their assertions are unqualified and often unquestioned. The problems arising out of house staff training derive largely from the fact that it is not a curriculum but an apprenticeship. As such, house staff training relies on an informal, rather than a formal, process of education. The usual norms of assessing educational programs are therefore difficult, if not impossible, to apply. House staff do not spend their time in classrooms. They are assessed by the Chiefs of Service or Directors of Medical Education in the teaching hospital, and they are tested by the examinations of the national specialty certifying boards. However, the education itself is largely a practical learning experience.

"Service" to the hospital and "education" may thus be synonymous. One hospital may require a great deal of work but give superb training; another may require fewer hours on duty but have less to offer the inquiring student. It is not service itself, but the *type* of experience that distinguishes an excellent from an ordinary apprenticeship. Moreover, the same position may provide good training for one physician (for example, one who gets on well with his superiors) and poor training for another (who does not). Stereotypes based on the notion of service alone must therefore be rejected.

At the same time, the apprenticeship format places enormous emphasis on the interpersonal skills brought to the job by the individual physician. Studies of the learning experience of USMGs in university settings have consistently stressed the importance of discussion of cases and theories with staff and colleagues; more time is spent in such conferences than with patients.[3] It follows that one measurement of a good teaching program is the degree to which informal contacts are encouraged. Stereotypes that ignore the importance of informal learning opportunities must also be rejected. Rather, we can argue that the most "exploited" resident may be the physician with the fewest opportunities to discuss cases on a free and open basis and the fewest opportunities to learn through teaching other students.

FMGS IN A WORKING SITUATION

A vignette of conditions in an actual hospital puts these considerations in a real context and helps clarify the ambiguities of the FMG's position. Redhurst hospital[4] is a mid-size, 400-bed community hospital that provides the only general hospital services to a relatively prosperous, middle-class town in the Northeastern United States. Almost all the town's physicians have attending privileges at the hospital—that is, they may admit and treat their private patients at Redhurst. Almost all are American graduates in private practice.

The hospital employed a house staff of 47 physicians in 1972–1973, only one of whom was a USMG, a woman resident in pathology. There was also one American who had been to Germany for medical school (a USFMG). The remaining 45 house staff, including the chief resident, were FMGs: there was a cluster of 14 from India, seven from South Korea, five from Taiwan, four from the Philippines, three each from Pakistan and Iran, and the remainder from Ceylon, Italy, Germany, Lebanon, Greece, the United Arab Republic, and Japan. Counting the lone USMG, 11 of the house staff were women, a higher proportion than the average figure among FMGs. Two of the male physicians had wives who were also physicians (FMGs) but were not working at the time.

The nature of graduate education in a community hospital does not encourage group cohesion. The hospital's Director of Medical Education provides a central point of reference for all FMGs and is regarded highly for his kindness and generosity. However, daily work is organized in different departments. Attending physicians admit patients and instruct the FMG. The FMG thus works with a large and shifting group of physicians, who are his teachers, "Everyone is a loner," (an FMG from the UAR), and it is a "pretty lonesome existence" (an Indian).

No special arrangements were made for the FMGs entering the American hospital system. The hospital orientation program included a presentation by Chiefs of Specialty Services explaining their own specialty, and arrangements by townspeople to take FMG wives around the town, pointing out the shopping centers. In this hospital, as elsewhere, it seems to have been tacitly assumed, first, that the large proportion of FMGs was a temporary phenomenon and therefore that no special arrangements were called for; second, that the mystique of graduate medical education requires its participants to cope with unexpectedness right from the beginning. Each individual was expected to find out how to behave, what to do, and how the hospital worked. An attending surgeon at Redhurst put this succinctly in describing American education as a "moving train" that new doctors have to jump on while it is going at top speed.

FMGs who cope best learn how to "be nice," particularly to nurses who have a key role as interpreters: an American attending physician may turn to an American nurse to explain the action to a new FMG. They must learn other subtleties of American life, among them the fixation of American doctors on time ("the Anglo Saxon temperament for punctuality"), the acceptance and social importance of alcohol (hard to understand for individuals from nondrinking cultures), and American attitudes about children and parenthood.

Some ingrained patterns must be discarded. For example, one Indian FMG at Redhurst noted that American culture trains the young professional to be aggressive and forceful, not deferential. The intern in India does not smoke in the presence of a senior, shows respect obviously, and stands up when he comes into the room. These characteristics are regarded by USMGs as signs of inferiority, lack of confidence, and weakness. Physicians coming from societies in which there are large numbers of women doctors, and where nurses have established roles as "doctors' helpers" must also readjust themselves to the sex stereotyping and class stereotyping that govern relations between American doctors and nurses. All these adjustments form part of a network of skills that together ensure "proper"—that is full—communication between FMGs and the American physicians to whom they are informally apprenticed in the house staff experience.

The FMGs at Redhurst felt themselves vulnerable in the American system, accepted without being assimilated. A number wanted to move to larger university units, but had been unable to get jobs, reinforcing their feelings of inferiority. Weak points of individuals were exploited by

American physicians. Thus a Japanese intern who had difficulty with English was referred to as a "Dodo" by the attending staff. (He moved on to a successful research position.) A Taiwanese graduate who could not cope left Redhurst after 4 months. An Indian physician said, "No matter how bright an FMG is, he is always starting his [American] career with a score of minus 100 when compared with his American counterparts. The FMG must somehow work his way back to zero before he can hope to gain 'points.' " Several noted the correspondence between a high proportion of FMGs on a house staff and a rating of that hospital program as being of poor quality. There was a general desire to move toward hospitals predominantly staffed by USMGs.

This vignette is illustrative in several respects. First, Redhurst, as a hospital of entry of FMGs, demonstrates the "cooling out" process we have noted;[5] 18 of the 47 house staff were first-year interns. FMGs learn that they are not to participate in the United States as "full physicians." By this, we mean that FMGs do not have a natural right to participate fully in all medical activity. They are aliens who must prove themselves. They learn that they are generally regarded as inferior and that they may have to set their professional sights at a relatively low level.

Second, the teaching relationship of apprentice and practitioner is fluid and unstructured; the practitioners take little or no formal responsibility for seeing that the FMG is properly trained. Rather, the apprentice must teach himself by exploiting all teaching possibilities. In some respects, the situation is almost an adversary relationship. If someone fails, this is felt to be a reflection on that individual, not a breakdown in hospital selection procedures nor a failure in the teaching process. Such observations are equally true for the experiences of USMGs.

Third, such experiences are accepted by the majority of FMGs as a necessary trade-off for the technical skills of modern specialists. Most of the observations of teaching at Redhurst, including the presentation of cases at Grand Rounds, buttressed the role of attending physicians as superior, house staff as inferior: a pact that FMGs appeared to have accepted. Only one departmental chief (a fulltime hospital staff physician) taught in an atmosphere of enjoyment and mutual respect, and this situation stood out from the others. As a result, FMGs tend to rationalize their experiences in terms of two distinctive criteria. As far as specialist training is concerned, there is general praise for the opportunities made available. There is, at the same time, considerable bitterness over personal relationships; overlying both is the ladder of perfection on which the FMG is situated, constantly comparing and being compared to American physicians.

The hospital's view of the role of house staff adds to the ambiguities.

Redhurst appears to have house staff in some departments but not others as a direct result of practitioners' interest. Thus there were residencies in pathology and in general surgery, but not in radiology or anesthesiology. FMGs fulfilled a role in terms of useful service to the institution (providing weekend and evening coverage, for example), but they also provided opportunities for American attending physicians to feel superior. By having a "staff" within the institution, the private practitioner strengthened his own links with the hospital. By teaching, he exercised and developed his own interests. A staff of FMGs was also less threatening than one of USMGs. Not only were the FMGs more vulnerable and less aggressive, they were less of a threat as future competition. By reinforcing the image of the inferiority of FMGs, the attending physicians were also warning them away—however unconsciously—from potential private practice in the area.

Such considerations must be borne in mind in interpreting the roles of FMGs in the American system. Yet although the context is one of multifaceted experiences, the *responsibilities* of FMGs can be documented by an analysis of our study data. The first questions to be examined are whether even the bare-bones stereotypes are appropriate with respect to hours of work and duties.

If unaffiliated hospitals required house staff to work longer hours than major teaching units, we could say that these hospitals receive a relatively greater service benefit from FMGs. If FMGs were shown to work demonstrably longer hours than USMGs or USFMGs, we would have a prima facie case for stating the FMGs are more frequently used for stand-by duties, relieving attending medical staff of additional presence in these institutions. These are not unimportant questions in current policy debates. If, for example, the services now performed by FMGs are to be done in the future by USMGs, we must know whether the duties of the two groups are, in fact, similar. If special programs are to be developed for those FMGs who continue to come to the United States, it is essential to know what FMGs now experience.

WORKLOADS

Respondents were asked to estimate the number of hours they worked each week, including "on-call" time and study time. They were also asked the number of nights on-call in the previous 4 weeks (excluding weekends), and the number of weekends on-call in the previous four, their current service assignment, and patient workloads. The results are given in Table 8.1. It should be noted that these data are self-perceived, that is, they report what house staff *said* they did, not necessarily what they actually did. The findings thus represent a combination of actual experiences and perceptions.

The table shows that FMGs claim shorter working weeks than USMGs, but report similar standby duties (nights and weekends). FMGs are responsible for fewer patients on both inpatient and outpatient units.

TABLE 8.1   WORKLOADS OF FMGS, USMGS, AND USFMGS, SELECTED INDICATORS

	FMG	USMG (Percents)	USFMG
Reported hours worked per week			
0–80	46.9[a]	33.1	26.5
81 or more	53.0	66.8	73.5
Number of nights on call in past 4 weeks			
0–4	34.5	35.6	19.0
5–8	36.9	42.1	55.5
9 or more	28.5	22.3	25.5
Number of weekends on call in past 4 weeks			
0–1	46.1	51.7	51.7
2	41.3	31.1	38.4
3–4	12.6	17.2	9.9
Current service assignment			
Inpatient	89.5	82.6	80.5
Outpatient/ER	10.5	17.5	19.5
Number of beds assigned for those on in-patient services			
None	32.0	28.7	26.5
1–20	46.4	40.7	27.6
21 or more	21.7	30.5	46.3
Number of patients seen per day for those on outpatient/ER services			
0–10	43.4	33.6	18.8
11–20	37.7	39.0	42.8
21 or more	18.8	27.5	38.1
Percent Base (N)	(690)[a]	(133)	(42)

[a] Percentages are weighted; N is unweighted.

Both USMGs and FMGs tend to work 81 hours or more a week and had been on-call for five or more nights and two or more weekends in the previous 4 weeks.

Table 8.2 shows that interns also worked longer hours than residents, with the least hours worked by those in research fellowships and similar positions. USMG interns reported longer hours than FMG interns, and USMG residents longer hours than FMG residents. The differences between USMG and FMG work weeks were thus consistent, except with respect to research positions.

TABLE 8.2   WORK WEEK BY TYPE OF TRAINING POSITION

			Percentage in each category reporting work weeks of 81 hours or more			
	FMG	Percent base (N)[a]	USMG	Percent base (N)	USFMG	Percent base (N)
Interns	64.5	(115)[a]	83.1	(35)	100.0	(3)
Residents	53.2	(485)	63.0	(86)	74.2	(34)
Research fellows and others	26.5	(90)	25.0	(12)	0	(5)

[a] Percent base figures include the total number o respondents in our sample in each category.
Percentages are weighted; N is unweighted.

These crude figures cannot be interpreted without allowing for possible differences in type of hospital and specialty because of the enormous variation in working conditions in different locales. The differences might be explained, for example, by the fact that FMGs are more likely to work outside major teaching units, in which workloads are generally more demanding than in other units.

Tables 8.3 and 8.4 indicate, however, that the differences are not directly attributable to type of hospital affiliation or major specialty. Table 8.3 shows that the differences in hours of work between FMGs and USMGs hold consistently over each type of hospital affiliation. Two-thirds of the USMGs in major teaching units, but only one-half of the FMGs, note a working week of 81 hours or more. Although a substantial minority of FMGs claim the long hours, the average FMG in a major teaching hospital has a shorter work week than the USMG (USFMGs work the most). The table also indicates that there is little difference in the workloads of FMGs in affiliated and nonaffiliated hospitals.

The number of nights and weekends on-call shows little variation by hospital affiliation for either group. Summing up, it appears that assigned duties such as nights on-call and weekends on-duty are experienced similarly by both USMGs and FMGs and by house staff in affiliated and nonaffiliated institutions. Hours of work and responsibility for patients are, however, subject to considerable variation. These may reflect choice, hospital expectations, and/or the time made available to house staff by seniors and colleagues.

TABLE 8.3   REPORTED HOURS WORKED PER WEEK BY TYPE OF HOSPITAL AFFILIATION

| | Percentage in each category at hospital who report a work week of 81 hours or more | | |
	FMG	USMG	USFMG
Hospital affiliation with a university			
Major teaching unit	53.0 (358)[a]	67.8 (103)	78.4 (28)
Limited use teaching	49.2 (115)	66.5 (19)	65.0 (5)
Graduate training only	58.0 (28)	100.0 (12)	0 (0)
Nonaffiliated	54.2 (165)	66.7 (6)	58.9 (7)
	NA = 24	NA = 3	NA = 2

[a] Percentages are weighted; *N* is unweighted.

Table 8.4 shows that, in general, USMGs also report longer hours than FMGs in each major specialty group. Exceptions in our study group were house staff working in obstetrics and psychiatry. For both USMGs and FMGs the shortest working weeks were reported in psychiatry and in the group of specialties that provide hospital-based support services: anesthesiology, pathology, and radiology.

Analysis by specialty groups within each of the categories of affiliation emphasizes the differences in work weeks between American graduates and FMGs. USMGs show a consistent pattern of longer hours than FMGs within each specialty group in each type of hospital affiliation. If nothing else, these findings suggest that FMGs are not required to work longer hours than USMGs; moreover, nonaffiliated hospitals put no greater demands on house staff that do university institutions.

TABLE 8.4 REPORTED HOURS WORKED PER WEEK BY SPECIALTY

	Percentage of respondents reporting a work week of 81 hours or more in each primary specialty group.[a]					
	FMG Percent	base (N)	USMG Percent	base (N)	USFMG Percent	base (N)
Primary specialty group						
Pediatrics	74.5	(65)[b]	79.4	(7)	0	(2)
General/family practice	62.2	(32)	100.0	(3)	100.0	(2)
Surgical specialties	60.9	(159)	87.9	(28)	75.8	(8)
Internal medicine and related specialties	60.2	(166)	84.9	(41)	93.4	(10)
Obstetrics/gynecology	57.8	(58)	50.0	(8)	93.1	(7)
Hospital-based specialties (anesthesiology, pathology, radiology)	31.1	(112)	46.8	(23)	36.0	(5)
Psychiatry	26.0	(62)	14.2	(13)	0	(2)

[a] Excludes respondents whose specialties were "undecided," "unspecified," or other than in these groups (36 FMGs, 10 USMGs, 6USFMGs).
[b] Percentages are weighted; N is unweighted.

However, the actual number of hours claimed by all groups is high compared to studies done on the more reliable time-log basis. A recent Institute of Medicine study noted an average work week of 65½ hours for all house staff, including stand-by time, considerably less than that of our data.[6] It is interesting, however, that work weeks reported on our study are high in all types of hospital affiliation and that the patterns are internally consistent among specialties. If there is a bias, it is systematic: heavy workloads are reported in all types of affiliation and by specialty group within affiliation.

Approximately one-fifth of both USMGs (19.5 percent) and FMGs (20.3 percent) said they were given too much responsibility, but there was no relationship between this claim and the number of hours worked per week. Of the USMGs who claimed that too much responsibility was being assigned to them, 58 percent worked 81 hours or more a week, a lower proportion than for USMGs as a whole. For FMGs, too, there was no association between work week and perceived degree of responsibility. Lacking evidence to the contrary, the different workloads may be ascribed to real differences in the time spent in various hospital activities by USMGs and FMGs—recognizing the tendency of both groups to inflate the number of hours worked per week. We conclude that there is, in any event, no outright "exploitation" of FMGs in terms of longer hours of work or on-call duties.

THE FMG AS A "LESS-THAN-FULL PHYSICIAN"

One possible explanation for longer working weeks by USMGs than FMGs is that the latter are in fact given less to do—or that less is expected of them. We asked our respondents in two separate questions whether they were given too much or too little responsibility. The results are shown in Table 8.5. More than one-fourth of the FMGs claimed that they were indeed being given too little responsibility, a much higher proportion than for USMGs. It would appear that, for these physicians, self-assessment of capabilities is not matched by delegation of clinical work by superiors.

Other findings strengthen the argument. Table 8.1 shows that USMGs tend to be responsible for more patients than FMGs. The USMGs were also more likely to work in outpatient departments and emergency rooms, in which more clinical autonomy may be called for than on in-patient units. Only 10 percent of the FMGs were assigned to outpatient or emergency work at the time of survey; an additional 1 percent performed some outpatient work as part of their in-patient assignments. Since the survey was administered in May and the hospital training year ran from the previous July, these low figures cannot be ascribed to gentle treatment or closer surveillance by hospital staff of a new crop of FMGs in their first few weeks of training. Clearly, interns and residents were not being used by hospitals in 1974 primarily as a source of staffing for outpatient departments (OPDs) and emergency rooms.

The majority of both FMGs and USMGs reported that they had done some OPD or emergency work within the previous year. However, FMGs did not appear to be assigned any special responsibilities for ambulatory care; rather, the reverse. Only 1.5 percent of the FMGs were working solely in emergency rooms at the time of the survey; another 2.7 percent were working in the combined ambulatory care settings (emergency and OPD), and 5.4 percent were in outpatient departments only.

FMGs in nonaffiliated hospitals and those affiliated for graduate training only were no more likely to work solely in outpatient and/or emergency care than were those in major teaching units. FMGs in hospitals with a limited affiliation were least likely to work in ambulatory settings: only 3.6 percent of the FMGs in such hospitals were assigned entirely to the emergency room and/or the OPD. Thus all house staff in general, and FMGs in particular, appear to be receiving little responsibility for—or instruction in—ambulatory care.

Within each category of service, in-patient and outpatient, USMGs carry more patients than FMGs. Almost one-third of the USMGs on in-patient duties said they were responsible for the routine care of 21 patients or more; this was true for little more than one-fifth of the FMGs.

TABLE 8.5   ASSESSMENTS OF INDIVIDUAL RESPONSIBILITY

	FMG	USMG (Percents)	USFMG
Respondents report too			
much responsibility	20.3[a]	19.5	16.6
Sick patients, R unsupervised	9.9	14.6	10.6
Too much work, other	10.4	4.9	6.0
Respondents report too			
little responsibility	25.8	14.7	19.2
By attending and private MDs; for admissions and discharges; for ordering tests	17.0	11.8	7.9
Other, including lack of responsibility generally, and in specific departments	8.8	2.9	11.3

[a] Percentages are weighted.

It may be that FMGs prefer a slower patient intake than USMGs. For some, communication may be difficult and may slow down the patient interview; others may be used to a more leisurely pace. Harrison concluded from similar findings that FMG preference is a basic reason for different patient responsibilities,[7] but it is quite possible that the differences also result from assessment of the relative capabilities of individual staff by supervising physicians. The FMG may be given fewer cases to handle. It remains true, however, that FMGs have rather less responsibility in the hospital than USMGs in terms of the number of patients they see.

The hours of work and the number of patients seen are still, however, crude indicators of actual responsibilities and tasks. Table 8.6 takes the analysis one stage further by reporting house staff assessments of the amount of responsibility carried or the frequency of a task in specified work situations. This table is interesting in that it plots out areas in which FMGs are distinguished from USMGs in their self-perceived roles in the American hospital.

TABLE 8.6   SELECTED HOSPITAL ACTIVITIES OF RESPONDENTS

	Percentage reporting in each category		
	FMG	USMG	USFMG
Maintenance of hospital activities			
"Great" deal of responsibility for management of patients on nights and weekends	64.7[a]	75.6	78.7
"Great" responsibility for decisions about outpatient care	55.8	61.8	68.5
"Often" manages patient from admission to discharge	54.8	68.8	62.2
"Great" responsibility for decisions on patient admissions	45.5	46.5	46.6
"Often" starts IVs	42.6	34.6	52.4
Often or sometimes does "scut work," such as daily blood counts and urine and stool examinations	37.4	54.9	54.4
Sometimes does other "scut work,"	35.5	51.7	43.7
Technician/secretary or orderly's work	27.2	41.4	33.1
Other	8.3	10.3	10.6
Sociocultural responsibilities			
"Often" decides on patient discharge	47.5	70.1	60.3
"Often" has access to information on patient's economic and social activities	41.5	57.9	56.3
"Great" responsibility for dealing with patients' relatives	35.5	62.8	57.5
"Great" responsibility for decisions on discharge	33.6	52.4	56.8
Supervision of staff			
"Often" teaches house staff	38.3	57.6	53.6
"Often" teaches other staff	26.2	29.1	44.4
"Great" responsibility for supervision of staff	11.1	26.8	31.3

Table 8.6 (*Continued*)

	Percentage reporting in each category		
	FMG	USMG	USFMG
Delegation by superiors			
"Often" talks with consultants	74.2	85.9	82.1
Attending "often" available	70.9	82.7	87.3
"Often" works as assistant to attending MD	52.5	36.0	61.3
"Often" works alone with previous instruction	58.4	61.9	65.5
"Often" works alone without previous instruction	18.3	9.6	15.0
Percent Base (N)	(690)[a]	(133)	(42)

[a] Percentages are weighted; N is unweighted.

The table divides the responses into four major classifications that are germane to the house staff experience. The first, maintenance of hospital activities, covers duties the house staff perform as a service to the institution that are necessary to keep the hospital going. If house staff were not there, the staffing patterns of the hospital would have to be changed. These duties include managing patients on nights and weekends and daily in the hospital (for which fully trained physicians would otherwise take responsibility) and tasks that might otherwise be performed by technicians: starting intravenous fluids (IVs), for example.

The second classification includes other tasks performed by a "full physician," that is, one to whom a complete range of professional responsibilities has been given. These center on the exercise of professional judgment—in clinical situations (for example, in deciding when a patient should be discharged) and in social situations (for example, talking to patients' relatives). These roles are grouped under the generic label of sociocultural responsibilities.

The third and fourth categories show the respondent's place in the hospital hierarchy. Both the supervision of staff and the degree to which responsibilities are delegated suggest the value placed on the FMG or USMG in terms of acceptance as a "full physician."

The tables show that decisions about outpatient care and in-patient admissions are quite similar, but that USMGs are more likely than FMGs to be responsible for patients on nights and weekends and to manage patients from their hospital admission through to discharge. FMGs say they are somewhat more likely to start IVs. However, general "scut work" (a favorite term of interns and residents, incorporating anything felt to be inappropriate to their status) is clearly of more concern to the USMGs. Over one-half of the USMGs said they did scut work at least "sometimes." Examples include:

> Paper work which could be done by a secretary. A lot of physically running-down X-rays, lab reports (A USMG).

> Plate cultures at night because there are no technicians then (A Canadian FMG).

> We pull beds to transfer the patients for operations or to different rooms. . . Secretary work. . .We print everything for the patients—Labels—for blood and urine samples (An FMG from Spain).

The table shows that FMGs report similar responsibilities for patient admissions as do USMGs. A rather similar pattern is followed with respect to decisions about outpatient care. On the other hand, FMGs have significantly less responsibility than USMGs (or USFMGs) in making decisions concerning the discharge of patients from hospital, in dealing with patients' relatives, and in supervising other medical staff. FMGs also claim less frequently than the other groups that they are given a "great deal of responsibility" for the management of patients on nights and weekends.

These differences affect the relative importance of these responsibilities as part of the general duties of each group. Thus, for USMGs, management of patients on nights and weekends drew the greatest number of responses as an area of great responsibility; dealing with patients' relatives came next, followed by decisions about outpatient care and decisions on the release of patients. For FMGs too the management of patients on nights and weekends was of first importance, although this was reported as a "great" responsibility by less than two-thirds of the FMGs compared to three-fourths of the USMGs. Decisions about outpatient care came next for FMGs, followed by decisions on hospital admissions; dealing with patients' relatives came fourth. These findings suggest a different array of duties for FMGs and USMGs.

More generally, Table 8.6 shows that both groups (FMGs and USMGs) see themselves as having an important role in maintaining the hospital's daily activities. Even under these "maintenance" functions, however,

USMGs report greater responsibility than FMGs. In areas of "sociocultural" responsibilities the gap widens. Relatively few FMGs are called on to exercise clinical judgment with respect to when a patient might be discharged or to deal with the patient's social situation. FMGs are far less likely to teach other house staff than USMGs and have less responsibility for staff supervision. Both groups report considerable access to superiors (consultants and attending staff) and are expected to work alone with previous instruction. Almost one-fifth of the FMGs also report that they often work without prior instructions. However, FMGs consider their role more frequently than do USMGs as being that of an assistant to attending physicians, rather than one of equivalent status.

DIFFERENCES BY TYPE OF HOSPITAL SETTING

Some of these differences can be explained by the differential distribution of USMGs and FMGs by type of hospital. In general, house staff have less responsibility for patient admission and discharge, dealing with patients' relatives, and managing patients on nights and weekends in nonaffiliated hospitals than in major teaching units. In the large university hospital, patients are admitted to university teaching services staffed by fulltime hospital personnel: house staff have a relatively autonomous role under the supervision of departmental supervisors. In the community hospital with little or no university affiliation, the traditional pattern continues to be one in which the attending physician (typically in private office practice) admits patients under his or her direct care; the resident is responsible to the attending physician and thus to individual, rather than departmental, procedures. As a result, the house staff is less autonomous.

FMGs in university settings have more responsibility for the admission of patients than FMGs in any other type of unit. In other respects too the major teaching unit may demand more by way of day-to-day hospital activities than the nonaffiliated unit. FMGs in university hospitals have more responsibility than other FMGs for outpatient decisions, managing patients from admission to discharge, working on nights and weekends, and undertaking "scut work" such as daily blood counts and stool examinations. On the other hand, FMGs in nonaffiliated units are much more likely to set up IVs.

Coupled with additional responsibilities for patient supervision in the university hospital are additional responsibilities in the sociocultural areas. FMGs in university hospitals have more responsibility for deciding when a patient is to be discharged than FMGs in any other type of unit, affiliated or nonaffiliated (although they claim that they "often" decide on discharge at a rather similar rate). The university unit also provides more opportunity for reviewing economic and social information concerning patients and for interviewing patients' relatives.

For example, FMGs in nonaffiliated hospitals said they had a "great responsibility" for managing patients on nights and weekends 57 percent of the time compared to 68 percent for those in major teaching units. Similarly, decisions on admission of patients ranked as a "great responsibility" for 41 percent of the FMGs in nonaffiliated hospitals compared to 51 percent in university units; on release of patients, 23 percent compared to 41 percent, and on dealing with patients' relatives, 29 percent compared to 39 percent.

Other dimensions can also be observed. As might be expected, FMGs in university settings teach other house staff and medical students far more frequently than FMGs in other types of unit. Only 8 percent of the FMGs in major teaching units said they "never" taught house staff and medical students, compared to 30 percent of those in hospitals with limited affiliation and 43 percent of those in nonaffiliated units. Those in nonaffiliated hospitals were also least likely to teach other health personnel and were somewhat less likely than those in university units to supervise staff.

Finally, FMGs in major teaching units are much more likely to work alone, with prior instructions, than those in nonaffiliated units. On the other hand, those in nonaffiliated units were much more likely than the others to be left on occasion in complete charge of patients *without* instructions. Almost three-fourths (73 percent) of the FMGs in nonaffiliated hospitals said they worked alone without previous instruction "often" or "sometimes" compared to little more than one-half of the FMGs and USMGs in major teaching units (55 percent and 54 percent, respectively).

These patterns undoubtedly reflect the greater size of house staff and other fulltime staff in university units and the departmental structure of administration. In a university service supervision is delegated down a departmental hierarchy. In a hospital relying largely on private attending physicians and with a smaller house staff, individual interns and residents may, on occasion, have no immediate supervisor to turn to. Since the prevailing pattern for FMGs in nonaffiliated hospitals is that of acting as deputy to the attending physician, the occasions on which house staff act alone without instruction reflect times at which the private physician is unavailable—for example, on nights and weekends.

It should be stressed that these distinctions are not merely a factor of "affiliation" versus "nonaffiliation." Similar patterns of responsibility are found in hospitals with limited university affiliation—which are also largely staffed by community physicians—as in nonaffiliated units. For example, responsibility for the discharge of patients was claimed as a "great responsibility" by 26 percent of the FMGs in hospitals with a limited affiliation compared to 23 percent in nonaffiliated hospitals and 41 percent in major teaching units. Clearly, the FMGs in nonaffiliated hospitals and in affiliated hospitals outside the major teaching university units feel they have less responsibility for clinical decision making than do their colleagues in university hospital settings.

Table 8.7 brings together the findings on selected responsibility reported by FMGs and USMGs in major teaching units and in hospitals with a limited university affiliation. This table shows that differences in responsibility are in part a function of the hospital setting. However, in

TABLE 8.7   DIFFERENTIAL RESPONSIBILITIES OF FMGS AND USMGS IN MAJOR UNIVERSITY TEACHING UNITS AND IN HOSPITALS WITH LIMITED UNIVERSITY AFFILIATION, SELECTED INDICATORS

| | (Percentages) | | | |
| | Major Teaching units | | Units with limited university affiliation | |
	FMG	USMG	FMG	USMG
"Great deal" of responsibility for patient admissions	50.9[a]	51.6	36.9	20.8
"Great" responsibility for patient discharge	41.1	55.9	25.5	37.6
"Often" manages patients from admission to discharge	58.5	64.8	50.3	88.0
"Great deal" of responsibility for outpatient decisions	59.0	65.0	50.7	41.6
"Great" responsibility for dealing with patients' relatives	39.3	65.7	31.6	55.1
"Often" teaches house staff and medical students	48.4	62.5	31.4	32.9
"Often" teaches other health personnel	28.3	29.6	32.3	16.1
"Often" talks with consultants	76.3	84.3	80.3	92.0
"Often" acts as assistant to attending MD	49.8	32.6	61.4	62.4
Percent Base (N)	(358)[a]	(103)	(115)	(19)

[a] Percentages are weighted; N is unweighted.

both types of hospital FMGs report different experiences from the USMGs.

In the major teaching units, FMGs state much less often than USMGs (and USFMGs) that they have a great deal of responsibility in the discharge of patients from hospital, dealing with patients' relatives, and medical teaching (although not teaching of nonphysicians). Thus 41 percent of the FMGs in university units claimed a "great responsibility" for release of patients compared to 56 percent of the USMGs in those units; 39 percent of the FMGs noted dealing with relatives as a prime task compared to 66 percent of the USMGs; 48 percent of the FMGs taught medical students or house staff compared to 63 percent of the USMGs. USFMGs' patterns followed or exceeded the responsibility levels of USMGs.

These findings could be explained by differences in interpretation of what is, indeed, a "great deal" of responsibility. It can be argued that FMGs with several years of clinical experience behind them may expect a greater responsibility than new USMGs, and that they feel capable of considerable autonomy. However, it is to be noted that the lower levels of responsibility for FMGs fall only in certain areas. FMGs in the major teaching units were as likely as USMGs and USFMGs to take a "great responsibility" for managing patients on nights and weekends, admitting patients, and making decisions about outpatient care. The three groups also claimed a similar frequency in the routine management of patients in hospital and in "scut work," such as daily blood counts and urine and stool examinations. It can be concluded that with respect to the day-to-day operation of a university hospital, including 24-hour coverage and decisions affecting outpatient care, FMGs have responsibilities and duties similar to those of USMGs.

At the same time, however, FMGs report less activity in areas based largely on interpersonal communication: with medical staff in the hospital and to a lesser extent with students and patients. USMGs spend more time discussing cases with consultants, supervising staff, teaching medical students, and communicating with patients and patients' relatives. These findings do not seem to reflect a different perception of the relative technical competence of FMGs and USMGs on the part of supervising physicians. FMGs are left to work alone, with or without previous instruction, at a rate similar to USMGs. Rather, it appears either that supervising staff see FMGs as performing a different role and different functions, or that FMGs are reluctant to take the responsibility of a "full" physician.

Data from our hospital case studies and from the USFMGs lead us to conclude that the distinctions derive from perceptions of the FMG by hospital superiors. Supervisors treat USFMGs as if they were USMGs, not FMGs, in dealing with the discharge of patients and with relatives, in supervising other staff, and in teaching medical students. This may be because USFMGs, starting at a presumed disadvantage to USMGs, make particular efforts to be visible and helpful to supervising physicians. It is more likely to derive from the fact that USFMGS are Americans. Whatever the reasons, USFMGs as well as USMGs in major teaching units report greater responsibilities in areas of sociocultural activities and interpersonal communication than FMGs. It is reasonable to suppose that it is in these areas that USMGs and USFMGs spend a greater number of hours than FMGs, accounting for a relatively longer work week.

USMGs in hospitals with a "limited" affiliation also appear to be given (or to take) relatively more responsibility than FMGs in the management of patients in hospital, including responsibility "on-call," and have greater access to socioeconomic information about patients. These differences may reflect a greater degree of trust placed in USMGs by attending physicians. Whatever the reason, they highlight the different roles of FMGs and USMGs in the same setting. In short, two processes are at work. University units are distinctive from all other units in the degree of clinical responsibility and teaching duties. At the same time, USMGs have greater responsibilities than FMGs in areas relying on interpersonal communication, irrespective of the training setting.

We conclude that these various differences are not directly attributable to technical competence—if so, FMGs would be given far less clinical responsibility than they are on nights and weekends. Rather, they reflect, on one hand, assessment of the FMG's cultural competence, and on the other, reflection of the FMG's status in the hospital. In both respects, the FMG is regarded as a "less than full" physician.

ARE FMGS EXPLOITED?

Differences can exist without there being invidious distinctions or discrimination. The question remains as to whether FMGs are in fact "exploited" by the American system.

Our findings show that FMGs are not "exploited" in terms of long hours or heavy responsibilities. On the average, FMGs put in fewer hours and claim less by way of responsibilities and duties than members of the other groups. FMGs in nonaffiliated hospitals, moreover, appear to fill quite similar roles to those in affiliated hospitals outside the major university units. Nonaffiliated hospitals appear to "exploit" FMGs in these terms no more than anyone else.

Charges that FMGs do "scut work" and that this is particularly rife in nonaffiliated hospitals are also questioned by our data. FMGs in major teaching units are most likely to complain of "scut work," but so are USMGs. Of all groups, interestingly, the USFMGs were particularly sensitive to "scut work," such as daily blood counts, urine and stool examinations; FMGs complain least. It may well be that these differences reflect different perceptions of what is, or is not, appropriate to the role and dignity of an American physician; USMFGs, especially concerned about their status, may resent any request to do routine work.[8] This observation does not deny our basic findings that FMGs complained of "scut work" less frequently than other physicians.

Table 8.8 shows another area—salaries—in which there is no evidence of overt exploitation of FMGs. The highest salaries reported were by USFMGs, the lowest by USMGs. These differences were not obviously explicable by the operation of the job market. One might expect, for instance, that university units, knowing they could rely on prestige to draw their staff, would pay less than nonaffiliated units, and this would account for different salaries among the groups. In fact, the average salary reported by FMGs in major teaching units was higher than that in other types of hospitals. Wishful thinking may have affected the replies, with USFMGs in particular inflating their salaries to what they feel to be a more appropriate level—a reflection, perhaps, of their concerns over status. Conversely, USMGs may have depressed their salary levels. In any event, the figures show no pattern of monetary discrimination against either FMGs or USFMGs. As far as exploitation is concerned, we would have to look for evidence from sources other than workloads or salary levels.

We have, however, shown differences in activities between FMGs and both USMGs and USFMGs. The data suggest that these are the combined result of the clustering of FMGs outside major teaching units in settings in

TABLE 8.8   REPORTED SALARIES

	FMG	USMG	USFMG
Annual Salary			
Up to $10,999	30.5	44.9	17.7
$11,000–12,999	37.6	32.1	34.8
$13,000 or more	31.9	23.0	47.4
	100.0(690)[a]	100.0(133)	100.0(42)

[a] Percentages are weighted; *N* is unweighted.

which clinical responsibility is less freely delegated, and of a relative unwillingness by superiors to delegate responsibility to FMGs in decisions affecting patients. The effect of this is to give FMGs, on the average, a less complete apprenticeship than USMGs and less clinical autonomy than individual FMGs might be used to or have expected in coming to the United States. An Indian physician in our study expressed a frustration with American training that is by no means unique: "We are not given the responsibility we deserve. . .We are not treated even as doctors sometimes. I feel sometimes like cheap labor—being exploited."

The idea of FMGs as "cheap labor" is widespread.[9] Our findings suggest that FMGs are not "cheap" labor if the alternative is replacement by USMG interns and residents, assuming such USMGs to be available. This may be the case in the future, as more graduates are supplied from American schools. However, if the alternative to FMGs is replacement by fully trained physicians (e.g., those in private practice), the employment of FMGs at apprenticeship salaries for a supposedly temporary period is clearly beneficial to the American system. As far as FMGs are concerned, however, the critical factor is not the development of economic yardsticks, but the feeling that in one way or another FMGs are second-class citizens in the American system. The varying levels of responsibility open to FMGs reinforce this attitude through internship and residency training.

Other more subtle factors also undoubtedly apply. Those who come to the United States with substantial experience choose deliberately to take a backwards career step in entering (or reentering) apprenticeship training. FMGs are like fully trained American professionals who choose to "go back to school," unaware of the costs, in so doing, of reduced status. For FMGs this reduction is compounded by the additional and inescapable fact of being foreign, with respect (1) to having to cope with the uncertainties of an alien system and (2) being treated as a "stranger" by Americans.

Some physicians explained the difficulty they had in moving to a reduced status in the American system. A Chinese physician trained in Taiwan remarked, "In my country we were allowed to do everything, and it's almost nothing here." A Mexican physician in surgical training in a hospital staffed by private physicians noted that the "surgical procedures and care of the private physician is followed rather than my own," and that "I do not always agree with the private physician."

Such complaints are voiced by only a minority of FMGs, but the themes run through most discussions of FMGs by FMGs. Our findings reflect a somewhat schizophrenic view of the FMG's position: 80 percent of the FMGs agreed "strongly" or "somewhat" with the statement that American training programs are the best in the world (compared to 95 percent of the USMGs). At the same time, 61 percent of the FMGs thought that American programs were an "excuse to staff hospitals"; the comparable figure for USMGs was 26 percent.

The two statements are by no means incompatible. As observed, a good apprenticeship requires delegation of responsibility and progressive work, and a hospital with staffing needs may provide both. Nevertheless, there is a problem in reconciling the role of the apprentice with the demands of a hospital service system when physicians on the staff are unable or unwilling to grant the apprentice full status. "Full" status implies that the apprentice is fully accepted and will, when trained, be an equal member in the local community of physicians. The ambiguity in the FMG's position is that complete acceptance as an apprentice implies a tacit commitment to practice in the United States as an American physician—and neither the FMG nor the local community of physicians may be willing to go this far.

Training physicians through an on-the-job system also leads to some bitterness among FMGs who feel thay are providing essential care to the American population while being viewed as less privileged—if not less competent—than American physicians. An editorial in a New York-based Indian publication made the point in 1974 in claiming racial discrimination against Indian and Asian FMGs, "who, in our opinion, are doing an excellent job of providing good quality medical care to all American citizens."[10] Our study did not seek evidence of racial discrimination, and this charge appeared infrequently in unsolicited comments. What did appear, however, was an undercurrent of "differentness," a feeling that however hard the FMG tries, it is difficult, if not impossible, to "catch up," that is to become fully accepted as an American physician.

We conclude, then, that FMGs are not exploited in terms of excessive hours of work, poor salary, or massive service expectations—at least in comparison to USMGs. We would prefer to dismiss the word "exploitation" altogether and analyze instead the implications of the observable differences between the roles of FMGs and USMGs. In terms of what FMGs actually do in American hospitals, our findings show that FMGs provide substantial coverage of in-patient services, including substantial off-duty support to the hospital's fully trained physicians.

The extent of such services can be measured, in one way, by the huge sums of money the United States would have to spend to provide sufficient manpower to replace the services of FMGs.[11] However, such exercises do not take into account the value of the American experience to the individual FMGs. We stress that most FMGs were happy with their specialist training experience.

Our findings do lead us, however, to question the nature and value of the house staff apprenticeship as a vehicle for the education of foreign exchange students. It may indeed be impossible to have a successful apprenticeship when the apprentice is, supposedly, not to remain in this country after training; American role models may be inappropriate. In one sense, the FMGs might be seen as "missionaries," preparing to take American medicine overseas. However, the teachers to whom FMGs are apprenticed are not oriented toward overseas missions. They are largely American private practitioners who may see FMGs almost entirely in two contexts: as temporary visitors who will leave and thus do not need full socialization into American medicine, and as hospital employees whose role is to provide supporting services.

The role of the FMG-as-apprentice poses educational dilemmas as well as questions of hospital responsibility, and it is to the educational questions we turn next. Here we must observe that the patterns of responsibility of house staff reveal differences in the perceived role and status of FMGs and USMGs. These differences should not be overstated. There are thousands of FMGs in fulltime practice in the United States who have clearly made a successful transition; we have shown, too, considerable upward mobility for FMGs in the American system. Nevertheless, as a group FMGs are stigmatized and regarded as "less-than-full" physicians. Their responsibilities reflect this stigmatization.

NOTES

1. Debate over the relative competence or "quality" of FMGs compared to USMGs provides a useful illustration. A number of studies have noted that FMGs have a relatively high failure rate on standardized tests, but there is a lack of demonstrable connection between such findings and competence per se. See Kathleen Williams and Robert Brook, "Foreign Medical Graduates and their Impact on the Quality of Medical Care in the United States," *Health and Society*, Milbank Memorial Fund Quarterly (Fall 1975), 549 and Aaron Lowin, *FMGs? An Evaluation of Policy-Related Research, op cit*, pp. 47–86.

2. See Mumford, *Interns, op cit*. These aspects of the internship (or the first-year residency which is replacing it) are reinforced and glamorized in the popular literature.

3. See, for example, Henry E. Payson, Eugene C. Gaenslin, Jr., and Fred L. Stargardter, "Time Study of an Internship on a University Medical Service," *New England Journal of Medicine* (1961), *264*: 439–443; Henry G. Payson and Jack D. Barchas, "A Time Study of Medical Teaching Rounds," *ibid*, (1961), 273: 1468–71; William Gillanders and Michael Heiman, "Time Study Comparison of Three Intern Programs," *Journal of Medical Education* (1971), *46*: 142–149; Robert S. Brown, "House Staff Attitudes Toward Teach-

ing," *Journal of Medical Education (1970)*, *45:* 156–59; Stanley Crosbie, "How Residents Apportion Work Time," *Hospitals* (1971), *45:* 60–63.

4. The name of the hospital is fictitious. Materials are drawn from one of a series of hospital studies we conducted, prior to the main study, in 1972.

5. See Chapter 7.

6. The Institute of Medicine of the National Academy of Sciences came up with an average work week of 58 hours, plus 7.5 hours on stand-by time. Only 12.9 percent of the FMGs in our study reported a work week of 60 hours or less, together with 10.7 percent of the USMGs. Crosbie found an average workweek of 69.2 hours for residents in hospitals affiliated with the University of Colorado Medical Center: Stanley Crosbie, "How Residents Apportion Work Time," *Hospitals* (1971), *45:* 60–63. Gillanders and Heinman, above, found a work week of 80–85 hours per week.

7. Barbara Harrison, *Foreign Doctors in American Hospitals*, p. 53.

8. See Harrison, pp. 49 ff.

9. See, for example, E. Fuller Torrey and Robert L. Taylor, "Cheap Labor from Poor Nations," *American Journal Psychiatry* (1973), *1304:* 428.

10. "Indian Physicians—A Maligned Minority," TransIndia, Oct. 7, 1974.

11. One estimate of the savings in educational costs to the United States in 1972—by not having to provide basic medical education to interns and residents who came from abroad—was $536 million with respect solely to the contributions from less developed countries. The Far East reported $405 million of this total. Whelan, *Brain Drain*, pp. 177–80.

THE EDUCATIONAL EXPERIENCE___

The physician apprentice is both worker and student. In Chapter 8 we conclude that FMGs are not exploited as workers in an employment situation. This chapter examines the educational experience in more detail. We argue that the quality of American graduate education is, on the average, lower for FMGs than USMGs, because of (1) their differential placement in the educational system; (2) their differential treatment, even where training settings are similar; (3) the ability of FMGs, as "strangers," to make full use of the opportunities available to USMGs who are, inevitably, "insiders" in the system. Cultural factors are intrinsic to the learning process, yet they have often been ignored in the research literature.

In an educational process that is largely informal, FMGs lean toward formal learning methods. In a structure that clusters FMGs for training largely with other FMGs, adequate models are unavailable on which residents can pattern all aspects of training and thus succeed as "American physicians" on a basis equal to USMGs. Moreover, the cultural heterogeneity of many house staffs discourages close communication and interaction among the apprentices themselves, thus affecting another aspect of the learning experience.[1] Finally, the pattern of training FMGs in hospitals staffed largely by private attending physicians (whether these are university affiliated or not) formalizes the role of the FMG as the physician's assistant and affects his or her choice of future career. Cumulatively, these patterns describe different learning environments for FMGs and USMGs.

WHAT DO RESIDENTS LEARN?

The relative value and appropriateness of the graduate medical education received by FMGs and USMGs has been difficult to measure because there are few yardsticks of what residents actually learn and are supposed to learn between graduation from medical school and recognition as a fully trained physician. Examinations by the specialty certifying boards can measure knowledge and reasoning ability, but it is well recognized that factual knowledge is only part of the physician's training during the 3- or 4-year graduate apprenticeship. Otherwise, a physician's education might be completed in a classroom, rather than in a lengthy practical experience.

A recent study of pediatricians by Burg and Wright suggests that the resident learns in three distinct areas. The first and most obvious area is knowledge. The resident must also acquire what the authors call "physical skills," such as the proper method of undertaking a physical examination or resuscitating a patient. Finally, the resident learns an important set of behavioral skills or attitudes. These include history taking and interviewing techniques, the development of motivation to continue learning, appropriate reaction to stress, and "integrity." [2] These three areas might be redefined in terms of the physician as scholar, technician, and professional.

How much weight should be given to each area in any particular specialty is still a matter for definition. Burg and Wright note that, at least in pediatrics, the specialty board tests knowledge, but must rely largely on the recommendation of program directors in the teaching hospitals for judgments on technical and professional abilities. This observation has two ramifications. First, specialty board examination results cannot be used to evaluate the total learning procedure; second, the resident is dependent on his local program chief for a good recommendation as a technician or professional. There is thus considerable subjective evaluation in the performance of residents in two out of three important learning areas, whereas knowledge can be evaluated through objective tests.

Alpert and others have stressed that technical skills are the most important element of learning during a university hospital internship, with most of the learning taking place on the wards and most of the teaching done by fulltime staff, including residents.[3] Brown also emphasized the importance of learning from other residents in a study of house staff at the University of Virginia hospital: the residents in this study claimed that half their training was received from fellow house staff, whereas another one-fifth of their time was spent teaching and supervising others.[4] Crosbie found residents at hospitals affiliated with the University of Colorado Medical Center almost fully engaged in practical experiences.[5] Little time was spent in formal study or research. Gillanders and Heiman also found that house staff in a university unit had little time to spend in studying the medical literature, while spending significantly more time in formal patient rounds than their counterparts in a Public Health Service hospital.[6]

These studies offer a picture of graduate medical education in the university setting based on practical learning rather than formal learning experiences. House staff avail themselves of the opportunity to pattern their skills—including knowledge, development of theories of disease, technical abilities, and professional behavior—on the model of other fulltime staff working in the same setting. Presumably, the evaluation of the resident by the program director reflects the degree to which the resident conforms to the prevailing model of excellence established in that particular institution. The model will, however, consist of the three elements of knowledge, technical competence, and professional behavior.

Assuming that the preceding arguments are valid, it follows that it is extremely important for the resident to perceive and accept the model prevailing at his or her teaching hospital and to be willing and able to participate in the hospital's learning methods. Notably, the resident must be able to learn from, and to contribute to, practical situations. The resident must demonstrate the acquisition of knowledge and "behave like an American physician." In short, the resident must demonstrate cultural competence.

It is this last area that may pose the most difficulty to a foreign-trained physician and in which he or she may run up against intractable problems of perception. The observation that FMGs tend to be readily accepted by American physicians as assistants, far less as junior colleagues, has important organizational ramifications. Not least, the FMG is less able than the American graduate to benefit from colleague networks, through which private practices tend to be established.[7]

Besides these professional considerations, there are educational ramifications. If the hospital is indeed an environment for learning rather than a direct teaching experience, and if interns and residents are expected to define their own roles and situations in this environment, to develop their own rationale for what they do, and their own system of "exchange relationships" between themselves and other students to benefit most from their experiences,[8] the FMG who is viewed differently from a USMG is disadvanged as a student compared to his American peers.

It may be remarked, finally, that the FMG who is regarded as having a low level of cultural ability will experience additional difficulties as an immigrant. Generally, the process of assimilation into the culture of the American hospital is more difficult for FMGs than USMGs, because FMGs spend less time in informal communication with other staff than do their American peers.

FORMAL AND INFORMAL EDUCATION

The finding that FMGs make less use than USMGs of informal learning experiences and rely more frequently on formal processes, holds irrespective of the type of hospital or training milieu. USMGs learn more through teaching others and by discussing cases with their peers, whereas FMGs are more likely to attend meetings, to listen to their chief of service, and to study in the hospital library.

The basic patterns are given in Table 9.1. Approximately 80 percent of the FMGs reported that they used their hospital medical library "often" compared to 53 percent of the USMGs. FMGs were also more likely to attend formal meetings: record and fatality meetings, clinical-pathological conferences (CPCs), tissue committees, and X-ray conferences. However, the FMGs and USMGs attended grand rounds (basic teaching by faculty around selected patients) and patient rounds at similar rates. It can be hypothesized (1) that both groups considered bedside teaching (and its extension into grand rounds) as the ideal learning experience, (2) that there were formal or informal pressures on house staff to attend grand rounds, but that such pressure was not exerted equally with respect to the other meetings.

The USMGs, on the other hand, reported rather more informal discussion opportunities with teachers and peers than did the FMGs: 83 percent of the USMGs said that an attending physician was often present or available to work with them (compared to 71 percent of the FMGs); 86 percent often talked over cases with consultants (74 percent of the FMGs), and 60 percent engaged in medical teaching (38 percent of the FMGs).

In each respect, the differences are not attributable to the distribution of

TABLE 9.1   ELEMENTS OF GRADUATE MEDICAL EDUCATION

| | Percentage in each category | | |
	FMG	USMG	USFMG
Library			
Often uses hospital medical library	79.9[a]	52.8	70.2
Rounds and meetings			
Often attends grand rounds	62.0	64.2	74.1
Often attends patient rounds	75.6	78.7	86.8
Attends record and fatality meetings conducted at least once a month	66.5	54.4	56.9
Attends CPC at least once a month	73.9	60.1	76.2
Attends tissue committees at least once a month	42.6	30.8	39.8
Attends X-ray conferences at least once a month	62.0	43.3	59.1
Discussion opportunities			
Attending physician is often present or available to work with R or to give instruction	70.9	82.7	87.3
Often talks over cases with consultants	74.2	85.9	82.1
Often teaches interns, residents, and medical students	38.3	59.6	53.6
Percent base (N)	(690)[a]	(133)	(42)

[a] Percentages are weighted; N is unweighted.

respondents in different types of hospitals, nor—in the case of formal meetings—to the availability of opportunities. USMGs and FMGs reported that the various committees were available in their hospitals to a similar degree. The distinctions arise out of the fact that the FMGs (and USFMGs) were much more likely to attend such meetings than the USMGs, even in the same type of hospital. For example, 87 percent of the FMGs in major teaching units said they attended CPCs at least once a month, compared to 67 percent of the USMGs in such units (and 89 percent of the USFMGs).

FMGs also stated more frequently than USMGs that there were other meetings they regarded as important that they were unable to attend because of time: 57 percent of the FMGs said they were prevented from attending meetings because of time, compared to 46 percent of the

USMGs. These patterns suggest that meetings have a greater significance for FMGs than for USMGs in the process of graduate education.

The use of the hospital library is also strikingly different among the various groups. The library holds a central place in the FMG's education in all types of training institutions: 81 percent of the FMGs in major teaching units described themselves as frequent library users compared to 52 percent of the USMGs (and 57 percent of the USFMGs) in these units.

The distinction in formal learning experiences between USMGs and FMGs thus appears to be the product of individual learning patterns rather than intrinsic to a particular teaching situation, at least as measured by level of affiliation. Although USMGs may use formal learning situations to reinforce and extend the knowledge gained in informal conversations with superiors and peers, FMGs appear to use this process in reverse, drawing on knowledge from texts and meetings as the resource for bedside situations.

It can be argued that for at least some FMGs, the formal learning situation is the one they are most used to. Medical education may mean didactic or "book learning," rather than the strong clinical experience that is supposedly the root of American medical education. Thus the FMG faced with a particular problem may be more inclined to seek information from a book or from a lecturer than from a staff physician or a fellow resident. On the other hand, the FMGs in our study were, on the average, several years out of medical school. Even if their pattern of undergraduate medical education were one of large classes and other formal sessions, one would expect the intervening postgraduate experience of the FMG, having focused on clinical experience, to have brought the physician into constant conversational contact with peers around specific clinical problems and cases. Although our data cannot prove causal relationships one way or the other, FMGs may seek information from books and other formal learning experiences because informal contacts are not accessible to them—or because they do not like to ask.

Other findings support this observation. It is striking, for instance, that USMGs learn far more frequently from other residents than do FMGs. Table 9.2 shows that almost one-half of the USMGs said they learned a great deal from residents, but only one-fifth of the FMGs. In part this may be because there are more residents available for USMGs to talk with: the average USMG and USFMG in our study worked on a service with five residents (and one intern) on the usual day shift, compared to an average of three residents (and one intern) for the average FMG. However, this difference does not fully explain why USMGs learn more from residents.

TABLE 9.2   LEARNING MODELS FOR HOUSE STAFF IN MAJOR TEACHING
UNITS

	(Percentages)		
	FMG	USMG	USFMG
Learned a great deal from			
Chiefs of service	40.0[a]	28.6	60.2
Private physicians	24.6	28.1	40.3
Residents	21.1	46.1	43.2
Nurses	0.4	3.4	0
Patients	44.1	62.3	40.5
Formally evaluated by			
Chiefs of service	84.9	84.0	100.0
Private attending physicians	46.4	45.2	53.9
Fulltime hospital physicians	66.8	73.7	81.7
Senior residents	45.4	47.4	55.4
Percent base (N)	(690)[a]	(133)	(42)

[a] Percentages are weighted; N is unweighted.

Moreover, the USMGs also reported that they learned more than
FMGs from nurses, whose average daily presence is the same. (Nurses
were not regarded, however, as a primary teaching source for any group).
Finally, USMGs claim that they learn far more from patients than do
FMGs. For residents and patients the differences are substantial. Since
USFMGs follow the pattern for USMGs in these respects, the findings
suggest strongly that the distinctions in informal learning patterns are
largely cultural in nature, that is, that American citizens communicate
more easily with other staff, nurses, and patients and thus can draw on
them more fully for needed information.

All these differences hold by the various types of hospital affiliation. In
major teaching units, for example, 85 percent of the USMGs said they
learned a "great deal" or "fair amount" from residents, 27 percent from
nurses, and 80 percent from patients. Comparable figures for FMGs in
major teaching units were 65 percent, 10 percent, and 68 percent. Perhaps
alarmingly, 13 percent of all the FMGs said they had learned "nothing"
from residents, 48 percent said thay learned nothing from nurses,
whereas 14 percent said they learned nothing from patients.

Instead, FMGs rely more often than USMGs on guidance from the chief
of the service to which they are assigned—another example of learning
through a formal process. Chiefs of service were cited most frequently by

FMGs (78 percent) as a source of learning, whereas residents were cited by the largest group of USMGs (83 percent). These distinctions do not follow formal responsibility for teaching as reflected in responsibility for evaluating the work of interns and residents (Table 9.2). The differences do hold over different types of hospital affiliation.

Although FMGs rely more often on formal patterns and USMGs on informal patterns of learning, USFMGs are in the position of drawing substantially on both systems. USFMGs use the medical library far more than USMGs, and they learn substantially from chiefs of service. In these respects, the USFMGs rely, like the FMGs, on formal learning mechanisms, but at the same time the USFMGs also utilize informal opportunities to a far greater extent than FMGs. Their relations with nurses, patients, and other house staff resemble those of USMGs.

The findings show, therefore, three patterns of instruction utilized by the three groups. These patterns exist in hospitals at all levels of university affiliation. On the average, the USMG learns most from the peers, his immediate superiors, and his students; the FMG relies more on meetings, independent study, and guidance by his service chief; the USFMG, identified to some extent with both groups, makes use of both systems.

LEARNING WITH OTHER FMGS

The majority of FMGs receive their American graduate medical education in a training milieu in which most of the house staff are FMGs; indeed, approximately one-half of the FMGs are in training settings in which FMGs comprise more than three-quarters of the staff. Only one-seventh train in situations in which more than three-quarters of the house staff are American graduates or USFMGs. Thus relatively few FMGs have the USMG as a prevailing model on which to pattern their own skills and behavior. USMGs, in contrast, are almost always trained with a majority of USMGs.

One must be careful about making qualitative judgments about training from these findings. Theoretically, at least, the "American" model —in which the majority of house staff are USMGs—may not be a useful pattern for foreign physicians. Many FMGs presumably come to the United States for American skills, not to be transformed into an American physician; that is, they may desire two elements of American graduate education, knowledge and physical skills, but only some elements of the third, professional attitudes and behavior. Other elements of professional role development may be more appropriately acquired in their home countries. (One element of professional attitudes that it may be undesirable to encourage in developing nations is the USMG's strong preference for private practice; another is reliance on expensive machinery.)

However, FMGs in training with other FMGs are far less satisfied with their American experiences than those training in an "American" setting. Table 9.3 shows that FMGs in training in hospitals in which less than one-quarter of the house staff is foreign consider that they enjoy rather better treatment in the United States system than do their peers in training with a great majority of FMGs. Although FMGs in all situations consider American training to be the best in the world, the responses to particular experiences vary considerably, with marked differences in viewpoint at each end of the scale. Thus 72 percent of FMGs in the most "Americanized" situations feel that American training is providing skills for their country of medical education to a great extent, compared to 39 percent of those training in an all-FMG situation.

Those in the latter position are, conversely, far more likely to consider that American training programs are "an excuse to staff hospitals and are not really for training" than those in the former situation. Indeed, a majority of FMGs in all classifications except where FMGs represented less than one-quarter of graduate trainees considered that American training was a means of staffing rather than training, an interesting

TABLE 9.3   FMGS' VIEWS OF U.S. EDUCATION BY PROPORTION OF FMGS ON HOSPITAL STAFF

| Percentage of FMG interns and residents on house staff | Percentage in each category agreeing to a "great extent" that | | | |
	Training provides skill for CME[a]	R is not treated as well as USMGs	R is treated better than other FMGs	Percent base (N)
0–25[b]	71.9	44.1	42.6	(118)[b]
26–50	52.6	58.6	30.8	(105)
51–75	60.4	56.5	29.1	(113)
76–99	46.6	69.0	22.0	(191)
100	39.4	63.6	24.3	(99)
All FMGs	52.7	60.4	28.2	(626)
				NA = 64

[a] Country of Medical Education
[b] Percentages are weighted; N is unweighted.

sidelight on FMG perception of their American education. Most USMGs refuted the statement. Overall, only 26 percent of the USMGs considered that American training programs were an excuse to staff hospitals, compared to 60 percent of FMGs. However, USMGs in training in situations in which three-quarters or more of the house staff were FMGs also considered that educational programs were primarily for staffing.

These findings suggest that the desired training setting for both groups is one in which a substantial proportion of house staff is American trained. FMGs in particular seek a model in which the great majority of the house staff are USMGs.

The rationale for this model is not necessarily that technical training varies in the different settings, but that FMGs are *treated differently*. Generally, both FMGs and—in particular—USMGs are firmly of the opinion that FMGs are not given training equal to that of USMGs (75 percent of all FMGs and 92 percent of USMGs agreed with this statement). The most satisfied members of both groups are found in hospitals in which less than one-half of all trainees are FMGs.

These differences are clearer when the responses are divided into those who "agree strongly" and "agree somewhat." In hospitals in which less than one-quarter of the staff are FMGs, 29 percent of FMGs "agreed strongly" that FMGs, in general, are given unequal training compared to USMGs. The comparable figure for those in all-FMG situations was 55 percent. In short, FMGs are most likely to be given training perceived as equivalent to that of the USMG in settings in which the USMG is in the majority. The smaller the proportion of FMGs in training in a particular institution, the greater their chance of an "American" education—and of being treated as an American.

The findings in Table 9.3 indicate that these perceptions derive from the respondents' own training circumstances. FMGs in hospitals in which a great majority of house staff were FMGs rated their own treatment compared to that given to USMGs, USFMGs, and other FMGs, as relatively much worse than that given to their counterparts in largely "American" training settings. In settings staffed wholly with FMGs, 64 percent of the FMGs said they were not treated as well as USMGs, 52 percent thought they would not be treated as well as USFMGs, and only 24 percent thought they were treated better than other FMGs. Comparable figures for FMGs in settings staffed with three-quarters or more USMGs were 44 percent, 26 percent, and 43 percent, respectively.

In plain terms, FMGs feel that they get the most appropriate education for their own countries and the best deal in terms of treatment by other staff when they are training with USMGs; the worst situation occurs when they are training with other FMGs. Since most USMGs are in training in major university units, the most desirable pattern for training in terms of the variables considered in this section is usually that of the major teaching unit.

The degree of contentment is, however, related to the proportion of FMGs and not to affiliation per se. FMGs responded to the question of whether FMGs were given equal training to USMGs at similar rates in all types of hospital affiliation. American training programs were regarded as excuses to staff hospitals to the least extent in hospitals affiliated for graduate training only and to the greatest degree in hospitals with the lowest level of affiliation (for limited use teaching).

We conclude that the nature of American training requires an adequate number of American role models from whom FMGs and other house staff can learn; a desirable proportion is at least three to one. Lacking such models, FMGs may be deprived of essential elements in their training as American physicians. As a secondary effect, the FMG in a situation in which most trainees are USMGs is more likely to be perceived by senior staff as a junior colleague than in situations in which FMGs are the rule, where he is given less to do. Third, the predominance of USMGs provides a firm, homogenous base for the "house staff culture" in the hospital. Instead of feeling isolated, the FMG is part of a tightly woven group, with its own slang, patterns of behavior, and humor. Since interactions and communication—among peers as well as between house staff and seniors—are so important in the physician's education, the FMG working in relative isolation from the American house staff culture is at a disadvantage to his peers. We stress again that such observations do not relate to the technical aspects of training per se, but to the behavioral skills and attitudes that are integral to the process of graduate medical education; yet without full assimilation into the hospital training process, opportunities for technical education may also be reduced.

THE ROLE OF PRIVATE ATTENDING PHYSICIANS

Two sets of considerations have been raised in this chapter in comparing the education of FMGs with that of USMGs. FMGs tend to utilize formal learning methods to a greater extent than USMGs, who in turn rely to a greater degree on informal learning processes. At the same time, FMGs trained with a large majority of USMGs are most content with their treatment in the American training system. We would argue that they also receive the best training. There are, however, other differences in the training situation offered by American hospitals that must be taken into account in assessing the FMG's experiences in American graduate education. Here we look further at training settings in terms of two distinctive patterns of hospital organization.

The importance of the social structure of the hospital in defining the role relationships of physicians (and others) is well established in the sociological literature.[9] American hospitals are extraordinarily diverse, and the resident on a university hospital service fulfills a different role from that of the resident in a community hospital staffed largely by private practitioners.

The university ward service, like the public hospital service, is a relatively autonomous treatment unit. Patients admitted to such units come under the care of the fulltime hospital staff. Although the patient may be discharged to the care of a private physician, treatment in hospital is the responsibility of a hierarchy of staff physicians. The house staff forms part of the hierarchy, and learning is transferred through an organized set of relationships. For the sake of convenience we describe this relatively autonomous, organized teaching setting as a "bureaucratic" model to distinguish if from the very different situation of learning in a hospital in which patients are largely under the care of private physicians, and the house staff is, as a result, less tightly organized.[10]

The private practitioner model in its purest state is one in which all patients in a hospital are admitted and remain under the care of a private physician, who has an unpaid hospital appointment as a member of the attending staff. In this situation members of the hospital house staff work on an ad hoc basis with a series of different practitioners and conform to individual methods of treatment and behavior. It is more difficult for the fulltime hospital staff to establish overarching hospital codes and practices. Although residents in a bureaucratic model may determine the treatment of a patient in hospital in accordance with institutional goals and policies, residents in the private attending situation must heed the wishes of independent practitioners.

In both situations the resident is an apprentice, but in the first he is an apprentice to a *system*, in the second an apprentice to *individuals*. We call the second model the "assistantship" model to stress the fact that the resident acts in each case as a private physician's personal assistant.

Many teaching hospital situations include a mix of patients, some under the care of private physicians, some under the care of fulltime staff. However, as Table 9.4 shows, a substantial proportion of FMGs are trained in a milieu that is predominantly a "bureaucratic" model or an "assistantship." Almost 30 percent of the FMGs in our study were in training programs in which no patients were admitted by private attending physicians, that is, in a bureaucratic setting. At the other end of the scale, 30 percent of FMGs were in hospitals in which at least three-

TABLE 9.4 DISTRIBUTION OF HOUSE STAFF BY PERCENTAGE OF PATIENTS ADMITTED BY PRIVATE ATTENDING PHYSICIAN

Percentage of private admissions	FMG	USMG	USFMG
0	28.8	26.9	21.8
1–25%	14.2	30.9	11.3
26–50%	16.6	19.1	21.8
51–75%	10.6	9.2	21.2
76–100%	29.8	13.9	23.9
Total	100.0(602)[a]	100.0(122)	100.0(36)
	NA = 88	NA = 11	NA = 6

[a] Percentages are weighted; *N* is unweighted.

quarters of the patients were under the care of private physicians, that is, in an assistantship setting.

USMGs, more often than FMGs, tended to train in situations that were wholly or predominantly bureaucratic. Thus 58 percent of the USMGs were in training settings in which at least three quarters of their patients were "staff" responsibilities (i.e., 0–25 percent private admissions). The comparable figure for FMGs was 43 percent; for USFMGs, 33 percent. USMGs also tended to train less often under the tutelage of private physicians. Only 23 percent of USMGs were in programs in which a majority of the patients were admitted to the care of private physicans (51–100 percent private admissions), compared to 40 percent of the FMGs and 45 percent of the USFMGs.

These distributions in part reflect the distribution of the various groups into hospitals with various types of university affiliation. USMGs, most notably, are clustered in the major teaching units. However, the association among the variables is far from a perfect "fit," because a university may have its own fulltime ward services and also maintain a close connection (or even ownership) of hospitals in which local physicians admit and serve private patients.

The distribution of the FMGs in our study group provides a case in point. One-half of the FMGs training in major teaching units said that the great majority of their patients (75 percent or more) were service patients: one-quarter said that most (75 percent or more) were private patients; the other one-quarter reported a mix. These patterns were different from those reported in hospitals with limited university affiliation where there

TABLE 9.5 FMGS IN TWO TYPES OF TRAINING MILIEU

Learning roles and activities	(Percentages)	
	Bureaucratic model — *no* patients admitted by private attending physicians	Assistantship model— 76–100% patients admitted by private attending physicians
Roles and responsibilities		
"Often" works alone with previous instruction	71.3[a]	46.9
Has "great" responsibility for outpatient care	69.4	35.9
Takes "great" responsibility on nights and weekends	67.9	52.8
Has "great" responsibility for admissions	65.7	18.4
"Often" manages patients from admission to discharge	62.3	44.7
Has "great" responsibility for discharges	52.7	8.2
"Often" has access to patients' socioeconomic information	50.6	30.4
Has "great" responsibility for dealing with patients' relatives	49.1	16.0
"Often" works as assistant to attending MD	46.3	61.8
"Often" starts IVs	36.0	43.0
"Often" does "scut work"	21.0	4.5
Social interactions		
"Often" uses medical library	79.1	86.8
Formally evaluated by hospital MDs	79.1	44.5
Learns a "great deal" from patients	55.7	42.1
Learns a "great deal" from chiefs of service	44.9	36.3
"Often" teaches medical personnel	40.4	24.3
"Often" teaches other health personnel	35.8	17.6
Is formally evaluated by private attending MDs	23.9	61.6
Learns a "great deal" from attending MDs	14.1	22.8
"Often" supervises other staff	15.5	4.0

Table 9.5 (*Continued*)

Learning roles and activities	(Percentages)	
	Bureaucratic model – *no* patients admitted by private attending physicians	Assistantship model— 76–100% patients admitted by private attending physicians
Perceptions of education		
U.S. training provides skills for U.S. medical practice to "great extent"	77.7	58.5
U.S. training provides skills useful in CME to "great extent"	44.9	52.9
Agrees "strongly" that U.S. training is the best in the world	40.1	29.1
Agrees "strongly" that FMGs are not given equal training to USMGs	36.9	51.5
Is given too much responsibility	23.6	15.7
Is given insufficient responsibility	15.6	46.6
Percent base (N)	(147)[a]	(191)

[a] Percentages are weighted; N is unweighted.

tended to be relatively more private patients, and in nonaffiliated units, where private patients were the norm. Nevertheless, one-quarter of the FMGs in the nonaffiliated units reported that the great majority of their patients (75 percent or more) were admitted to "service"—that is, largely bureaucratic—settings.

An analysis of our data shows that the organizational structure of the educational settings is an important indicator of the type of educational opportunities available to different FMGs. The data are shown in summary form in Table 9.5 with respect to the two paradigm settings. The differences are striking in certain respects: in the wholly bureaucratic setting (i.e., in programs in which house staff see only "service" patients), FMGs have greater responsibility for patient care, learn more from hospital staff and patients, and are more likely to consider their education as good preparation for American medical practice, than their counterparts in the predominantly assistantship settings (i.e., where they see mostly private patients).

There is no evidence that FMGs in assistantship situations take sub-stantial responsibility while the private physician attends to other duties or pleasures; quite the reverse. Almost one-half of the FMGs in the assistantship situation complained of too little responsibility; few com-plained of too much. Areas of substantially less responsibility than in the bureaucratic situation include night and weekend duties, determining patient admission and discharge, patient management from admission to discharge, responsibility for dealing with patients' relatives, access to socioeconomic information, and outpatient care. House staff in the assis-tantship model also work alone less often, do less "scut work," and are given less supervisory and teaching responsibilities. They complain more often that FMGs are not given equal training to USMGs, are less certain that American training is the best in the world and that their training is fitting them for American practice, but are somewhat more likely to claim that their training is providing skills usable in their country of medical education.

The overall picture of training in these settings is one of far greater communication and responsibility in what we have called the bureau-cratic model, that is, in teaching settings in which the fulltime staff is responsible for patient admissions. One notable finding is that, although FMGs in assistantship settings are usually evaluated formally by attend-ing physicians, relatively few say they learn a great deal from these same physicians. Thus 62 percent said they were formally evaluated by attend-ing staff, but only 23 percent reported that they learned a great deal from them.

The general picture of the assistantship model is of a much more fragmented system of learning than in the tightly knit social structure of the bureaucratic setting. A majority of FMGs in assistantship situations said they often worked as assistants to attending physicians, took great responsibility for patients on weekends, but not at other times, and felt that FMGs were not given training equal to USMGs. In comparison to the bureaucratic setting, the FMGs in assistantship settings also reported less communication and interaction with other members of the hospital com-munity.

These general patterns were also observed for USMGs in the differ-ent situations. Recognizing the importance of responsibility and social interaction in house staff education, we conclude that the bureaucratic model offers greater opportunities for acquiring knowledge, physical skills, and attitudes than does the private assistantship situation.

Table 9.5 compares the training settings at the extremes of the range of bureaucratic-assistantship situations. In terms of the *ideal* training locale, as perceived by house staff, the most advantageous situation appears to be one in which between one-quarter and one-half of all patients are admitted by private attending physicians, that is, a predominantly bureaucratic model with some chance of private admissions. FMGs in this particular mix have a much higher chance of managing patients from admission to discharge than in the solely bureaucratic model; they attend grand rounds and patient rounds more often, do more teaching of medical students, learn much more from medical staff, residents, and chiefs of service, and are less likely to claim that FMGs are given inferior training or that training programs are an excuse to staff hospitals. FMGs in these settings are also the most likely of all groups to say that their training is providing skills for their own countries to a great extent.

THE EDUCATIONAL PROCESS

If graduate medical education is indeed a patterning process, with substantial emphasis on learning physical skills by observing and being instructed by other physicians and on professional attitudes and behavior, the training milieu is of the utmost importance—more important, perhaps, than the competence of individual teachers or the caliber of students. We have observed that FMGs are less happy with their training in situations in which a large majority of house staff are FMGs. We conclude that these findings reflect a causal relationship: that is, FMGs in these situations are deprived of sufficient models on which to pattern their own skills and behavior. At the same time, they are regarded by attending physicians as assistants rather than as junior colleagues. Thus the opportunities for patterning are also less readily available. FMGs are driven to rely more than they would otherwise on formal patterns of education. Since apprenticeship learning depends largely on informal opportunities and relationships, the average FMG is automatically in an inferior training situation to that available to the USMG.

The role of patients admitted by private physicians adds a further dimension to these distinctions. Technically, almost all patients admitted to American hospitals are now "private" patients; the old charity wards disappeared with the advent of private health insurance, Medicare, and Medicaid. However, although the patient may be regarded as a private patient, the staffing models that provide the milieu for training interns and residents vary considerably, according to the responsibility for care of an individual patient within a given service setting. FMGs trained in units in which most patients are admitted by private physicians work more often as assistants and have less responsibility than FMGs in hierarchical or bureaucratic settings. These points are a function of the setting rather than the distribution of FMGs in that the patterns exist equally for USMGs in different settings.

Since responsibility is a key element both in the learning process and in being acknowledged by seniors as a junior colleague, we may conclude that FMGs dealing largely with private admissions are in an inferior teaching milieu to those in bureaucratic settings. Since more USMGs than FMGs are in predominatly bureaucratic settings, we also conclude that USMGs are again, on the average, in the more advantageous training situations.

These differences, moreover, tend to hold by specialty: 23 percent of the FMGs training in the specialties of internal medicine were in assistantship situations (75–100 percent private admissions) compared to 12 percent of USMGs in those specialties; 16 percent of the FMG pediatricians, and none of the USMGs; 48 percent of the FMG surgeons compared to 35 percent of the USMGs; and 28 percent of FMGs in the hospital-based fields of anesthesiology, pathology, and radiology, compared to 7 percent of the USMGs. In obstetrics/gynecology the proportion was the same (23 percent); however, more USMGs than FMGs were in wholly bureaucratic situations (no private patients). Psychiatry was unusual in that there were virtually no trainees in predominantly private situations, USMG or FMG, a reflection of the pattern of training in public psychiatric hospitals. Generally, FMGs as a group appear to be in less advantageous teaching settings, irrespective of medical specialty, than their peers who are USMGs.

These findings raise serious questions about the nature of training available to FMGs and more generally about the content and quality of graduate medical education, which deserve detailed analysis in the field. One would expect, for example, that house staff trained in different settings would, after a period of years, perform differently in standardized tests, such as the certifying examinations of the specialty boards. Such studies have not yet been carried out, although there is a general impression that different results are apparent in the graduates of different hospital programs.

For USMGs the situation has been difficult to measure, because other factors intervene that make causal influences unclear. Notably, it is argued that USMGs follow careers along one of a number of well-defined "tracks"; the best medical students go to the best teaching programs and subsequently get the best test results.[11] It is not clear from such a process (assuming that it does exist) how far the final result is affected by the graduate experience and how far by the initial "sorting" of USMGs into different hospital programs.

With respect to FMGs, however, the type and nature of the graduate experience may in fact be critical, since well-defined "tracks" do not exist in any qualitative sense for the great majority of FMGs, with respect to which physicians enter graduate education in which programs (see chapter 4). Even if we move from arguments based on the relative value or quality of different hospital programs, our findings show that the context of graduate medical education they receive is, on the average, different from that of USMGs. The mix of responsibilities, availability of interaction with other house staff, superiors, and students, and perceptions of FMGs by other physicians create a learning environment—an atmosphere—that is different for many FMGs from that available to the USMG.

EDUCATIONAL EXPERIENCE AND CHOICE OF CAREER

One final and rather different element of the educational experience should also be observed. If graduate medical education is indeed a process of observation of, and modeling on, superiors, one would expect the career choices of house staff to follow the career patterns prevailing in particular institutions. It follows that the type of hospital may influence the future careers of graduate trainees.

Table 9.6 shows that, at least to some extent, FMGs are drawn to, or influenced by, particular American training settings with respect to their career aspirations. FMGs heading for careers as faculty or in research positions are more likely to be found in hospitals with the greatest degree of university affiliation (major teaching units and hospitals with limited affiliation) and least likely in nonaffiliated hospitals. Private practice, however, is not specific to university affiliation per se.

Section B of the table shows, however, that a preference for private practice is clearly related to the role of private attending physicians (the proportion of private patients admitted to hospital units), whereas training in a more "bureaucratic" setting is related to a continuing career as a fulltime staff physician. Thus 48 percent of FMGs in the assistantship model (76–100 percent private admissions) said their career preference was for private practice, and only 12 percent preferred fulltime hospital staff positions. In contrast, 35 percent of those in more bureaucratic models (0–25 percent private admissions) preferred private practice, whereas 26 percent preferred hospital staff positions. Those choosing other careers were similarly distributed in both training situations.

These findings, coupled with our findings on the educational experience, lead us to conclude that FMGs are influenced by prevailing patterns in their teaching hospitals in two important ways. First, FMGs are dis-

TABLE 9.6 TYPE OF PRACTICE PREFERRED BY FMGS IN SELECTED
TRAINING SETTING

A. Hospitals by type of university affiliation

| | Level of affiliation | | | |
	Major teaching unit	Limited use	Graduate training	Nonaffiliated
Private practice	40.6	32.1	45.4	49.0
Faculty/research	34.9	39.3	20.8	16.9
Fulltime hospital staff	19.7	20.3	25.3	24.8
Government and other positions	4.6	8.3	8.4	9.2
Total	100.0(358)[a]	100.0(115)	100.0(28)	100.0(165)

B. Hospitals by proportion of private admissions

| | Percentage of private admissions | | | |
	0–25	26–50	51–75	76–100
Private practice	35.2	45.7	43.3	48.2
Faculty/research	31.2	27.3	38.2	32.4
Fulltime hospital staff	25.6	22.3	14.5	11.5
Government and other positions	7.9	4.7	4.0	7.9
Total[b]	100.0(238)	100.0(91)	100.0(82)	100.0(191)

[a] Percentages are weighted; N is unweighted.
[b] Excludes 26 FMGs who said the question was not relevant to their work,
12 who "didn't know", and NA = 50.

tributed into training settings that provide less responsibility, on the
average, than that expected of USMGs. Since graduate education is based
on close contacts, including delegation of responsibility between senior
and junior staff, FMGs are found in the least advantageous training
situations.

As a second effect, these patterns push FMGs into different types of
careers. It is notable that approximately half of the FMGs trained in
"assistantship" situations say that they too will become private practitioners. One cannot help but ask whether these physicians, who are
given the least responsibility during training, are most appropriately
trained for future roles in which they will assume a great deal of responsibility as independent practitioners, that is, they will practice largely

outside organized settings in major cities in their own countries or in the United States.

CONCLUSIONS

This chapter has developed the theme of the FMG as a "less-than-full" physician. Our findings suggest that this concept has widespread implications and cumulative effects. Because FMGs tend to be regarded differently from USMGs, the nature or their graduate education is also different. This is so because of the apprenticeship mode of learning, and the tripartite expectations of the learning experience: competence in knowledge, techniques, and professional behavior.

The latter, professional and/or cultural competence, is of overriding importance, because it is a critical gateway to other forms of learning. The resident who is not perceived as a "full" physician has fewer opportunities for informal discussions and consultations and is given less clinical responsibility. Cumulatively, therefore, the FMG may not only be perceived as culturally less competent than the USMG, he or she may also receive a less than optimal graduate educational experience. These two processes have a self-fulfilling effect for at least a substantial minority of FMGs. Thus the physician who is regarded as less "competent" may, in the end, be less competent by having a lesser education.

From the point of view of developing American policies for the education of foreign physicians, there is a need to define the basic purposes of the experience for different individuals. FMGs coming for specialized training to prepare them for university teaching or research are presumably best served in university hospitals in the United States, but a substantial proportion of the FMGs in our study who looked toward university careers were training outside the university units. Either they were mismatched (in which case the allocative system is imperfect) or their career expectations were unrealistic (in which case, perhaps they should not have entered the United States). Either conclusion suggests the need to develop a more rational system of international exchange.

The present system of allocating substantial numbers of FMGs to hospitals staffed predominantly by private attending physicians may also encourage FMGs to consider private practice in the United States as a future career. This may be a benefit to individual FMGs for whom private practice in major cities in the home country may already be overcrowded and academic medicine uninteresting or impossible to achieve. It may also benefit the American populations these physicians will eventually serve. We make no value judgments here as to what is "best," but we stress again that immigration policy should be developed in an informed context, with respect to the specific purposes of exchange and permanent migration.

From the point of view of individual physicians, we see a recurring pattern of relative isolation woven into the educational experience. FMGs come into the United States as aliens and continue along a path of alienation. They are neither fully assimilated into the American hospital social system, nor are they, on the average, as likely as USMGs to train in programs in which a tightly knit social structure is achieved (i.e., in relatively bureaucratic training settings). These patterns deserve scrutiny with respect to American obligations for the graduate education of foreign physicians. They also have ripple effects on the total experiences of individual migrants as they live in, and adjust to, the United States.

NOTES

1. On the importance of cultural homogeneity as a condition of close interaction between house staff, see Patricia L. Kendall, "The Learning Environments of Hospitals," in Eliot Freidson Ed., *The Hospital in Modern Society* New York: Free Press, 1963, pp. 195–230; M. M. Dasco, L. Antler, and H. A. Rusk, "Foreign Medical Resident Training in the United States", *Annals of Internal Medicine (1968)*, 68:1105–13.
2. Frederic D. Burg and F. Howell Wright, "Evaluation of Pediatric Residents and Their Training Programs," *Journal of Pediatrics (172)*, 80: 183–89.
3. Joel J. Alpert, Joseph Youngerman, Jan Breslow, and John Kosa, "Learning Experiences during the Internship Year: An Exploratory Study of Pediatric Graduate Education," *Pediatrics* (1973), 51: 199–205.
4. Robert S. Brown, "House Staff Attitudes Toward Teaching," *Journal of Medical Education* (March 1970), 45: 156–59.
5. Stanley Crosbie, "How Residents Apportion Work Time," *Hospitals, J.A.H.A.* (1971), 45: 60–63.
6. William Gillanders and Michael Heiman, "Time Study Comparisons of Three Intern Programs," *Journal of Medical Education*, (1971), 46: 143–49.
7. The classic work on such processes remains Oswald Hall, "The Informal Organization of the Medical Profession," *Canadian Journal of Economic and Political Science* (February 1946), 12: 30–41.
8. These themes are developed by Stephen Miller, *Prescription for Leadership: Training for the Medical Elite*, Chicago, 1970.
9. See, for example, Rose Laub Coser, "Authority and Decision-Making in a Hospital," *American Sociological Review* (1958), 23: 63; Melvin Seeman and John Evans, "Stratification and Hospital Care I: The Performance of the Medical Interne," *Ibid.*, (1961), 26: 67; Emily Mumford, *Interns: From Students to Physicians, op cit*, Chapter 9, "The Uses of Diversity," and passim.
10. Roemer and Friedman have developed a typology of hospital medical staff organization based on a five-step scale from "very loosely structured" to "very highly structured." In the latter it is noted that the organizational framework takes pre-

cedence over medical individualism in the structure of medical staff relationships; however, doctors entering such environments accept the constraints imposed by highly structured organizations, and relationships are relatively peaceful. The investigators found that friction in hospital–doctor relationships was most evident in the hospitals classified in the middle of the range, that is, in hospitals with partially structured medical staff organization. These findings are interesting to our study because internship and residency training normally takes place in these two types of organization. The "highly structured" categories (Roemer and Friedman's types IV and V) correspond to some degree to our classification of a "bureaucratic" setting, whereas our "apprenticeship" model is more like their types II and III. Our classification is, however, based on the proportion of private patients on in-patient services, as reported by our respondents, whereas theirs is based on the number of salaried medical staff.
Roemer and Friedman find the optimal model, as far as hospital performance is concerned, to be one with a medical staff organized under type IV, that is, with a relatively strong bureaucratic structure. Our findings suggest that such settings are also optimal for graduate medical education. Milton I. Roemer and Jay W. Friedman, *Doctors in Hospitals: Medical Staff Organization and Hospital Performance*, Johns Hopkins Press, Baltimore, 1971.

11. See for example, Fremont J. Lyden, H. Jack Geiger, and Osler L. Peterson, *The Training of Good Physicians: Critical Factors in Career Choices*, Commonwealth Fund Book, Harvard University Press, Cambridge, 1968, pp. 223–24 and passim.

10

LIFE IN THE
UNITED STATES_____

Hospital work dominates the lives of interns and residents. Long work hours and "immersion"methods of training make this inevitable. For the nearly 40 percent of FMGs who live in the hospital and/or with other house staff, hospital life and life in the United States are virtually synonymous.

Earlier chapters indicate that FMGs and USMGs experience hospital life differently. In this chapter we examine the non-work experiences of FMGs to show how this affects their ability to absorb training and provide services. Our conclusions parallel earlier chapters: although the formal aspects of the FMGs' situations provide them with amenities comparable (and in some cases, superior) to those of USMGs and USFMGs, FMGs are systematically more isolated culturally and socially from mainstream America and mainstream medical America. Outside the hospital, like other immigrant groups, FMGs are organized along ethnic and religious lines. This inhibits their ability to participate fully in the life of their hospital settings and makes it difficult for them to become fully socialized, culturally competent physicians.

ORIENTATION PROGRAMS

Most entrants to graduate medical education, whether USMG, USFMG, or FMG, begin their American training with a formal orientation program (Table 10.1). FMGs, entering the United States at different times of the year and thus not always able to meet the usual July 1 beginning date, were most likely to miss orientation programs.

TABLE 10.1   FORMAL ORIENTATION AT FIRST U.S. HOSPITAL

	FMG	USMG	USFMG
Yes	64.5	74.2	60.3
No	33.0	25.3	39.7
Missed program	2.0	0.5	0
	100.0% (685)[a]	100.0% (133)	100.0% (42)
	(NA=5)		

[a] Percentages are weighted; N is unweighted.

However, this difference is less noteworthy than the fact that more than one-quarter of each group said they had received no formal orientation.[1]

Formal Orientation to the Hospital

In many respects the content of orientation programs is similar for each of our respondent groups. Virtually all orientation programs informed house staff of their daily schedule, introduced them to the Chief of Service for whom they would be working in the hospital, and presented an explanation of the hospital's rules and regulations (Table 10.2). FMGs were somewhat less likely to be introduced to their fellow house staff than were USMGs and USFMGs, although the difference is not significant. Thus the administrative relationships in the hospital appear to be quite thoroughly covered.

Other aspects of orientation suggest, however, some potentially serious deficiencies. One of every five USMGs and FMGs reported that their orientation program did not cover the hospital's procedures for ordering drugs or diagnostic tests. Although such information may be unnecessary for USMGs who have already spent considerable time in clerkships in American hospitals, it is presumably essential for FMGs for whom procedures may be quite different.[2]

Since those trained abroad may be unfamiliar with American usage, one might expect FMGs and USFMGs to be given special sessions on American terminology during formal orientation sessions. Thus their rates on these variables would be higher than for USMGs. In fact, the reverse is true. All the USMGs said that medical terminology and abbreviations had been explained to them during their orientation. In contrast, little more than one-half of the FMGs responding said that their orientation included an explanation of American medical terms and their uses.

TABLE 10.2   CONTENT OF HOSPITAL ORIENTATION PROGRAMS

	Percentage answering "Yes"		
	FMG	USMG	USFMG
In your orientation program were you			
Informed of daily schedule?	96.3[a]	91.7	93.1
Introduced to your chief?	95.2	93.9	100.0
Given an explanation of hospital rules and regulations?	90.2	89.2	86.2
Introduced to fellow house staff?	86.1	96.2	100.0
Informed of procedures for ordering diagnostic tests?	79.9	78.3	91.2
Informed of procedures for ordering drugs?	77.4	79.8	93.1
Informed about the city or town?	61.1	65.7	62.7
Given an explanation of U.S. medical terminology and abbreviations?	53.3	100.0	62.7
Percent Base (N)[b]	(428)[a]	(96)	(26)
	NA = 5		

[a] Percentages are weighted; N is unweighted.
[b] Includes respondents who reported formal orientation programs: 257 FMGs reported no formal orientation programs (including 20 who missed the program), as did 37 USMGs (one missed the program), and 16 USFMGs (zero).

In summary, formal orientation programs are not available to a substantial minority of new interns and residents. Many of those that do exist appear to be merely a way of greeting new staff rather than the means of transmitting patient care information. It would seem self-evident that all FMGs (and USFMGs) should be given formal teaching in the basic diagnostic and teaching practices pertaining in their institutions, including familiarity with the format and uses of all case records.

Lacking such information in formal orientation or teaching sessions, house staff must rely on informal channels of communication: they must pick up procedures as best and as fast as they can from other house staff in the hospital. In our case studies we found a relatively strong transfer system from the more senior to incoming staff, particularly where one group of FMGs initiates a new group into hospital customs and procedures and where all FMGs are from the same nation. However, such a process may work best at hospitals in which the majority of house staff are FMGs. In hospitals in which FMGs are in the minority or from diverse backgrounds, their initial lack of familiarity with the basic language of American hospital medicine may well emphasize the fact that FMGs are strangers and begin a continuing process of lack of communication and isolation of FMGs from other staff and assumptions that FMGs, being ignorant, are inferior.

Formal Orientation to American Culture

FMGs must, moreover, orient themselves simultaneously to professional customs in the hospital and to more general aspects of American life. They have a double burden of adjustment. Information about living and work conditions appears particularly lacking. When asked, "Did the orientation program fail to provide you with any information which you felt was needed?" one-quarter of the FMGs (26.2 percent) reported "Yes," a higher proportion than for the USFMGs (18.0 percent) and markedly higher than for USMGs (12.3 percent). FMGs are less *informed* through the orientation programs regarding patient care and less *satisfied* with orientation programs than are USMGs. One-third of the FMGs who complained said they needed more information about living conditions, including housing, transportation, and location of the hospital, and the American "life style"; one-third cited the need for more specific information about the job; the remaining third cited numerous specific complaints.

The need of FMGs for cultural information should be stressed, because this is part of the natural milieu of the American physician. As noted, hospitals often do not inform FMGs about house staff living conditions before they arrive. This deficiency, for a sizable minority of FMGs, is not rectified once they are in the United States. Less than two-thirds of the orientation experiences of our respondents included information about the city, or town, in which they were to live (Table 10.2). Two-thirds of the FMGs (67.4 percent), USMGs (64.5 percent), and USFMGs (66.0 percent) were given some information about housing, but all groups said that they received this predominantly from friends. Most of the FMGs who were not given information from friends or through orientation programs were of the opinion that available information was inadequate or nonexistent. They had to find housing on their own, were disappointed, or felt deceived by the information they had been given.

Many other crucial non-hospital-specific bits of information were lacking for many FMGs. The one out of every two FMGs who complained of knowing too little about the social and economic characteristics of patients (Chapter 5) may lack knowledge relevant to decisions about patient care. In this regard FMGs felt they needed more prior information about subjects such as health insurance, patient's living conditions, psychological and race differences, and the general mix of the patient population. Such knowledge is important not only as a basis for providing patient care, but also as a means of communication as a member of the medical profession. The need for knowledge of cultural terminology is as important here as it is in familiarity with medical usages and terms. In the hospital, terminology forms a kind of language or code to which the acolyte must have access. Without it, he or she is not fully equipped and cannot be treated as an equal. Suppose, for example, that an FMG in the first few days of hospital work is asked by an attending physician or social worker whether a patient has Blue Cross. The FMG is at a tremendous disadvantage if he or she does not even know what Blue Cross is. This lack of cultural competence may unfairly affect colleagues' judgments of technical medical competence. Because of a cultural lack, an FMG may be assumed to be ignorant in areas in which he or she has in fact great capabilities.

This distinction between "cultural" and "technical" competence is critical. Beginning with relative ignorance of the American professional context, the FMG faces American training with certain disadvantages: an increased likelihood of being in hospitals of lesser prestige, of being trained with other FMGs rather than with a majority of USMGs, thus making socialization into American medicine more difficult, of facing immediate problems of daily living in seeking housing and transportation, and of ignorance of the terminology of American medicine that has become second nature to the USMG. These reflect the lack of cultural rather than technical competence but block FMGs from immediate entrance into the professional world of their medical peers.

Orientation in the Use of English

For many FMGs communication is hampered by having to converse in a foreign language—English. One-third of our respondents decided to come to the United States despite doubts about their English abilities.

This hesitation appears to have been realistic. More than one-fifth of the FMGs said that English had caused them difficulty in communicating with members of the health, professions to a "great" or "moderate" extent; an additional 20 percent said it caused difficulty to a "small" extent. In short, only one-half of the respondents reported no difficulty with English as a means of communicating with their American peers or in dealing with patients.

As might be expected, the greatest difficulties were experienced by those whose medical education was received in a language other than English. Two-thirds of of the graduates from Japan and South Korea reported that English deficiences had caused problems with colleagues. FMGs from South and Central America, Thailand, Taiwan, Syria, and Iran also expressed relative difficulties. West German graduates, taught in German, were an exception to the general rule. Those instructed in English during medical school, on the other hand, reported virtually no difficulty communicating with the staff of an American hospital or with patients. These included graduates from Canada, Sri Lanka, the United Arab Republic, India, Eire, Pakistan-Bangladesh, and the Philippines.

The findings indicate some cause for concern, not only in the adjustment of particular groups to the American system but also in their immediate relationships with patients. More than one-third of the FMGs from the Latin American countries of Argentina, Brazil, Colombia, and Mexico said that the English language had caused "moderate" or "great" difficulty in dealing with patients, and about two-thirds of the FMGs from these groups said they had experienced difficulties to at least a "small" extent. Japanese and South Korean graduates had an even greater language barrier. Four-fifths of the Japanese graduates and nine-tenths of the South Korean graduates noted at least some English language problems in dealing with patients, as did four-fifths of the Thai graduates. Graduates from Syria also experienced problems in communicating with patients, with only one-fourth saying they had had no difficulties. FMGs in some specialties experience greater difficulties than others (Table 10.3). Professional relationships were most affected among FMGs in obstetrics/gynecology, hospital-based specialties, psychiatry, and family medicine. Relationships with patients were most affected among psychiatrists, family practitioners, and surgeons.

These patterns probably reflect the combination of two overlapping factors: (1) the relative status of a specialty and (2) the relative reliance in each specialty on language as a means of diagnosis and treatment. Status considerations may be especially important for the specialties of internal medicine. As we have observed, internal medicine is a relatively competitive field. This means that the poorer English speakers may not be selected to positions in this field and that those who are selected may have a greater opportunity to mix with USMGs (and thus to gain language familiarity) than do FMGs in other fields. The hospital-based fields are, on the other hand, relatively uncompetitive, with reverse implications. In specialties such as psychiatry and general/family practice, status considerations may be less important than the need for an easy rapport with patients. FMGs in psychiatry reported more difficulties in communication with patients to a greater extent than those in other specialties.

Although the differences among specialties are interesting, they do not alter the basic finding that the English language is perceived as a major problem by FMGs not trained in English-speaking medical schools.[3] Lack of familiarity with English is perhaps the major stumbling block in FMG adjustment to the American medical system. However, it is simplistic to separate language from the more complex cultural differences that separate FMGs from USMGs and from FMGs of other nationalities, and that slow their adjustment to the American medical system. The next section of this chapter focuses on cultural differences between USMGs and FMGs.

TABLE 10.3   FMGS REPORTING ENGLISH LANGUAGE DIFFICULTIES BY SPECIALTY

	Percentage in each specialty reporting difficulty with profession[a]	Percentage in each specialty reporting difficulty with patients[b]	Percent base (N)
Obstetrics/gynecology	36.5[c]	17.0	(58)[c]
Hospital-based specialties	29.0	17.2	(112)
Psychiatry	26.7	22.2	(62)
General/family practice	24.4	18.8	(32)
Surgical specialties	21.7	18.0	(159)
Pediatrics	21.4	13.6	(65)
Internal medicine	15.0	12.7	(166)
Other—unknown	19.4	13.9	(36)
All specialties	22.4	16.1	(690)

[a] English caused problems with professional staff to a great or moderate extent.
[b] English caused problems with patients to a great or moderate extent.
[c] Percentages are weighted; N is unweighted.

CULTURAL DIFFERENCES BETWEEN USMGS AND FMGS

Compared to USMGs, FMGs are a heterogeneous group: their backgrounds, personal situations, and work situations are substantially more diverse that those of their American-trained counterparts. One of the consequences of this diversity is that FMGs, as individuals, are often isolated in their work roles. The probability that a given FMG will encounter a fellow physician with a similar background and similar work situation is far lower than for a given USMG.

This situation translates into difficulties in establishing close relationships with interns and residents from different backgrounds, and into feelings and experiences of social and occupational isolation. The primary adaptive strategy FMGs employ (probably unintentionally) to counter this isolation is the clustering of national groups. FMGs, like most other job seekers, use convenient information networks to find their jobs. For an FMG's first position, such networks often consist of fellow countrymen who have worked in the United States and who place them in hospital settings in which other house staff trained in the same nation are located. Thus when one visits some American hospitals one will find given hospitals exclusively or predominantly staffed with Turkish citizens in some instances, Filipinos in others, and South Koreans in others. Although this does blunt somewhat the isolating effects of informal and probably unintended practices within hospitals, FMGs remain isolated from the mainstream of American medicine and American cultural life. This can be seen both in the comparison of their work situations with those of their American-trained counterparts and in their day-to-day interactional patterns[4]

The variable in our study with the clearest cultural reference is the religion of the groups of medical graduates.[5] Differences among the groups are marked. The modal religion for USMGs is Protestantism. Of USMGs stating a preference, 75 percent are Jewish or Protestant.[6] Seventy percent of the FMGs are either Catholic or members of a non-Western religion such as Hinduism, Confucianism, or Buddhism. Of FMGs stating a religious preference, 86 percent are Catholic or of non-Western religions. Furthermore, many Catholic FMGs are not Roman Catholic but Eastern Orthodox Catholics. To the extent that religion is an indicator of cultural orientation, USMGs and FMGs come from substantially different worlds.

These differences in religion can be interpreted on a number of levels. In terms of the formal ties of these individuals to the larger societies, very different areas of contact are open for the two groups. Church groups often serve as means of introduction to communities for newcomers: in fact, as discussed later in this chapter, church groups were the community organization to which the greatest number of the interns and residents in our sample belonged. To the extent that FMGs or USMGs or their families are members of such groups, they are introduced to very different segments of American society. This difference gains additional importance from the fact that FMGs are newcomers to American society and will thus be especially vulnerable to the impressions of American culture they receive during their medical training.

It is safe to presume that these religious differences also imply differences of outlook and personal style. That is not to say that differences in religion in themselves indicate these other differences; however, they are parts of different types of cultural formations. These religious differences become particularly useful for interpreting the different patterns of social interaction of different groups. European FMGs whose religions more closely parallel those of the USMGs exhibit friendship and social patterns similar to those of USMGs. Asian and Middle Eastern FMGs exhibit different patterns that might be ascribed to differences in cultural background and cultural preferences. The marked religious differences between USMGs and FMGs give clues to the dimensions of cultural cleavages between these two groups.

A second dimension that indicates differences in personal situations between USMGs and FMGs is their social status in their country of origin. Our data indicate that within their own societies, FMGs are born to relatively higher social classes than are USMGs, that FMGs are relatively more encapsulated in a physician subculture, and that they are more likely to have spent their secondary school years in a large population center central to the activities of elites in their countries. In their own cultural context, FMGs are probably more strongly linked to centers of power and privilege in society than USMGs. The social-cultural background of FMGs, therefore, has two impacts on their experiences in the American health care system: (1) It gives them different experiences and separates them socially and culturally from their USMG counterparts and (2) It threatens the strong identity of personal privilege and superiority that their experiences in their country of medical education have reinforced. The sharp contrast between their privileged positions in their home countries and their general assessment that they are not as well treated as USMGs, is likely to have marked effects. On one hand the contrast may cause some to question their own self-evaluations and feelings of competence but to continue to work within the American system; on the other hand, it may cause others to withdraw and feel simultaneously alienated and superior and bitter at American discrimination. These patterns go a long way towards explaining reports of seeming incompetence and lack of confidence among some FMGs in American hospitals and a corresponding lack of interest in hospital social life.

Residence and Family

Only a limited amount of data is available in our study on residential patterns. We asked all respondents whether they lived in a building in which other interns or residents lived. Thirty-seven percent of the FMGs, 16 percent of the USMGs, and 34 percent of the USFMGs replied that they lived in a building with other interns and residents. These differences, reflecting a cleavage between FMGs and USMGs, have at least two possible explanations: (1) The higher proportion of FMGs living with other interns and residents could reflect their desire to integrate themselves more fully into the American medical mainstream; (2) A more plausible explanation to us is that the overrepresentation of FMGs in buildings in which house staff live reflects difficulties dealing with residential problems. Many FMGs in our sample reported housing difficulties. This is probably a symptom of the differential ability of FMGs and USMGs to make their way easily in the United States. At the time of our study 66 percent of FMGs were married with children. On the other hand, only 37 percent of USMGs had children. The cultural pattern of not marrying and/or having children late or not at all—which has been so widely discussed in American social science and popular literature—is far more characteristic of the American-trained physicians than of foreign-trained physicians.

Another myth about foreign-trained physicians is clearly dispelled by our data. Only 5 percent of the FMGs have spouses and/or children continuing to reside in their countries of origin. The stereotype of the male FMG who leaves his entire family abroad and comes alone to the United States to work and study is appropriate for only a very small proportion of hospital house staff.

Family life can cushion difficulties of assimilation FMGs may experience at work, and it can reinforce cultural ties. Furthermore, through spouse's work and children's schools it can provide additional opportunities for cultural assimilation.

However, the fact that most FMGs have families and that most USMGs do not, further underscores differences in the kinds of social networks in which these two groups are likely to be involved. Unmarried people or childless couples have very different needs from those of married couples with children who are trying to establish their new identities as adults and simultaneously cope with the rigors of child rearing. This results in married couples with children, childless married couples, and single adults often operating in very different social worlds. If foreign-trained physicians operate more in the world of the married with children and American-trained physicians in non married or married-without-children settings, an additional pressure results, further isolating American-trained and foreign-trained physicians from each other.

Organizational Membership

Our data on cultural orientation and marital status show marked differences between FMGs and USMGs that antedate their training experiences. The contrasting social lives of FMG and USMGs are, in large part, a reflection of these differences. FMGs and USMGs have different patterns both of organizational membership and of contacts with individuals.

Panel 1 of Table 10.4 shows the number of nonprofessional organizations to which each of the groups of interns and residents belonged. Organizations included religious, social, nationality, sports, and hobby and crafts groups. In all three cases, the dominant pattern is nonparticipation, largely because the work schedules of interns and residents allow little time for such activities. Almost two-thirds of all interns and

TABLE 10.4   ORGANIZATIONAL MEMBERSHIPS OF INTERNS AND RESIDENTS

	FMG	USMG	USFMG
Nonprofessional clubs			
No membership	77.9	59.9	58.6
One membership	17.5	30.2	30.8
Two or more memberships	4.6	9.9	10.7
Total	100.0%	100.0%	100.0%
	(688)	(133)	(42)
	(NA = 2)		
Professional clubs			
No membership	39.6	53.2	38.5
One membership	37.9	22.8	42.6
Two or more memberships	22.5	24.0	18.9
Total	100.0%	100.0%	100.0%
	(690)	(133)	(42)

[a] Percentages are weighted; N is unweighted.

residents claimed that they did not belong to any nonprofessional organizations. Participation was strongest among USMGs and weakest among FMGs. Panel 2 of Table 10.4 indicates the pattern of professionally related organizational memberships. These included American, state, and specialty medical associations as well as associations representing FMG physicians. Such opportunities often readily present themselves at the work place, and slightly more than 50 percent of the sample report membership in a medically related organization. Although the percentage and differences are not large, the patterns of participation reverse those of the previous table. USMGs participate least in these organizations and FMGs participate most.

These seemingly contradictory findings may be seen as futher evidence of the relative social isolation of FMGs and their corresponding attempts to make up in professional terms for the results of this isolation: FMGs are blocked from full partipation in the life of their communities through cultural differences that separate many of them from the predominant patterns of their communities. Their relative lack of participation in non-work related organizations is a further indication of this isolation. To counteract isolation and to attempt to "catch up" with their American-trained counterparts, FMGs participate in professional organizations somewhat more than USMGs. Memberships in professional organizations often serve as certification of professional status. In their desire to be recognized as professionals and to receive a good United States professional education, such certification is important for FMGs. Furthermore, this certification is of special importance for the large proportions of both FMGs and USMGs who try to switch hospitals during their training.

Contacts with Individuals

Problems of FMG assimilation and/or alienation are a central theme of this book. In this chapter we see how these problems are reflected in cultural differences and differences in family status, residence patterns, and organizational memberships. Now we examine these problems in the context of friendship patterns and personal contacts.

Table 10.5 indicates that, when compared with each other, FMGs have more contact with other FMGs, and USMGs have more contact with other USMGs (panels 1 and 2). USMGs report seeing other USMGs away from work on the average of once a week; they see FMGs approximately once per month. The overall pattern is

1. Each group interacts more within itself than it does outside the group.

TABLE 10.5 EXTRA WORK SOCIAL CONTACTS OF INTERNS AND RESIDENTS

	FMGs with				USMGs with		USFMGs with		
	USMGs	FMGs	CME[b] graduates	U.S. families	USMGs	FMGs	USMGs	FMGs	CME graduates
Daily	6.4	11.6	15.0	9.5	15.0	2.1	22.5	5.3	7.7
Once per week	19.1	22.0	31.8	25.8	50.2	4.4	27.2	22.5	13.0
Once per month	21.7	23.5	22.6	27.3	26.3	19.0	22.5	15.4	18.3
Less than once per month	28.7	23.6	15.8	28.3	6.8	38.9	10.7	27.8	17.8
Never	24.0	19.3	14.7	9.2	1.7	35.6	17.2	29.0	43.2
	100.0%	100.0%	100.0%	100.0%	100.0%	100.0%	100.0%	100.0%	100.0%
	(688)[a]	(689)	(689)	(688)	(133)	(133)	(42)	(42)	(42)

[a] Percentages are weighted; N is unweighted.
[b] Country of Medical Education

2. Overall, USMGs report more extrawork contact with other house staff than do FMGs.

3. USFMGs, although falling between the two groups, are closer to the USMGs' pattern of interaction.

FMGs were also asked about the amount of the contact they had with graduates of their country of medical education and the amount of contact they had with American families (columns 3 and 4). They report that such contact takes place only on the average of once per month for both these types of individuals.

FMGs' extrawork social lives, as reported by our respondents, are surprisingly isolated. Social life that is measured on a monthly basis for the groups with which most social interaction takes place is clearly not active. In posing these questions, respondents were asked, "In life outside of the hospital, how often do you see other house staff who are FMGs—daily, once a week, at least once a month, less often than that, or never?" All the alternatives were presented, and FMGs consistently responded that they had little contact. These findings indicate, both in absolute terms and compared to USMGs, that FMGs are socially isolated not only from mainstream America (represented by contact with American families), but also from American peers and even FMG and country of medical education peers. This finding points to a significant source of problems for the training of FMGs and their provision of medical services, especially if one presumes a close relationship between levels of social integration, work performance, and learning abilities. This pattern of isolated and encapsulated social interaction indicates that the FMGs' relatively inferior experiences in hospital work settings may be the symptom and the result of a pervasive syndrome of isolation, stigmatization, and stratification of interns and residents outside, as well as inside, the hospital on the basis of cultural differences. Table 10.6 probes this more deeply.

Panel 1 of Table 10.6 shows differences among FMG racial–cultural groups in terms of social contact as measured by total amount of reported contact and percentage of foreign friends.[7] This table suggests that White FMGs have more social interaction than do Blacks or Orientals, with Indians having markedly less social interaction than the other groups. In addition White FMGs have a larger proportion of American friends than Indians or Blacks, and Orientals have the largest proportion of foreign friends. This seems to indicate that those FMGs who are most like American citizens—White FMGs—acculturate most readily to American life.

Since patterns of social contact appear to be affected by racial-cultural type, one might also posit that FMGs who speak English well would be

TABLE 10.6   SOCIAL CONTACT OF FMGS

Racial cultural type	Amount (Percentage)			Percentage foreign friends				
	Low	High	Total	All U.S. Friends	Mixed	All foreign	Total	Percent base (N)
White	46.2	53.8	100.0[a]	11.8	54.2	34.0	100.0	(350)[a]
Black	52.1	47.9	100.0	3.3	44.9	51.8	100.0	(28)
Indian	61.7	38.3	100.0	1.9	45.4	53.7	100.0	(96)
Oriental	52.4	47.6	100.0	5.1	28.6	66.3	100.0	(216)

English skill	Amount (Percentage)			Percentage foreign friends				
	Low	High	Total	All U.S. friends	Mixed	All foreign	Total	Percent base (N)
Excellent	53.8	46.2	100.0	10.1	53.8	36.1	100.0	(244)
Good	52.3	48.7	100.0	5.8	36.3	58.9	100.0	(285)
Fair/poor	51.2	48.8	100.0	0.8	31.8	68.4	100.0	(156)
								(NA = 5)

[a] Percentages are weighted; N is unweighted.

more assimilated than those with poor English. Panel 2 of Table 10.6 indicates that FMGs with different levels of English skills have approximately the same overall amount of social contact, but that the people with whom they have this contact are somewhat different. Excellent English speakers have the most American friends, and poor English speakers the least. FMGs who have mastered English and those who continue to have language difficulties are equally likely to have fuller social lives. However, excellent English speakers are much more likely to include American citizens in their social worlds; poor English speakers are more likely to have contact only with foreigners. Poor English speakers are not isolated from other FMGs, but, as expected, they are relatively isolated from American culture.

Tables 10.5 and 10.6 show that FMGs do not have extensive social contacts with American citizens and that, as individuals, they are relatively isolated during their American medical training. Furthermore, among FMGs, non-Whites and poor English speakers have less contact with American citizens.

CONCLUSIONS

The substantial differences between USMGs and FMGs in terms of cultural background, social origins, and initial orientation to the American health care system parallel findings indicating differences between FMGs and USMGs regarding informal aspects of hospital experiences. FMGs are relatively isolated from the mainstream of both American medicine and culture. This isolation is further indicated by their limited organizational participation and their social contacts. However, an FMG who is ascribed to be of a racial-cultural group typical of American culture and who has mastered English is more likely to have social contacts with Americans, as commonsense would suggest.

Although it is impossible to demonstrate conclusively through this study, it is possible that, even if all else was equal these differences would produce medical training and provision of medical services by FMGs inferior to the training that would result if suitable orientation programs, English training, living situations, and work situations were created to minimize the differences between the FMGs and the American milieu and/or to build on the strengths and experiences of FMGs. Similarly, it is likely that social and cultural alienation outside the hospital produces feelings of separateness, defensiveness, and a questioning of personal identities among FMGs that weaken their confidence and ability to perform and learn effectively as interns and residents in American hospitals.

These are important elements in considering the continuing question facing many FMGs while they are training here: To go back to their own country, or to stay in the United States. Ease of assimilation into American life may make a future career here a happy prospect. On the other hand, isolation suggests the haunting possibility of continuing alienation from mainstream medicine and American life.

NOTES

1. USMGs and USFMGs training in hospitals not affiliated with universities were more likely to miss orientation programs than their counterparts in affiliated hospitals. FMGs in nonaffiliated hospitals were less likely to miss orientation programs than FMGs in affiliated hospitals.
2. Higher proportions of USFMGs reported that their orientation included information about procedures for ordering drugs and diagnostic tests. One explanation for this may be that hospitals take special pains to introduce USFMGs into their house staff positions, perhaps considering that they have a greater need of such information than FMGs, who are generally more experienced. However, this explanation does not account for the difference observed between USMGs and *both* USFMGs and FMGs in the coverage of information about American medical terminology and abbreviations.

3. Joy Parkinson, *Manual of English for the Overseas Doctor*, London: Churchill Livingston, 1976 attempts to alleviate this problem in the United Kingdom. Although some American hospitals have made modest attempts at producing such a manual, no such comprehensive volume exists in the United States.

4. We cannot pretend to make a full comparison of the social and cultural situations of American- and foreign-trained house staff. The main thrust of this research was to document the work situations and mobility patterns of these two groups. The volume of information needed to probe these areas forces us to omit items describing belief patterns, personal styles, dress patterns, eating patterns, recreational preferences, and other cultural and social characteristics which we observed at first hand in our hospital case studies. However, certain questions probing the personal situations of our respondents do enable us to sketch a picture of the differences between USMGs and FMGs on selected dimensions.

5. For a discussion of religion that indicates its centrality for individual cultural orientations, see James E. Dittes, "Religion: Psychological Study," in David L. Sills, Ed, *International Encyclopedia of the Social Sciences*. Vol. 13, New York: MacMillan, 1968, pp. 414–421.

6. USFMGs appear to be a special group of American citizens who are disproportionately Catholic and Jewish compared to USMGs. See Chapter 2.

7. The total amount of reported contacts was calculated by summing, for each respondent, the amount of contact reported in the four categories of interaction in Table 10.5. The percentage of the individual's three closest friends who were citizens of countries other than the United States was calculated from answers to the question in which the individual indicated his three closest friends in the United States and their nationalities.

11

THE DECISION TO REMAIN
OR TO RETURN_____

Three options are open to the FMG who has completed postgraduate medical education in the United States: (1) return to his or her country of medical education, (2) stay in the United States, or (3) migrate to some third country.[1]

This decision, like the original decision to come to the United States, has often been treated as if the choice were made at one point in time, and the dynamics of the decision often have been illustrated by the use of the "push-pull model." As in Chapter 3, we find that using the "push-pull model" focuses the decision process on the countries that represent migration options, rather than on the meaning of the migration decision within the life and medical career of the FMG. Therefore we have organized our discussion of the FMG's decision to remain in the United States or return to his or her country of medical education to reflect the dynamics of the medical career. We first discuss the motivations for remaining in the United States or returning to the country of medical education. We then discuss, in sequence, the manner in which differences in general personal situations, individual work situations, and career plans are related to FMGs' decisions to remain or return.

MOTIVATIONS FOR REMAINING OR RETURNING

All FMGs were asked whether they had decided to leave the United States or remain after their training. Of the total FMG responses, 273 answered that they had decided to remain ("stayers"), 340 answered that they had decided to leave ("leavers"), and 75 answered that they were undecided. When these figures are "weighted" to allow us to generalize to the whole population, we find 44.5 percent who have decided to remain, 44.6 percent to leave, and 10.9 percent undecided.[2] Table 11.1 presents the responses of the "stayers" and the "leavers," ranked according to the percentage of each group indicating the relevance of each motivation.

The motivations reported by the stayers for remaining in the United States bear an initial resemblance to those reported in Chapter 3 for coming to the United States for postdoctoral training. The list is headed by desires for better medical facilities and research opportunities, followed closely by the attraction of the economic prospects of the United

TABLE 11.1   MIGRATION MOTIVATIONS FOR STAYING IN OR LEAVING THE UNITED STATES[a]

"Stayers' " Motivations	Percentage	"Leavers' " Motivations	Percentage
Better medical facilities	93.2[b]	Family in CME	93.2
Better research opportunities	88.4	Should serve CME	91.5
Economic prospects	86.0	Moral obligation	80.9
Prefer U.S. life style	74.6	Dislike U.S. life	67.3
Private practice opportunity	67.8	No work in U.S.	31.4
To become U.S. citizen	67.7	Legally required by U.S.	28.5
Politics in CME	67.4	Avoid U.S. draft	22.1
Family likes U.S.	66.0	Legally required by CME	18.3
Better education for children	58.4	Trouble getting U.S. license	14.5
No socialized medicine	52.4		
Percent base (N)	(273)[b]	Percent base (N)	(340)

[a] Data are not included for "undecideds," $N = 75$. NA = 2.
[b] Percentages are weighted; N is unweighted.

States. However, the rest of the motivations (all cited by well over one-half of the stayers) mix family preferences and career preferences in a manner quite distinct from the motivational pattern characterizing the decision to come to the United States.[3]

The decision to stay in the United States includes both career and family considerations. This is a broader range of concerns than characterized the original decision to come to the United States. Simply coming to the United States for postgraduate education is a relatively simple matter, an episode to be reconciled with career plans, not necessarily a decision leading to a lifetime commitment. Deciding to stay in the United States as a true "immigrant" represents a long-term commitment for which the plans of a lifetime may have to be reoriented. Thus, although most FMGs may end up staying in the United States after completing training, their reasons for coming to the United States may often have been based on quite different considerations. After examining the motivations of the leavers, we attempt to identify some of the factors associated with this decision to return or remain.

The desire to be reunited with family is the prime reason cited by FMGs for not remaining in the United States. This was also a concern for the original decision to come to the United States. However, the next two motivations for going home, feeling an obligation to serve the people of the FMG's country of medical education and feeling a moral obligation to return, were not relevant to the original decision to seek training in the United States. These responses to moral imperatives—the first related to the FMG's role as physician, the second to his other role as citizen—become relevant at the end, rather than the beginning, of the FMG's postgraduate training. Temporarily migrating to the United States for advanced medical training is usually consistent with an FMG's sense of patriotic duty; however, permanently abandoning one's homeland may be a violation of this trust.

Legal requirements to return and work difficulties in the United States motivated only a minority of the leavers. However, a stated dislike for aspects of American life was cited by two-thirds of the leavers as a reason for returning to their country of medical education. Alienation from American culture is thus an important migration motivation. When this alienation from American culture is viewed in conjunction with other judgments about the United States and the country of medical education, an intense double bind is visible for certain FMGs. This double bind consists of (1) simultaneously feeling affection for one's CME and feeling apprehensive about returning there to practice medicine, and (2) simultaneously experiencing career security in the United States and feeling personally alienated from its culture. This double bind, as discussed in

Chapter 3 and in the next section, is an important strain during United States graduate training for FMGs from certain nations.

To summarize our findings regarding the aggregate pattern of migration motivations: stayers indicate a broad motivational basis for remaining in the United States. Of primary importance is the desire for better career oportunities, but a preference for American lifestyles and a concern over the politics of one's country of medical education are also of major importance. Leavers, on the other hand, have a narrower range of motivations. Most important is a desire to be reunited with family, followed closely by feelings of moral obligation to the country of medical education. Also of significance is a stated dislike for aspects of American culture, with legal requirements and work problems in the United States of relatively minor importance.

MIGRATION PLANS AND COUNTRY OF MEDICAL EDUCATION

The decision to remain or return is affected by the simultaneous operation of three types of job market. These markets are (1) an international market for a limited number of teachers, researchers, and specialists, (2) the United States medical manpower market, and (3) the markets in individual countries of medical education. In making career decisions, FMGs continually assess oportunities in all three markets. Perhaps the most crucial indication of a given FMG's employability and interest in each of these three markets is the country and medical school in which the FMG received undergraduate medical training. If an FMG has received a superior medical education, employability in all three markets is increased. If there is a high demand for physicians together with good wages and a stable, attractive professional and political climate in an FMG's country of medical education, the FMG will be more interested in the market there and less interested in the international or United States markets.

FMGs trained in nations with superior medical training and an attractive professional climate will be in great demand. They will be interested in all markets, especially that of their CME. A well-trained FMG from a nation with an unattractive professional climate tends to be more interested in jobs outside the CME. A substantial minority of our sample were not trained in distinguished medical schools. These were more likely to be interested in returning to their CMEs if political conditions there were stable and physician demand were expanding. To the extent that either of these conditions did not hold, they focused on other markets, especially that of the United States, because they were located in the

United States and jobs were available for physicians here. The job prospects of FMGs from different types of CMEs are presented in Figure 11.1.

Medical Education in Countries
of Medical Education

		Superior	Undistinguished
Professional climate in Country of Medical Education	Attractive	Good prospects and interested in all markets, especially Country of Medical Education	Best prospects in Country of Medical Education market
	Unattractive	Good prospects and interested in international and U.S. markets	Limited prospects likely to stay in United States

Markets: International
      United States
      Country of medical education

Figure 11.1. Job prospects for FMGs from different Countries of Medical Education

Table 11.2 reports the migration plans for FMGs from nations with six or more respondents in our study group. CMEs with high proportions of "leavers" are generally those in which the demand for physicians was high in 1974 (e.g., Thailand) and/or had expanding economies (e.g., Japan, South Africa, Mexico, Iran, and Brazil). CMEs with high proportions of "stayers" were generally those with socialized medical systems (e.g., Eastern Europe, Cuba, and the United Kingdom) or were experiencing serious political and social turmoil (e.g., Ceylon, the Philippines, South Korea, and India). CMEs that have attractive professional climates and provide superior medical education were in the middle of the distribution, reflecting the greater freedom of choice available to FMGs from those nations (e.g., Canada and West Germany).

However, the quality of medical education and professional climate in the CME provide only a partial explanation of FMG migration plans.

TABLE 11.2   FMG MIGRATION PLANS AND COUNTRY OF MEDICAL
EDUCATION

	Percentage planning to return to CME Leavers	Percentage planning to stay in U.S. Stayers	Undecided	Total N
Thailand	87.0	9.1	3.9	100.0 (44)[a]
Japan	86.5	13.5	0	100.0 (11)
South Africa	79.8	20.2	0	100.0 (8)
Syria	74.8	8.4	16.8	100.0 (10)
Mexico	65.6	24.9	9.5	100.0 (26)
Colombia	62.4	33.3	4.2	100.0 (18)
Iran	60.3	27.3	12.4	100.0 (43)
Brazil	59.6	15.6	24.8	100.0 (20)
Canada	55.6	38.8	5.6	100.0 (14)
Spain	54.2	37.3	8.5	100.0 (21)
Lebanon	54.3	45.7	0	100.0 (11)
Argentina	51.5	48.5	0	100.0 (21)
Pakistan– Bangladesh	46.2	42.9	10.9	100.0 (36)
Peru	45.4	39.8	14.8	100.0 (12)
West Germany	42.5	57.5	0	100.0 (11)
Ireland	41.3	58.7	0	100.0 (11)
India	40.3	43.2	16.4	100.0 (41)
South Korea	40.0	53.8	6.1	100.0 (30)
United Kingdom	36.8	63.2	0	100.0 (9)
Philippines	36.7	54.4	8.5	100.0 (47)
Egypt (UAR)	34.5	46.3	19.2	100.0 (16)
Taiwan	34.4	40.7	24.9	100.0 (62)
Ceylon	29.4	63.0	7.5	100.0 (18)
Cuba	6.8	93.2	0	100.0 (11)
Eastern Europe	4.4	89.3	6.3	100.0 (23)
Other	45.5	40.5	14.0	100.0 (116)
Total	47.2	41.3	11.5	100.0 (690)

[a] Percentages are weighted; N is unweighted.

Many other considerations are important, especially the perceptions and
motivations of the individual FMGs, introduced at the beginning of this
chapter. Tables 11.3 and 11.4 report the migration motivations of stayers
and leavers of the same 15 countries discussed in Chapter 3 and reported
in Table 3.7.

TABLE 11.3 MIGRATION MOTIVATIONS OF STAYERS AND COUNTRY OF MEDICAL EDUCATION

(Percentages of Stayers in each CME indicating each motivation for remaining)

	Quality U.S. medical Facilities	U.S. research prospects	U.S. economic prospects	Likes U.S. culture	Private practice in U.S.	To become U.S. citizen	Political and social problems in CME	Family likes U.S.	Education of children in U.S.	No socialized medicine in U.S.
West Germany	100.0[a]	56.2	0	56.2	100.0	43.8	12.4	56.2	12.4	56.2
Spain	100.0	100.0	74.4	100.0	73.3	100.0	86.7	100.0	26.4	87.8
Colombia	88.3	100.0	76.5	76.5	65.0	23.5	23.5	76.5	88.3	35.2
Peru	100.0	62.1	100.0	61.1	88.9	22.1	50.0	61.1	22.1	50.0
Argentina	100.0	92.3	100.0	84.7	84.7	84.7	57.3	57.7	42.3	42.3
Brazil	100.0	81.9	100.0	18.1	18.1	18.1	63.8	18.1	18.1	36.2
United Kingdom	84.7	31.7	100.0	69.3	100.0	69.3	54.0	69.3	15.3	69.3
Thailand	100.0	100.0	100.0	56.2	100.0	43.8	56.2	100.0	100.0	12.4
Philippines	100.0	94.9	100.0	84.7	77.9	64.4	98.3	69.5	83.0	44.2
Egypt–United Arab Republic	73.0	73.0	73.0	84.7	65.3	92.3	92.3	15.3	34.7	57.3
Iran	95.9	100.0	81.6	85.7	85.7	67.3	55.1	73.5	73.5	59.2
Taiwan	96.0	92.0	89.0	85.0	62.0	76.0	82.0	82.0	62.0	52.0
South Korea	97.1	97.1	100.0	72.5	69.6	57.3	81.9	48.5	60.8	52.5
India	100.0	95.5	87.4	68.2	68.2	72.6	38.6	74.3	49.8	70.4
Cuba	63.3	80.1	56.6	80.1	86.7	93.4	100.0	69.9	80.1	86.7
All CMEs	93.2	88.4	86.0	74.6	67.8	67.7	67.4	66.0	58.4	57.4

[a] Percentages are weighted.

231

TABLE 11.4 MIGRATION MOTIVATIONS OF LEAVERS AND COUNTRY OF MEDICAL EDUCATION

(Percentage of leavers in each CME indicating each motivation for returning)

	Separation from family and friends	Should serve CME	Moral obligation to return	Dislikes U.S. culture	No work in U.S.	U.S. legal obligation to return	Avoid U.S. draft	CME legal obligation to return	Trouble getting license
West Germany	100.0[a]	100.0	50.0	100.0	0	0	0	0	0
Spain	100.0	42.1	40.7	74.0	40.7	51.9	7.4	0	7.4
Colombia	49.9	100.0	100.0	69.9	6.2	12.5	37.4	6.2	18.7
Peru	100.0	100.0	63.0	62.5	37.0	31.5	21.0	21.0	0
Argentina	100.0	100.0	100.0	83.8	5.4	0	21.5	21.5	5.4
Brazil	100.0	100.0	87.0	56.5	30.5	43.5	34.8	17.3	65.3
United Kingdom	100.0	100.0	100.0	100.0	0	0	0	0	0
Thailand	95.2	90.3	87.6	52.4	20.7	23.4	13.1	20.7	5.5
Philippines	97.4	100.0	79.0	71.0	18.4	47.4	36.8	44.7	36.8
Egypt–United Arab Republic	100.0	100.0	100.0	100.0	100.0	0	0	0	0
Iran	100.0	95.9	95.9	80.5	29.9	38.9	18.6	39.2	24.7
Taiwan	73.6	97.3	97.3	64.3	51.4	27.0	12.2	8.1	29.7
South Korea	95.8	100.0	60.5	65.6	57.2	0	0	4.2	4.2
India	100.0	83.1	78.0	72.8	50.8	24.6	36.4	2.6	5.1
Cuba	100.0	100.0	100.0	0	0	0	0	0	100.0
All CMEs	93.2	91.5	80.9	67.3	31.4	28.5	22.1	18.3	14.5

[a] Percentages are weighted.

In 1974 the West German economy was expanding, and it offered an attractive professional and political climate. West German FMGs had the freedom to return to West Germany to good positions or to stay in the United States, another Western culture. Compared to individuals trained in other nations, interns and residents trained in West Germany were rather diffident regarding their decision to come to the United States; they expressed concern about separation from family and friends and the possibility of missing the job market at home, but relatively little enthusiasm for American medical facilities, salaries, and other aspects of American life (Table 3.7).

This diffidence continues to be reflected in their motivations for staying or leaving. West Germans are not pressed by the law, nor are they constrained by economics or politics. Stayers appear attracted by the opportunity to control their own careers, and leavers miss life in Germany.

Stayers are less impressed than any other group of FMGs by the culture and economic prospects of the United States. What does impress them most is the quality of American medical facilities and especially the opportunity to set up private practice.

FMGs returning to West Germany note standard motivations— separation from family and friends and feeling morally obliged, but for these leavers, life in the United States has apparently turned indicated a dislike for American culture.

The decisions of Spanish FMGs are somewhat more complicated to analyze because a substantial proportion are Cubans who migrated to Spain and received medical training there before coming to the United States. As a result, the responses of the leavers and stayers reflect distinct patterns.

The leavers reflect a pattern relatively close to that of the West Germans—relatively few reasons given for leaving, with separation from family and friends and a dislike of American culture predominating. The stayers, on the other hand, reflect a pattern close to that of the Cubans, with great importance placed on liking American culture, the desire to become a citizen, and political problems in the CME. It can be argued that Spanish-born FMGs pursue their self-interest as avidly as the West Germans, whereas Cuban-born, Spanish-trained FMGs see the United States as their only viable life alternative and only contemplate leaving (as was the case of one Cuban-born Spanish FMG and one Cuban FMG) when they find it impossible to obtain a medical license in the United States.

FMGs from Colombia and Peru were heavily influenced in their decision to come to the United States by advice from professors in their

countries of medical education. They continued to exhibit generally positive reasons for remaining in the United States or returning to their
countries of medical education. Compared to FMGs from other Third
World nations, few "stayers" felt alienated from the United States, and
few "leavers" were returning home reluctantly.

Colombians were more attracted to the United States for family
reasons, stating a relatively strong preference for American culture and
even indicating a marked desire to have their children educated in the
United States.

Peruvians were strongly attracted by American economic prospects, by
the opportunity to set up private practice in the United States, and were
moderately concerned about political and social problems in Peru. (In
1974, Peru's authoritarian socialist government had indicated an interest
in regulating medicine).

FMGs planning to return to Colombia and Peru were not particularly
motivated by a dislike for American culture but were more concerned
about moral obligations to serve their country of medical education and
looked forward to rejoining family and friends.

Argentine FMGs return to Argentina or stay in the United States at
more or less average rates; however, their migration motivations indicate
somewhat polarized reasons for these decisions. Argentine motivations
for leaving parallel those of West German and United Kingdom FMGs by
attributing much importance to a dislike of American culture and a strong
affection for their home culture.[4] Argentines staying in the United States,
on the other hand, indicate strong positive feelings toward United States
culture and are similarly positive about becoming American citizens. In
addition, Argentine "stayers" attribute the usual high importance to
economic and career prospects in the United States.

Table 11.4 indicates that a relatively high proportion of Brazilians plan
to return to their country of medical education. For Brazilians, the overwhelming motivation for staying in the United States lay in career prospects. The major motivations for returning were separation from family
and friends and moral obligations, with an unusually high proportion
reporting legal problems in the United States. Since Brazil's extensive
middle class and recent expansion of medical facilities provide incentives
for Brazilians to return home, this last finding probably indicated a
reluctance to deal with the labyrinthine legal complications that most
FMGs resolve to change visa status, get an American license, and avoid
the United States draft. Brazilians are probably more in a position to "do
as they please" than FMGs who must face returning to CMEs mired in
underdevelopment.

A relatively high proportion of United Kingdom physicians came to the

United States because of a perceived lack of career opportunities in their countries of medical education. These perceptions appear unchanged during their training in the United States, and a relatively high proportion intend to remain. Leavers were highly motivated by a dislike of American culture, separation from family and friends, and moral obligations to return. The leavers' dislike of American culture was paralleled among the stayers who indicated, with the West Germans and Brazilians, the lowest rate of preference for having their children educated in the United States. Stayers were unusually highly motivated by opportunities to set up private practice, the lack of socialized medicine, and economic prospects in the United States.

This dislike of some aspects of the United States and attraction by others indicates that some United Kingdom-trained FMGs were caught in a form of the double bind discussed previously. This also characterizes FMGs trained in countries such as Egypt, Iran, India, and South Korea, discussed later. FMGs from these countries have in common a strong positive feeling toward the culture of their CME and a disdain for American culture. This results in stayers remaining in the United States for career reasons despite apprehension about American culture; both leavers and stayers are distressed over separation from family, friends, and their homeland and are concerned about lack of career opportunities and/or political or social instability there. In the case of the United Kingdom, some respondents indicated that this apprehension focuses on an intense dislike for that country's system of socialized medicine.

FMGs from Thailand tended to be more positive than other Asian-trained FMGs about American culture and obtaining medical specialization in the United States as motivations for seeking an American education. Of all country groups, Thais indicate the highest rate of return to their country of medical education, probably because of job opportunities perceived to be available by members of this cohort because of the recent construction of medical facilities in Thailand. Since advanced medical training is necessary to obtain these jobs, Thai physicians were able to be positive about coming to the United States and also positive about returning home. The few Thais who chose to stay in the United States indicated normal personal attractions to American medical facilities and economic prospects but also indicated that their families were unusually highly attracted to the United States.

FMGs from the Philippines, the largest group of FMGs in the United States, were also positive about seeking an American medical education. This attitude was reinforced by their home government's designing medical education on the American model and encouraging advanced training there, because of the large community of Filipino medical personnel already living in the United States and the historical ties between the United States and the Philippines. Filipinos also indicated positive feelings toward the United States but stated more concern over political and social problems there than did any other national group except the Cubans. Filipino leavers indicated that family and feelings of obligation were the most important reasons for returning. The small proportion of Filipinos who decided to return home did, however, exhibit an unusually high incidence of work and legal problems as contributory factors to their migration decisions.

FMGs from the United Arab Republic and Iran—the two Islamic countries considered in this analysis—indicated the strongest double binds of any national groups. Although economic conditions in Iran may have resulted in Iranian-trained FMGs disproportionately planning to return home and U.A.R. FMGs disproportionately planning to stay in the United States, FMGs of both countries who chose to return home indicated a strong dislike of American culture as an important reason for their decision. Furthermore, all five of the FMGs from the United Arab Republic who decided to return home indicated that they could not find work in the United States, and an unusually high proportion of the Iranians reported work and legal problems. The double bind was most apparent among graduates from the United Arab Republic planning to stay in the United States whose major reasons for staying were political and social problems in their country and who indicated very little desire to have their children educated in the United States. For these two national groups it would appear that differences between Islamic and Western culture—those most noted by respondents concerned male-female relations and dietary prohibitions—had a strong impact on the feelings of these FMGs toward the United States.

Apart from the Philippines, the three nations that send the largest numbers of FMGs to the United States are Taiwan, South Korea, and India. FMGs from these three nations have remarkably similar aggregate response patterns. Like the Filipino FMGs, the stayers were strongly positive about the quality of American medical facilities, and economic prospects, and expressed little alienation from American culture. However, political problems were important reasons for Taiwanese and South Koreans staying in the United States (the survey was administered before India's 1975 constitutional crisis) whereas Indians were attracted by the private medical system in the United States.

Some evidence of a double bind was manifested by the leavers' average indication of dislike for American culture. However, separation from family and friends and feelings of moral obligation to their CME were the most important motivations for returning home. It would appear that, although a double bind is of some importance for FMGs from these Asian nations, it is less salient than for those raised in Islamic cultures.

As discussed in Chapter 3, Cuban FMGs exhibit a singular pattern of migration motivations. Table 11.2 shows that the only group whose migration plans parallel those of the Cubans are those FMGs trained in Eastern Europe (most of whom are political refugees). The one Cuban who plans to leave the United States indicated trouble in getting a license to practice medicine in the United States. Cubans appear to stay because of political and social differences with Communist Cuba and, as a result, have a pattern of responses that reflects total identification with the United States—a desire to become an American citizen, to set up one's own private medical practice, to have children educated in the United States, and a liking for United States culture. Cubans are the least able to "do as they please." Since opportunities for private medical practice in Cuba are virtually nonexistent, their responses reflect a pattern of total identification with American culture and medicine.

To summarize this section of the chapter: Although the quality of medical education and the professional and political climate affect to some degree the migration decisions of all FMGs, those trained in different nations do exhibit a variety of motivational bases for their migration decisions. In evaluating these migration decisions, it is particularly important to note how political and cultural considerations, both in the United States and the countries of medical education, are evaluated in terms of the career and family plans of these FMGs. FMGs take these contingencies into account and develop preferences for remaining in the United States or returning to their countries of medical education that minimize personal risk and discomfort and maximize opportunities for personal and career enrichment and advantages.

MIGRATION PLANS AND PERSONAL SITUATIONS

The personal situations of individuals such as the FMGs in our sample are circumscribed to some extent by their respective genders and social status. The proportion of women physicians is smaller in the United States than it is in many other countries. Therefore one might hypothesize that, because of their gender, female FMGs would find resistance to remaining in the United States and would return to their countries of medical education in greater proportions than male FMGs. The first panel of Table 11.5 indicates that this is not the case. In fact, male and female FMGs plan to remain or plan to return in virtually identical proportions.

Since in most parts of the world the father's status is the major determinant of family status, the father's education rather than that of the mother or some combination of the two spouses' education was taken as our indicator of social status of the family of orientation to which the FMG belongs.[5] The second panel of Table 11.5 indicates a nonlinear relationship between the father's education and the intention to return to the CME or remain in the United States. It is our interpretation that this pattern reflects different motivational patterns for FMGs of different social statuses. FMGs whose fathers are highly educated are more or less equally divided between those who intend to return home and those who intend to stay in the United States. Those who plan to return home envision good family and career prospects there and have often even formulated career plans before leaving for the United States. FMGs whose fathers have completed a moderate level of education are much more likely to stay in the United States where they perceive more opportunities for themselves and are better able to take advantage of those opportunities than if they returned home. Compared to more highly educated FMGs, fewer of them have established opportunities in their countries of medical education. FMGs whose fathers have the least education are most likely to return to their country of medical education, not because they anticipate opportunities but because they have not developed expertise to establish themselves advantageously in the United States, and their most reasonable alternative is to return home to begin medical practice.[6]

Another set of information that provides insight into differences between leavers and stayers is information about the FMGs' arrival in the United States. This includes the time at which the FMG decided to come to the United States, where the ECFMG exam was passed, the date of arrival in the United States, and arrival visa type.

The first panel of Table 11.6 indicates a pattern similar to that reported in Chapter 3 regarding when the decision to come to the United States was made. "Early deciders" were more likely to have a coherent plan that involved their receiving training in the United States and staying here. Those deciding late in medical school or immediately after medical school had a career plan that was more likely to have them returning home after completing their training abroad. Those who decided very late usually decided (as indicated in Chapter 3) because of concern with political and social conditions in their country of medical education and were likely to remain, not because of a long-term career plan, but because of the disruptive circumstances that led them to come to the United States.

The second panel of Table 11.6 indicates that the vast majority of individuals who took the ECFMG examination in the United States plan

TABLE 11.5   FMG MIGRATION PLANS AND PERSONAL
CHARACTERISTICS

			Percentages	
		Leavers	Stayers	Undecideds
Gender	Men	85.7	85.2	79.5
	Women	14.3	14.8	20.5
		100.0 (340)[a]	100.0 (273)	100.0 (75)
Father's Educa-tion	Completed college or pro-fessional school	48.9	45.3	45.1
	Completed secondary school, some college	23.0	37.6	27.9
	None or some secondary school	25.8	15.5	14.0
	No information	2.4	1.6	13.0
Percent base (N)		100.0 (340)	100.0 (273)	100.0 (75)

[a] Percentages are weighted; N is unweighted.

to stay permanently in the United States. Only a minority of those who took the ECFMG examination in their country of medical education or some third country intended to stay in the United States. This is further evidence of a coherent career pattern for stayers. Often (as discussed in Chapter 4) individuals who passed the ECFMG exam in the United States came to the United States on a tourist visa and took the test at the beginning of that stay. The FMG then explored job opportunities, and when notification of passing the exam was received, it was possible to begin work with little delay. Sometimes such individuals would engage themselves in work even before receiving the results of this exam, often following this strategy as a result of hospital encouragement. It appears that many FMGs have made an effort to learn details of the operation of American immigration and medical employment systems—the

TABLE 11.6   FMG MIGRATION PLANS AND ARRIVAL INFORMATION

	Percentages		
	Leavers	Stayers	Undecideds
When decided to come to U.S.			
Before medical school	3.9[a]	5.5	8.1
Early medical school	13.5	21.0	14.9
Late medical school	27.0	16.8	23.0
Right after medical school	25.8	11.7	27.0
1 year after medical school	29.7	45.0	27.0
	100.0	100.0	100.0
Where passed ECFMG			
USA	8.0	24.2	23.2
Country of Medical Education	67.8	52.6	55.2
Other	24.2	23.2	21.6
	100.0	100.0	100.0
Date of arrival in U.S.			
Before 6/70	11.7	33.8	18.1
6/70 to 5/72	36.6	43.6	54.0
After 5/72	51.7	22.6	27.9
	100.0	100.0	100.0
Arrival visa type			
Visitor	5.7	1.9	5.2
"H" visa	3.3	2.0	0
Exchange visitor	68.1	58.1	70.4
Student	2.4	2.4	3.4
Permanent resident	20.4	34.0	21.0
Refugee	0	1.6	0
Percent base (N)	100.0 (340)[a]	100.0 (273)	100.0 (75)

[a] Percentages are weighted; N is unweighted.

games–playing we have described—to minimize the loss of time and resources involved in setting up a medical career in the country of their choosing.

The clear relation between the date of arrival in the United States and migration plans is shown in the third panel of Table 11.6. Altogether 68 percent of those in our sample who arrived before June 1970 plan to stay, together with 47 percent of those arriving between June 1970 and May 1972, and 28 percent of those who arrived after May 1972. These figures are remarkably consistent with our earlier studies of return migration rates of FMGs in the United States.[7] The findings in our earlier studies point to the conclusion that, although less than one-third of

FMGs intend to stay in the United States on their arrival here, with the passage of time close to three-quarters of a given cohort of FMGs eventually remain in the United States.

This is an important finding. As FMGs learn more about the American medical system, become more and more involved in that system, over come their apprehension about American culture, learn about economic and career opportunities in the United States, and feel more and more distant from family and friends in their country of medical education, nearly one-half of each cohort change their minds from intending to return to the country of medical education to intending to stay in the United States. Such a decision is of great import for these individuals. It is a cause of great concern to them, not only during their internships and residencies but throughout their medical careers. Our field studies and Portes' study in Argentina[8] indicate that the options of practicing medicine in the United States or one's country of medical education are alternatives constantly considered by physicians throughout the world. Our findings on FMG experiences as house staff in the United States suggest that the process of graduate medical education, by socializing aliens at least to some extent, encourages FMGs to behave as immigrants. Thus the tendency to stay increases the longer the FMG remains here in the United States.

The fourth panel of Table 11.6 lists six types of visas. The types are ordered according to the proportion of leavers among FMGs who held each type on arrival in the United States. Individuals on visitors' visas are most likely to return, followed by individuals on H visas, individuals with exchange visitor visas, individuals with student visas, and individuals with permanent resident visas; finally, all individuals who entered the United States on refugee visas currently intend to stay in the United States. The most remarkable point here is that no matter what visa an FMG held on arrival in the United States—even an extremely restricted visa such as a visitor's visa or H visa—a substantial proportion of the FMGs now intend to stay in the United States to practice medicine. A second important finding is that so many individuals who originally entered the United States on exchange visitor visas now intend to stay in the United States.[9] With the passage of time, substantial numbers of individuals who originally came to the United States as exchange visitors adjust their visa status and remain in the United States permanently.[10] A third finding is that there is some correspondence between the initial visa obtained by an FMG and the FMG's eventual migration plans. For example, individuals who originally entered the United States on permanent resident visas are approximately 40 percent more likely to indicate during their postgraduate training an intention to stay in the United States than are individuals who originally entered the United States on exchange visitor visas.

MIGRATION PLANS AND WORK SITUATIONS

Leavers and stayers do not differ markedly with respect to selected aspects of their work situations. Furthermore, when there are differences, these may well reflect the way different work situations fit into the long-term career objectives of various FMGs, rather than the way these work situations may have affected the FMGs during their period of advanced training in the United States. The first two panels of Table 11.7 contrast leavers and stayers with respect to the size of the cities and the size of the hospitals in which they were working. Leavers were very slightly more likely to be living in metropolitan areas, and stayers were more likely to be living in provincial cities; leavers were more likely to work in large hospitals, and stayers were more likely to work in smaller hospitals. Panels 3, 4, and 5 of Table 11.7 show a weak tendency in leavers to be in advanced training in major teaching units and private hospitals. Similarly, there is a slight tendency for leavers to be located in training centers with relatively lower proportions of FMGs as interns and residents and for stayers to be located in training centers in which a higher proportion of interns and residents are FMGs. To a small degree, therefore, there is some evidence of the existence of a group of "true" exchange students working in the in the more desired training settings, and a group of "true" immigrants being assimilated through relativity humble work situations.

Yet these relationships are not strong enough to indicate that hospital sizes, types, and affiliations powerfully influence FMG migration plans. Rather they reflect that FMGs with different migration plans function as interns and residents in all medical work settings. However, our field studies indicated that the most coherent and durable long-term migration plans are held by a few relatively privileged FMGs who manage to get advanced training in large private hospitals that are major teaching centers in large cities and that have relatively small er proportions of FMGs among their intern and resident staff.

A final difference between leavers and stayers with regard to current work situations is their medical specialty, as shown in panel 6 of Table 11.7. Here there is an apparent trend of relatively more leavers in the specialties of surgery, medicine, and obstetrics/gynecology and more stayers with hospital-based specialties or going into general practice. However, further analysis shows that this difference is more a function of

TABLE 11.7   FMG MIGRATION PLANS BY SETTING OF TRAINING IN 1974

		Leavers	Percentages Stayers	Undecideds
City Size				
	Metropolitan area	72.3[a]	65.6	70.4
	Large provincial city	27.7	34.4	29.6
		100.0	100.0	100.0
Hospital size				
	1–499 beds	53.4	58.9	56.9
	500 or more beds	46.6	41.1	43.1
		100.0	100.0	100.0
Hospital Type				
	Major teaching	60.3	54.6	62.7
	Limited teaching	21.2	22.8	23.1
	Nonaffiliated	18.4	22.6	14.2
		100.0	100.0	100.0
Hospital affiliation				
	Private	65.4	57.8	66.7
	Veterans Administration	6.4	8.6	2.8
	Other Public	28.1	33.6	30.6
		100.0	100.0	100.0
FMG concentration				
	0–25% FMG	11.9	8.8	2.9
	26–50% FMG	9.0	10.1	8.7
	51–75% FMG	11.9	9.5	15.9
	79–99% FMG	34.7	39.2	58.0
	100% FMG	32.5	32.4	14.5
		100.0	100.0	100.0
Medical specialty[a]				
	Surgery	29.7	22.1	12.4
	Medicine	29.1	24.2	31.8
	Ob/Gyn	7.0	5.1	10.5
	Pediatrics	7.8	6.5	19.2
	Psychiatry	5.7	8.4	3.4
	Hospital spec.	14.4	26.3	11.4
	General practice	1.6	3.1	4.0
	Undec/other	4.8	4.4	7.2
Percent base (N)		100.0 (340)[a]	100.0 (273)	100.0 (75)

[a] Percentages are weighted; N is unweighted.

the way medical specialty is related to type of practice than it is of medical specialty in and of itself.

MIGRATION PLANS AND INFORMAL WORK SITUATIONS

Although the formal work situations of leavers and stayers are not markedly different, one can observe striking differences in certain more informal aspects of their work situations.

There were, however, no differences between leavers and stayers with regard to their English abilities. Interviewers' evaluations of the English abilities of FMGs resulted in virtually equal proportions of leavers and stayers being judged to be at each level of English ability indicated in panel 1 of Table 11.8. Interviewees also evaluated their own English difficulties with colleagues (panel 2) and patients (panel 3). Stayers and leavers reported similar levels of problems. This leads one to the conclusion that, although problems with the English language may greatly interfere with many FMGs' abilities to take full advantage of the training opportunities available or to provide medical services easily, problems with English are not a major determinant of FMGs' eventual migration plans.

Stayers and leavers reported marked differences in the types of personal contacts experienced in the United States. These are shown in panels 4–8 of Table 11. 8 and include contact with FMGs from the CME, contact with other FMGs, contact with American MGs, contact with American families, and numbers of American friends. Leavers had more contact with FMGs from the CME and other FMGs than did stayers, and they had less contact with USMGs and American families and had fewer American friends than did stayers. Although the level of contact reported by stayers was far below that reported by USMGs in Table 10.5, stayers are far closer to the USMG pattern than leavers. It cannot be determined whether patterns of social contact influenced the decision to remain or return or if, once this decision has been made, FMGs prepare themselves for their futures by orienting their social plans accordingly. However, it does appear that leavers and stayers demonstrate markedly different social patterns. Leavers have relatively more contact with FMGs, especially those from their country of medical education. Stayers have relatively more contact with American MGs and families and have more American friends than leavers.

Stayers are also more positive than leavers about their experiences in the United States as reported in their evaluation of their personal treatment. They are more likely to report that they are treated better than or the same as USMGs. Once again it is impossible to determine whether these responses indicate that different treatment was important in forming different migration plans or whether these perceptions were altered once migration plans had been made. However, we can safely conclude that there are differences in perceptions among FMGs with different migration plans. Those who are planning to stay in the United States appear to be more readily assimilated into the American social system.

MIGRATION PLANS AND PARTICIPATION IN VOLUNTARY AND PROFESSIONAL ORGANIZATIONS

This also differs markedly between leavers and stayers. Stayers are much more likely than leavers to be members of strictly professional organizations such as the American Medical Association or state medical associations. Here it is easier to infer that, once the migration decision was made, the stayers moved to consolidate a professional base by joining these professional associations. Differences between stayers and leavers are less sharp regarding membership in medical specialty associations and community organizations—organizations that combine professional, educational, and social purposes.

The hypothesis that stayers are simply "joiners" is rejected, because leavers are more likely than stayers to join medical associations for physicians from their country of medical education. FMGs are more likely to belong to this type of organization than any other kind of professional or community organization. There is thus a personal desire to maintain ties with home and the desire to keep all professional options open. Even among stayers, the option of returning home to practice medicine is not a closed alternative. Membership in such an organization makes this option more feasible if it is ever desired.

MIGRATION PLANS AND MEDICAL SKILLS ATTITUDES

Leavers and stayers are also different with respect to their attitudes toward the practice of medicine and the teaching of medical skills. This is shown in Table 11.9.

The first panel of Table 11.9 shows that leavers were more likely than stayers to think that they learned skills appropriate for their country of medical education in the United States. The second panel shows that stayers were more likely than leavers to think that they had learned skills in the United States appropriate for the United States; the third panel

TABLE 11.8   FMG MIGRATION PLANS AND INFORMAL WORK SITUATION

| | | Percentages | | |
		Leavers	Stayers	Undecideds
Interviewer evaluation of FMG English ability				
	Excellent	42.6[a]	43.4	25.1
	Good	37.3	39.0	44.6
	Fair/poor	20.1	17.6	30.3
		100.0	100.0	100.0
English problems with colleagues				
	Yes	49.3	48.2	49.4
	No	50.7	51.8	50.6
		100.0	100.0	100.0
English problems with patients				
	Yes	52.6	49.1	45.6
	No	47.4	50.9	54.4
		100.0	100.0	100.0
Contact with with FMGs from CME				
	Monthly	73.9	67.2	59.9
	< Monthly	26.1	32.8	40.1
		100.0	100.0	100.0
Contact with FMGs				
	Monthly	63.4	51.3	55.3
	< Monthly	36.6	48.7	44.7
		100.0	100.0	100.0
Contact with USMGs				
	Monthly	45.9	52.2	31.4
	< Monthly	54.1	47.8	68.6
		100.0	100.0	100.0
Contact with U.S. families				
	Monthly	58.9	68.1	58.2
	< Monthly	41.1	31.9	41.8
		100.0	100.0	100.0
Number U.S. friends				
	Many or some	46.5	57.4	38.7
	Few or none	53.6	42.6	61.3
		100.1	100.0	100.0

Table 11.8 (*Continued*)

		Percentages		
		Leavers	Stayers	Undecideds
Treatment compared with other FMGs				
	Better	25.3	31.3	27.0
	Same/worse	74.7	68.7	73.0
		100.0	100.0	100.0
Treatment compared with USMGs				
	Better/same	37.6	42.0	38.8
	Worse	62.4	58.0	61.2
		100.0	100.0	100.0
Joined AMA				
	Yes	11.6	24.8	11.0
	No	88.4	75.2	89.0
		100.0	100.0	100.0
Joined state medical association				
	Yes	7.3	18.0	9.7
	No	92.7	82.0	90.3
		100.0	100.0	100.0
Joined medical specialty association				
	Yes	23.7	34.9	23.8
	No	76.3	65.1	76.2
		100.0	100.0	100.0
Joined medical association for CME MDS				
	Yes	36.1	33.3	35.5
	No	63.9	66.7	64.5
		100.0	100.0	100.0
Joined community club(s)				
	Yes	18.1	26.5	19.5
	No	81.9	73.5	80.5
Percent base (N)		100.0 (340)[a]	100.0 (273)	100.0 (75)

[a] Percentages are weighted; N is unweighted.

TABLE 11.9   FMG MIGRATION PLANS AND MEDICAL SKILLS ATTITUDES

	Percentages		
	Leavers	Stayers	Undecideds
Learned skills in U.S. appropriate for Country of Medical Education			
Great extent	55.7[a]	48.0	52.1
Moderate or less	44.3	52.0	47.9
	100.0	100.0	100.0
Learned skills in U.S. appropriate for U.S.			
Great extent	61.7	72.8	65.7
Moderate or less	38.3	27.2	34.3
	100.0	100.0	100.0
Health needs of U.S. and CME are different			
Great extent	54.7	42.6	55.8
Moderate or less	45.3	57.4	44.2
	100.0	100.0	100.0
U.S. training should teach skills relevant to CME			
Great extent	58.1	44.6	60.1
Moderate or less	41.9	55.4	39.9
Percent base (N)	100.0 (340)	100.0 (273)	100.0 (75)

[a] Percentages are weighted; N is unweighted.

shows that leavers were more likely than stayers to indicate a feeling that the health needs of the United States and those of their country of medical education are different; the fourth panel shows that leavers were also more likely than stayers to feel that their American training should have taught them skills relevant to their country of medical education.

Most probably the leavers and stayers had internalized different attitude sets that better prepared them for acting on their respective migration plans. Although leavers' and stayers' migration plans indicate different careers for each group, each is likely to feel that it has learned skills necessary to implement its plans and that its experiences have been consistent with the programs of the educational institutions through which it has moved. Leavers feel that they should have been taught special CME-related skills in the United States, that they have learned such skills, and that the health needs of their country of medical education demand such skills. Stayers feel that they have learned skills appropriate to the United States and do not feel that American training should give special CME-related skills, nor are they as likely to feel that the health needs of the United States and their country of medical education are different.

These attitudes constitute another difference between leavers and stayers. Without a longitudinal design tapping attitudes at different stages of the FMG's career, it is impossible to determine whether leavers and stayers started out with different attitude sets. However, these findings do indicate differences in attitudes between leavers and stayers that are consistent with their eventual migration plans.

MIGRATION PLANS AND CAREER PLANS

The career plans of leavers and stayers differ markedly. Panel 1 of Table 11.10 indicates that stayers are much more likely than leavers to have changed their medical specialty sometime during their careers. Of these, 57 actually stated that they had changed their specialty to get the position they held at the time of the interview (panel 2).

This is a major difference between career patterns of stayers and leavers. Leavers are much more likely singlemindedly to pursue a coherent medical career. They are more likely to stick with one specialty and (as indicated earlier) decide to come to the United States in the normal course of completing their medical education and are more likely to obtain training in higher-prestige teaching institutions. These patterns are consistent with the desire by many leavers to return to a faculty or research position in their home countries; indeed such career pattern may be a condition of returning to such positions.

Stayers, on the other hand, are much more likely to adjust themselves and their careers to new opportunities. This flexibility may be good for the United States health care system, because such FMGs often change specialties to take jobs unfilled by graduates of American medical schools. However, if the distribution of specialties held by foreign medical graduates on arrival in the United States is in any sense a reflection of the health care needs of their countries of medical education, this changing of specialty to adjust to the United States medical system subverts one of the other objectives of the program of having FMGs receive advanced medical training in the United States. The result of their training does not refine skills the FMGs first learned in their CME undergraduate training. Rather, FMGs who have changed their specialties return to their CMEs or stay in the United States, having mastered quite different skills.

A second aspect of FMG career plans is reflected in the way FMGs regard the phenomenon of medical licensure. Panel 3 of Table 11.10

TABLE 11.10   FMG MIGRATION PLANS AND CAREER PLANS

	Leavers	Percentages Stayers	Undecideds
Ever had different specialty?			
Yes	32.6[a]	44.6	28.8
No	67.4	55.4	71.2
	100.0	100.0	100.0
Changed specialty to get current position			
Yes	5.6	13.2	8.1
No	94.4	86.8	91.9
	100.0	100.0	100.0
Has unlimited license			
Yes	21.0	55.5	26.3
No—will take exam	58.5	31.9	61.8
No—won't take exam	14.8	1.3	2.6
No—undecided	5.8	11.3	9.2
	100.0	100.0	100.0
Type of practice preferred			
Med. school faculty	35.4	16.1	11.0
Private practice	30.7	50.3	43.4
Hospital based	17.5	25.6	20.5
Research	8.3	4.0	8.9
Government position	3.4	0.6	4.9
Don't know/other	4.7	3.3	11.2
Percent base (N)	100.0 (340)[a]	100.0 (273)	100.0 (75)

[a] Percentages are weighted; N is unweighted.

indicates that, although stayers are much more likely than leavers to hold an unlimited license at the time of our interview, virtually all the FMGs—both the stayers and leavers—intend to take a medical licensing examination in the United States. Only 8 percent stated that they would not take the examination.

One reason that only 15 percent of the leavers indicate that they will not take a medical licensure examination is that, even though they plan to return to their country of medical education, having an unlimited license to practice medicine in the United States is viewed as a form of career insurance. Although their initial plans are to return to their countries of medical education, they are well aware that at some future time they may wish to return to the United States, either temporarily or permanently, to practice medicine. If they already hold an unlimited license to practice medicine in the United States, such a career would be considerably more feasible. In taking a licensing examination, there is nothing to lose but registration fees, studying time, and a little pride (if one were to fail). On the other hand, there is considerable career flexibility to be gained by passing this exam.

Another reason, curiously, may reflect the socialization aspects of American graduate education. FMGs may take the license because it is the expected "thing to do" at that stage of American graduate education, irrespective of their career expectations.

Panel 4 of Table 11.10 shows a clear divergence in the type of medical practice preferred by leavers and stayers. FMGs planning to take up government positions, to teach on a medical school faculty, or to carry out medical research are more likely to be leavers. FMGs planning to set up private practice or to base their careers in a hospital are much more likely to plan to remain in the United States. These distinctions are by no means absolute. Forty-seven of the stayers indicated an intention to be on a medical school faculty, and 88 of the FMGs planning to return to their CMEs indicated an intention to begin private practice there. Despite these overlaps, the distinction indicated here is one of the most consistent and fundamental between FMGs planning to return to their CMEs and those planning to stay in the United States.

When these data are viewed with the preferences of USMGs, one can see that the stayers prefer a type of practice that bears important similarities to those of USMGs because like the USMGs, they show a marked preference for entering private practice. Also, like the USMGs, approximately one out of every six stayers would prefer to be on the faculty of the medical school (compared to one out of every three leavers). A marked difference is that approximately one out of every four of the stayers plans to enter hospital-based practice, whereas only one out of every 12 of the USMGs plans to have this kind of practice.

We find, then, that stayers do not simply fill in the gaps left by USMGs, nor do they become carbon copies of United States-trained medical graduates. Rather, some are able to carry out medical practices similar to those of their American-trained colleagues, and others do take positions—usually hospital-based positions—that are not filled by American medical graduates or which are more accessible than private practice to FMGs, who are already members of the American hospital network.

CONCLUSIONS

This chapter builds on our previous findings by locating current FMG migration plans in the context of their long-term career plans. The decision to return or remain is in each case an individual decision designed to maximize personal benefit and minimize inconvenience. FMG migration plans continue to change through their medical careers. In Chapter 3 we saw that less than 30 percent of FMGs plan to stay in the United States when they first decide to migrate for advanced medical training; on arrival this figure increases to 33 percent; in this chapter and in our other studies we have learned that during graduate training this figure slowly increases to 75 percent.[11]

Motivations for remaining or returning are similar to those reported for the initial decision to migrate to the United States discussed in Chapter 3. The attraction of United States medical facilities and economic prospects in the United States are the most important reasons for FMGs deciding to remain. Separation from family and friends is the strongest motivation for returning, although a motivation not important in the decision to migrate—feeling a moral obligation to serve one's country—is also a major motivation for FMGs returning to their countries of medical education.

FMGs trained in different nations exhibit a variety of motivational bases for their migration decisions. Those trained in Western cultural areas and nations that offer an attractive professional environment are most likely to return to their countries of medical education. Some FMGs —especially those from non-Western cultural areas who are dissatisfied with political conditions at home—feel caught in a double bind in that they are alienated from United States culture yet see good job prospects here and simultaneously desire to return to their CMEs but see little chance of practicing medicine there in a manner consistent with their career expectations. In assessing the role of FMGs in the American medical system, it is important to ask whether such conflicted motivations affect FMG abilities to fulfill their potential as high quality medical practitioners—but this goes outside the scope of this study.

FMGs who plan to remain in the United States develop stronger links to the mainstream of American culture and medical system. This includes contact with USMGs and American families and informal experiences at work that resemble the experiences of USMGs. Some FMGs who plan to return to their CMEs are relatively more tied to fellow CME FMGs and feel poorly treated at work, others are among the most privileged and satisfied.

Generally differences between leavers and stayers are of degree rather than kind. Although stayers' families are somewhat more privileged, were in somewhat lower-status hospitals, spoke slightly better English, and belonged to more professional organizations, percentage differences rarely exceeded 10 percent.

The manner in which stayers and leavers relate to national and international medical manpower markets is clearer. Stayers were preparing themselves for American medical needs, with more than 75 percent entering private practice and hospital-based medicine. Leavers were most likely to prefer using their advanced training to gain a position on a medical school faculty.

Visas, although limiting free movement among medical manpower markets, were not insurmountable obstacles. More than one-half of the stayers had originally entered the United States with "visitor" status and many adjusted their visa status after arrival in the United States.

Licensing examinations, in addition to certifying medical competence, also functioned as "insurance policies" for FMGs. Whereas virtually all stayers plan to take these examinations, substantial proportions of leavers also had such plans. Holding a medical license makes returning to the United States a more viable future option.

To the extent that it is useful to "type" leavers and stayers, we suspect that there are two major subgroups of each. Among leavers we could identify a relatively high-status group whose plans to come to the United States and return home are consistent with a long-term coherent career strategy, and a second less-privileged group of FMGs who return home more from a sense of moral obligation rather than because of long-developed plans. This second group is not able to rely heavily on personal ties to help advance their careers either in the United States or in their CMEs. Among stayers, one group is more drawn by the attractions of American culture, material well-being, and the American medical system; another group resists strong desires to return home due to fears of being unable to practice medicine at a level equal to expectations generated in medical school and in the United States.

NOTES

1. Since less than 3 percent of our sample indicated plans to migrate to a third country, this alternative is not extensively discussed.
2. The responses in this chapter are "weighted" to allow generalization to the population of interns and residents in American hospitals in 1974. However, responses such as these, given during advanced training, should not be used as an indicator that between 70 and 75 percent of a given FMG cohort can be found in the United States up to 8 years after completing their postgraduate training. (See Haug and Stevens, *op. cit.* and Stevens, Goodman, and Mick, "What Happens to Foreign Trained Doctors Who Come to the United States?" *op. cit.*). A major point of this chapter is that career and personal situations affect migration plans throughout the FMG's career. The experiences of other cohorts of FMGs and the suggestion in Table 11.6 that the longer an FMG stays in the United States, the greater the probability that he or she plans to remain indicate that the 47.2 percent of our sample who reported plans to leave the United States is a substantial overestimation and will probably decrease over time.

3. These 10 motivations for staying and the nine reported for leaving are the entire set of motivations explicitly queried in the questionnaire. We do not attempt to use them to construct scales of migration motivations. Rather, they are the responses most frequently cited in our field studies and pretests.

4. This parallel is all the more understandable because many Argentine FMGs are first-generation children of European migrants to Argentina.

5. Robert F. Winch, *The Modern Family*, New York: Holt, Rinehart and Winston, 1971, Chapter 8. We recognize that, although this single measure is incomplete, it is substantially useful to assume for the purpose of this analysis that FMGs whose fathers have completed college or professional school are of higher status than FMGs whose fathers only completed secondary school or part of college, and that these, in turn, are of a higher social status than FMGs whose fathers have only had some secondary school education or less.

6. This interpretation underlines our feeling that FMGs vary markedly in their abilities to relate to an international network of medical practitioners. Some FMGs (and some USMGs) can formulate careers that routinely transcend national borders. The opportunities of others are more limited. Rather than choosing between choice posts in their country of medical education and choice posts in the United States, their decision may be between choice posts in the United States and mediocre posts in their country of medical education or mediocre posts in one or both locales. The social status of the FMG, as described by his family of orientation, is an important factor in explaining such variation. This is discussed further in Chapter 12.

7. See Haug and Stevens, and Stevens, Goodman, and Mick, *op. cit.*

8. Alejandro Portes, *op. cit.*

9. This reflects the pattern of visa adjustment discussed in Rosemary Stevens, Louis Wolf Goodman, Stephen S. Mick, and June Darge, "Physician Migration Reexamined," *Science*, October 31, 1975.

10. One consequence of American adjustment is that a kind of double counting inadvertently goes on because of migration and naturalization service procedures that count FMGs as entering the United States both when they originally come on exchange visitor visas and when they adjust their visas from visitor to permanent resident status. In the last 10 years this has resulted in the overcounting of approximately 15,000 physicians. This casts substantial doubt on many statistics that indicate precise numbers of foreign physicians in the United States.

11. See Stevens, Goodman, and Mick, *op. cit.*

12

CONCLUSIONS AND
POLICY INTERPRETATIONS

We have followed the migrant physicians from their backgrounds in their countries of origin and education, through medical school and (for many) other medical experiences abroad, to the decision to come to the United States, the way in which this was carried out, and their subsequent experiences in the United States and its health care system; finally, we have examined the FMG's career expectations. In each chapter we developed our conclusions on the nature of physician migration for different career stages and the range of experiences of individual physicians. In this final chapter we look at the implications of our conclusions for the health manpower policy questions and the intellectual questions regarding migration and the structure of occupations in the United States that motivated this study of the migration of physicians.

What have we learned about the process of migration of physicians that is of interest to policy debates? What role do FMGs play in the American hospital system? What myths and stereotypes do our findings confirm or repudiate? How do our findings affect the way we think about elite migration and the structure of occupations in the United States? What areas for change are suggested and/or possible?

PHYSICIANS AS MIGRANTS

Our study shows FMGs to be cautious, perhaps unrealstic, but resourceful migrants. Drawn from privileged groups in their own nations—the product of elite education in major cities—the individual physician feels equipped with readily transportable international skills. There is some naiveté attached to the assumption that medicine is a body of techniques and that the foreign physician seeking specialization will fall neatly into a system of American training that is only partly designed to impart such skills. Given the lack of information available to FMGs about American medicine and the problems of adjustment to American life, FMGs cope with considerable finesse.

From the beginning, the FMG is faced with double binds, conflicts, and uncertainties. It is difficult for these young physicians, most of whom have never lived abroad before, to anticipate the nature of medical education in the United States. American physicians going abroad would have similar difficulties. The confidence instilled by their relatively privileged social backgrounds may encourage physicians to see themselves as part of an international medical elite, part of a worldwide society of physicians. For most, however, privilege breaks down on coming to the United States because of the tenuous ties through which they are recruited for their positions as interns or residents. Few are recruited by American institutions identifying them as individuals and showing interest in their qualifications; few go under the protective umbrella of professional arrangements between an American university and a sponsoring agency in their own country; rather, the great majority make their own arrangements for American training through friends who are or have been in the United States for similar training, or through writing blind letters to unfamiliar hospitals listed in AMA or state directories.

The decision to come to the United States is not always crystal clear: a double bind is apparent in the constant weighing of opportunities in the home country with those in the United States. Such tensions are compounded by the system of entry for FMGs for training in American hospitals. Some enter in the classic pattern of earlier immigrants; they join friends who have already begun to unravel the mysteries of the American system and are steered to jobs known to be available. Others take their chances through a battery of letters, accepting whatever job is offered. In both cases, the physician enters as a supplicant and as an employee rather than as a graduate student. Jobs are available because they have not been filled by American physicians. At the point of entry to the United States, the physician becomes the "FMG," filling a residual role in the American system.

The various roles of an FMG—international professional jet setter, lowly exchange student, provider of medical services, recipient of post-doctoral education, immigrant seeking to "make it" in the United States, alien regarded as a "less-than-full" physician—create for these migrants a confusing array of images. We have shown that physicians come to the United States primarily for advanced training. In so doing, they seek to maximize individual career opportunities. However, in coming to the United States their professional context shifts. It is one thing to maximize career opportunities in the long term: for example, by justifying 5 years of training in an average or relatively non-prestigious American hospital as a means of gaining certification in a specialty, thereby enhancing opportunities for private practice and teaching on return to one's home country. It is another matter entirely to find oneself, in the short term, as "low man or woman" in the pecking order of physicians in the United States.

Generally, FMGs, being human, seek "occupational realization" with respect both to long-term and short-term career aspirations. Once in the United States, the FMG conforms to the professional culture of American medicine and accepts its norms as given. Those able to do so rise in the system; they seek jobs in university units, complex research-oriented institutions, other institutions highly regarded by USMGs and more senior FMGs. Those FMGs not able to rise tend to be unhappy with their status, if not with the technical aspects of training. At the same time, their self-image as advanced medical students subtly changes. FMGs in the United States measure themselves against USMGs rather than against their counterparts in their country of training. This comparison is painful for FMGs not merely because of differences in training, but more important, it is painful to the extent that a given FMG's cultural background differs from those of USMGs.

The apprenticeship nature of American graduate education reinforces this situation. Rewards and punishments of American training in the hospital reaffirm the American way as the only way of doing things. The FMG learns that previous experience is irrelevant and that technical competence alone is insufficient. To succeed, the FMG must act like an American physician and be accepted as an equal. In acquiring the necessary cultural competence to become accepted, the physician becomes de facto an American physician. It is not surprising, from only this aspect of the process of socialization, that the longer an FMG stays in the United States the more likely he or she will report a desire to remain here.

Yet ambiguities and uncertainties are also present. Many FMGs enter the United States reluctantly, with deep concerns about the American way of life, as well as with lack of knowledge of American social and professional customs. During their time in the United States, many of these physicians continue to be ambivalent about American life and their roles in it. Those who are clearest in their minds about whether they will stay in the United States (thus accepting their role as immigrants) and those who will definitely leave (accepting a role as international students) experience the least uncertainty. Our studies show, however, that relatively few FMGs have clear-cut career migration goals when they decide to come to the United States. Rather, the decision to stay in the United States or to leave is constantly reassessed. In terms of developing policies for physician education and training it is significant that the FMGs' experiences by the time of our study made the tendency to stay (including those who are undecided) outweigh the tendency to leave.

"AMERICANIZATION" AND INTERNATIONAL EXCHANGE

In looking at migration as a process, one must examine the various professional contexts of medicine the FMG experiences. The foreign physician is exposed to three such contexts concurrently: (1) the professional system of the home country, (2) the international context assumed in seeking to migrate, and (3) the professional system of the United States. Our findings suggest that the FMG retains relatively few ties with the professional system of the home country once he is in the United States. Migration is largely a matter of personal initiative.

Many FMGs have strong ties to fellow nationals in the United States. However, these are established because of social affinity and are not often a means of linking physicians to their societies at home. Such ties, and ties with established ethnic and cultural groups in the United States, may in fact have the opposite effect, reinforcing the FMG's tendency to stay. Our findings on the social interactions of FMGs with fellow nationals suggest that FMGs make their career decisions first and bolster or rationalize them by their subsequent behavior.

The international context of medical practice may seem glamorous and legitimate to the physician considering a period of study in the United States. In many countries, American training has a definite cachet. However, although the international context may seem a real one from the point of view of the physician in the home country, it vanishes once he or she is in the United States.

It may be unfair to call the American medical profession ethnocentric, but it is not entirely inaccurate. Perhaps because American medicine is regarded as the best in the world by most domestic practitioners (as both the USMGs and FMGs in our study attest), or perhaps because few American physicians have been extensively exposed to health conditions abroad, there is little awareness in the professional milieu of the activity of medical professions anywhere else. Moreover, it follows that if American medicine is "best," medicine elsewhere must be "worse." By being foreign in the United States, the FMG can claim no benefit as an "internationalist." Quite the reverse: the FMG is automatically disadvantaged in the American system. The American professional culture thus remains as the dominant context for FMGs once they have embarked on American training, and the FMG is stigmatized by this positioning.

It should be stressed, however, that this situation is neither inevitable nor immutable. One obvious implication of the migration process as we describe it is the potential for significantly relating to the other two contexts of professional decision making. The training of foreign physicians could be regarded in the United States as an international responsibility. If exchange visitors were recruited to, and taught in, international teaching centers of acknowledged eminence, those FMGs could develop their image (as well as their skills) as members of an international medical elite. Potential teachers and research workers, in particular, might be drawn to fellowships in university centers, where their particular interests and needs might be met. Although such fellowships would be possible for relatively few of the thousands of FMGs who seek to come to the United States each year, the very existence of such programs would provide a focus for international medical education and goals for foreign physicians that were clearly specified in program entry. The individual would know, quite clearly, whether the program he or she was to enter was an international fellowship or an American graduate apprenticeship.

Our findings lead us to conclude that the latter is inappropriate preparation for potential medical school teachers, particularly when the apprenticeship is taken outside major university centers, as is true for the majority of FMGs. Moreover, the apprenticeship requires foreign physicians to relinquish the norms of their own system to an unreasonable extent, assuming that the reasonable expectation is international exchange.

Recognized university fellowship programs could impart technical, specialized knowledge to a group of acknowledged ability drawn from all over the world *without* requiring immersion into American residencies. The international flavor of this enterprise would also be enhanced if it were also open to American students and if portions of the training took place in foreign medical schools in which students could be exposed to different forms of training and different health conditions.

Reinforcement of the professional context of the CME might also be undertaken by a more directive role by foreign governments and medical schools in organizing American training for graduates from their schools.

Linking agreements between the United States and foreign institutions, for example, could develop special foci for the training of nationals from special countries in the United States. The United States Immigration and Naturalization Service might only grant exchange visitor visas contingent on sponsorship of the visitor by foreign governments, schools, or another recognized agency—somewhat of an extension of current provisions, even as revised under recent law (P.L.94–484).

Such suggestions are not new, nor is it appropriate to dwell on them here. Furthermore, they do not begin to touch on problems of the organization of health care and the rural-urban maldistribution of medical and other resources that characterize most of the world's nations. Our conclusions lead us, however, to raise these limited considerations as potential policy implications arising from our findings. If, indeed, the various roles of FMGs are to be unraveled, it is logical to suggest a system of training in the United States that distinguishes the roles of international experts, exchange students, and immigrants.

As a device for the incorporation of immigrants into American society, it should be remarked that the hospital residency program appears to work relatively well. Foreign physicians are no more disadvantaged than any other group of immigrants, whose classic pattern of entry has been through relatively lowly jobs and whose classic success story has been one of upward social mobility. As a program designed to socialize physicians into American medicine half-way through their professional careers, the residency may indeed be an ideal portal of entry into American medicine and society—assuming permanent immigration is the goal.

We conclude, in short, that the functions of international exchange and immigration demand clearly defined organizational responses from American medical institutions. International exchange students should be taught in university centers which are internationally renowned or—at the very least—are sensitive to other countries' cultures and needs. Prospective immigrants, on the other hand, expecting to remain in the United States as hospital employees or private practitioners, are more appropriately placed in traditional American residency positions for rapid socialization as American physicians.

THE NEED FOR BETTER INFORMATION

This study suggests that many of the individual problems of the FMG arise because there is a single, undifferentiated training system and because FMGs are expected to make their way through this system unaided. The resulting migration patterns thus have little organizational rationality. For example, one physician coming for advanced training to return home a teacher may train in a community hospital with a superb capacity to teach American private practitioners; another, expecting to become an American private practitioner, may receive training with a strong research emphasis.

A system of training that differentiates among career paths could help individuals decide on their American hospital of training and even whether to come to the United States. Better information, particularly about the variety of opportunities offered in the United States and a hospital's expectations of foreign house staff, might also serve to stem some bitterness from unfulfilled expectations. The United States government or professional agencies, such as the Educational Commission for Foreign Medical Graduates, could aid foreign physicians through films and other materials on American training, offered by the U.S. Information Service and/or ECFMG examination centers.

That FMGs might benefit from better information is indicated not only by our findings of the inadequacy of information now available—in areas such as type and nature of hospital affiliation, opportunities, duties, and work expectations—but also by what we learned about the resourceful use by FMGs of those sources that are available, including medical school professors, physicians with American experience, and medical directors. It should not be surprising that physicians who have grown up in major cities throughout the world, in families that are largely professional, should cope well with the various "systems" that confront them in the process of migration.

However, we question whether the complexity of these systems is really necessary. Some foreign physicians may benefit by being able to manipulate the disorganized processes of examinations, visas, and job acquisition. If the primary purpose of migration from the American point of view is to encourage the survival of the fittest—fitness being defined as the ability to play the system—this process may be all to the good; but the Darwininian ethic is an odd criterion for international educational exchange. Our findings suggest that there is considerable mismatching of talents and interests between foreign physicians and American training opportunities. Moreover, some who migrate may benefit less from their American experience than others who consider migrating but never get here. Better information about job opportunities and training expectations, including variations among different types of American programs, would assist not only the many thousands of physicians throughout the world who consider coming to the United States, but also the American hospital system.

PRESSURE POINTS FOR CHANGE IN THE PROCESS OF MIGRATION

On the face of it the major United States visa programs appear to work roughly as intended at the point of access to the United States. Younger physicians still in training enter largely on exchange visas and older practitioners as immigrants. However, these distinctions break down after arrival. FMGs are adept players of the "visa game." A majority of FMGs in internships and residencies in the United States in 1974 had arrived initially on exchange visitor visas. At the time of the survey, most had changed to permanent resident (immigrant) visas and had gained the freedom to remain in the United States and to work indefinitely.

If there had been no opportunities for adjustment of visa status in our sample, only about 30 percent of the FMGs would have had the opportunity to stay permanently in the United States to work, compared to the 50 percent who said they wanted to stay or were undecided about staying beyond their period of training, and the 70 percent who will probably stay, should future visa arrangements allow them to do so. In permitting FMGs to stay, the American visa system has tacitly recognized most FMGs as immigrants irrespective of their initial visa status. This lack of clarity has certainly allowed FMGs to exercise initiative. At the same time, it has added to other confusions by not differentiating the roles of (1) exchange student and (2) immigrant expecting permanent residence. The lack of clarity in the training system has thus been reinforced by a lack of purpose in visa regulation.

We have noted, too, that there is no clear channeling of FMGs into different types of training programs according to initial visa status. Physicians coming into the United States as "exchange visitors" have entered hospitals affiliated with universities as well as hospitals without a university connection. There has been no overall supervision of training opportunities—not even simple evaluations in specific areas—to test how far the intentions of international exchange programs are in fact being met. Such activities are suggested because, as our data show, American training programs are not geared to the general health needs of other nations—particularly those of less developed countries. A listing of CME needs by our FMG respondents put administration, nutrition, communicable disease control, and maternal and child health services at the top of the list. These are not primary subjects for American graduate medical education.

The question is raised as to why the United States offers a large exchange visitor visa program—through which 4717 physicians entered the United States in 1974 and 2849 in 1975[1]—when the value of the program is unclear for the nations that supposedly benefit. In any event, our findings indicate that FMGs, aware of this discrepancy, shift when they can from exchange visitor visa status, thus enlarging their career options. Taking an American licensure examination provides a further basis for enabling the FMG to stay in the United States should this alternative prove desirable.

Besides gaining a visa, the prospective migrant must pass a qualifying examination. We have shown that this presented little difficulty to the FMGs who were interns and residents in 1974, although it may have provided an effective screen for others. Not only did most of our sample pass the ECFMG examination on their first attempt, but a substantial minority (one-seventh) gambled and entered the United States without their ECFMG examination, passing it after arrival. The ECFMG thus provides another games-playing situation, which, although troublesome for the 60 to 70 percent of the test takers who fail each sitting, constitutes a minor barrier for those who actually come to the United States.

A third barrier for prospective entrants is entry to the American hospital system—finding the first American job. Again, we have shown that FMGs cope as best they can with the limitations built into the system. The same process of weighing the options applies as in other aspects of migration. FMGs draw on all information available to them, from friends, relatives, professional acquaintances, and publications to gain their first appointment in an American hospital.

Among the array of decisions and barriers, there are two factors critical to the process of migration: the decision to come, which we have explained in terms of enhancing individual career opportunities, and success at arriving in the United States. The decision to come is largely voluntary, a reflection of the "new" professional migration. In one way or another, the foreign physician expects greater benefits from coming to the United States than from the professional opportunities for which training may have been received in the country of medical education.

The simple fact of arrival in the United States is more important than holding the ECFMG certificate, having a temporary visa, or coming to an appropriate job. Once here, the FMG is able to cope with situations to a greater or lesser extent. Indeed, for many FMGs migration continues while in the United States. A substantial minority of FMGs "play the American hospital system" and move from job to job in an upwardly mobile progression. Typically, as we have seen, the physician moves from one hospital to another in the same state and then moves to a more prestigious hospital elsewhere (although usually within the Northeast and Great Lakes states).

In terms of the policy implications arising from our findings on migration per se, the two essential "pressure points" are (1) influence over decisions to come and (2) influence over arrival in the United States. We have shown that the decision to come is arrived at after a complex balance of considerations in the home country and the United States. It is thus not easily influenced by change in any one of these: for example, by the introduction of financial bonds that must be posted before the physician can leave a country or reports of riots in the United States. *Perhaps nothing short of massive changes in the health and education systems of individual countries and changes in opportunities in the United States would affect the decisions of individuals to come to the United States to any major extent.*

The fact of FMG arrival in this country is, however, directly susceptible to decisions taken by the government of the United States and in the hospital market place. Our findings suggest that the changes in examination procedures for FMGs which are now being developed—the development of a new test to replace the ECFMG examination, to make a more challenging screen of technical knowledge and raising the standards of English proficiency—will prove to be relatively unimportant as a device to control (i.e., limit) the flow of new migrants. FMGs who come to the United States are self-selected; they should be able to cope quite well with more stringent requirements. Changes in United States visa regulations or restrictions on job opportunities are, however, critical to migration. Restrictions in immigration laws and a tightening of the job market suggest a steady decline in the number of new entrants.

With this decline the nature of the "system of entry" for FMGs, as we have described it, becomes all-important. What purpose *ought* FMG training to have in the United States? How should FMGs be trained?

FMGS IN THE AMERICAN HEALTH CARE SYSTEM

Our findings have shown that many FMGs enter the American system into training settings that are educationally, professionally, and organizationally different from those entered by most USMGs. The typical location of training for USMGs is major university teaching units. Most FMGs enter American training outside the major teaching units, in community hospitals with or without university affiliation. FMGs tend to enter smaller hospitals with fewer residency programs and less research emphasis than do USMGs. Moreover, the FMG typically enters a hospital in which the majority of the house staff are FMGs.

These distinctive patterns of entry into graduate medical education have some important implications. First, we have observed that, as manpower for American hospitals, FMGs serve as a strategic reserve. Their presence gives USMGs more flexibility in choosing jobs because they fill less desirable hospital house staff positions. For example, from 1972 to 1975, 44,269 physicians graduated from American medical schools.[2] Since the average length of graduate training is 4 years, these 44,269 USMGs should have been filling available internships and residency positions for 1975–1976. In fact, 68,122 positions were available.

American and Canadian graduates filled 65 percent of the available internships and residencies in 1974–1975. Thus over one-third of all positions were available for the employment of FMGs.

USMGs took first "pick," drawn to university hospitals and certain states. As a result, there were few jobs for foreigners in California (to take a major example) and relatively large numbers in New York. Thus the proportions of USMGs and FMGs in house staff jobs varies greatly among states and among types of hospital. In nonaffiliated hospitals, in particular, only one-third of available jobs were filled by graduates of American medical schools.

The presence of FMGs camouflages the decision-making effects of USMGs. If there were no FMGs and the existing system of allocating USMGs remained unchanged, states such as New York, Illinois, New Jersey, and Michigan would have critically large numbers of vacant positions. What would probably happen is that these states would insist on some kind of national "rationing" of house staff positions, so that USMGs were distributed more equally across the whole country. (This process is already becoming evident.) The availability of FMGs has delayed any such considerations, despite the fact that FMGs filled only 18,131 of the 23,855 positions not filled by USMGs in 1974–1975, leaving 5724 vacant.

It should be observed, however, that the number of American graduates is predicted to increase by more than 20 percent to 15,512 by 1981. This will make it difficult for all USMGs to count on the luxury of relatively unfettered residency choice, either of specialty or location. Unless the number of residencies is expanded, which seems unlikely given recent statements by organizations such as the AAMC[3] (but which is not supported by recent AMA statistics), USMGs will begin to replace FMGs in less "favored" institutions and states. The fact that the demand for FMGs as a strategic reserve is beginning to disappear is an important consideration in setting FMG immigration policy.

As the demand for FMGs decreases substantially, more USMGs will find themselves training in community hospitals, taught by private practitioners, in an educational milieu quite different from that in major teaching units—at least as it has been developed for the teaching of FMGs. Questions will inevitably be raised as to the nature of postgraduate training for USMGs. Our distinctions between the "assistantship" model of apprenticeship in community hospitals and the "bureaucratic" model of university teaching services deserve careful and continuing scrutiny as the balance shifts in the number of USMGs and FMGs. USMGs may be unwilling to accept the lesser degree of clinical responsibility we have observed for FMGs—and private practitioners unwilling to concede greater clinical autonomy to their house staff. Some clashes between house staff and attending physicians, avoided by the tacit acceptance of FMGs as "less-than-full" physicians, may flare up in such hospitals in the future. More generally, as USMGs take over positions previously held by FMGs, USMGs as a group will experience a much greater variation in training settings than has been true up to this point.

The role of the FMG as a "less-than-full" physician also deserves consideration. From the standpoint of the stratification of the medical profession, it has been convenient not to consider FMGs as being in any way interchangable with USMGs. Impressionistic criticisms of the poor English-speaking ability of FMGs and inferior competence have been useful devices to "place" FMGs as a group, in a distinct— inferior—category to USMGs. As long as FMGs are regarded as outsiders, their place in the American system in these least prestigious positions with relatively less responsibility can be rationalized. The "less-than-full" physician concept thus reinforces other tendencies to stratify postgraduate American medical training and place FMGs in less desirable positions.

We see, in effect, two related processes. In one the FMGs form a supposedly temporary strategic reserve to be drawn on in the absence of American practitioners. In the other, the role of the FMG in the system is that of the classic immigrant, taking available jobs and receiving the stigma of a "different" status. Problems arise because these two processes do not mesh perfectly. FMGs are not merely immigrants nor merely a strategic temporary reserve. Indeed, properly categorizing FMGs is a serious problem for the staff of hospitals to which they come.

There is thus a confusion of roles among FMGs themselves and a confusion of perceptions of the "FMG role" in the American hospital system. Moreover, the various ways of categorizing the FMG continue to mold FMGs' careers. Some FMGs behave in the American system as successful immigrants (this is most likely for those culturally most like American natives), but the majority continue their training outside major teaching units. All house staff, USMG and FMG, consider FMGs to be treated less well than USMGs. FMGs feel, in addition, that their primary immediate organizational purpose is to provide support and staff services for American hospitals.

CONTRIBUTIONS OF FMGS

Clearly, FMGs make substantial contributions to American hospitals, in some specialties more than others. Our data show FMGs in their first position in 1974 to be only half as likely to enter the medical specialties as USMGs and twice as likely to enter surgical fields. They also entered hospital-based fields, general/family practice, pediatrics, and obstetrics at a higher rate than USMGs. We have also shown some willingness among FMGs to change specialty fields. With the powerful lure of a job, it would seem then that the United States is attracting FMGs disproportionately into some fields and perhaps discouraging them from entering others. FMGs in the hospital-based fields of anesthesiology, pathology, and radiology were most likely to enter training in major teaching units, probably because these fields are relatively unpopular among USMGs.

The major contributions of FMG interns and residents are in in-patient support services, with relatively little contribution to out-patient and emergency services. Thus 90 percent of the FMGs were on in-patient assignments at the time of survey, with 10 percent doing ambulatory work. Virtually none of those on in-patient services had additional out-patient responsibilities.

Whatever the solution, the contributions of FMGs are large. In 1974–1975, there were 18,131 FMGs in house staff positions in the United States, of whom 15,181 were in affiliated hospitals and 2934 in non-affiliated programs. Assuming that FMGs earn their pay, they contributed approximately $250,000,000 of services to the American health care system in 1974–1975.

FMGs perform somewhat different functions in different types of hospitals. The key functions in all types are what we call maintenance of hospital activities (admissions, coverage at nights and weekends, routine patient care, out-patient decisions). FMGs in university settings are, however, often called on to exercise judgments in the areas of socio-cultural responsibility (discharge planning, discussion with patient relatives, access to patients, socioeconomic data), in supervising staff and teaching, and in the areas of delegated responsibility. However, in all types of hospital FMGs are given (or take) less responsibility for exercising *clinical judgment* and for negotiating with patients and their relatives: two important aspects of graduate medical education. We conclude that while the technical competence of FMGs is recognized and utilized by their superiors, there is reluctance to admit to their cultural abilities. Because FMGs are treated differently from American citizens (USMGs and USFMGs), their functions in the hospital are different.

Several important policy implications arise from our findings on the functions of FMGs in different hospital settings. First, it should be stressed that although there are important differences in FMG responsibility among categories of hospital affiliation, these are not, as is often assumed, between the "affiliated" and the "nonaffiliated" hospitals. The most important differences in FMG responsibility are between major teaching units and those with second-level university affiliation, that is, hospitals with "limited affiliation."

Second, it should be noted that many FMGs in major teaching units are those with the most experience in the American health care system. Our findings on the mobility of FMGs in American hospitals show that nonaffiliated hospitals have acted as "buffers" or "sorters" of new entrants. After a period of time the more talented and culturally competent FMGs move to more desirable locations. Major teaching units benefit from this process; other hospitals perform a screening function for FMG access to the American system.

FMGs in hospitals at any given point are not all necessarily at the same stage of their careers. Moreover, at least to some extent, the "entry" hospitals experience a double disadvantage as training institutions: they must initiate a continuous influx of new physicians into the American system, while maintaining the least talented, ambitious, or socially adaptable members of each cohort. This different training milieu and the different culture of community hospitals give FMGs who remain in such units not only a different training (one that, we argue, is less complete than that available to USMGs or to FMGs in major teaching units) but also different career expectations. FMGs trained by American private practitioners are more likely to follow their role models into private practice.

At the same time, the hospitals act to depress FMG expectations of success in the American professional system. There is a self-fulfilling prophecy in these events. For a combination of reasons, and in different ways, FMGs are expected to be different from USMGs; their experiences ensure that these differences exist. It should be observed, then, that (1) FMGs and USMGs in American training are not directly comparable in terms of their contributions to and benefits from the American experience; (2) differences do exist between FMGs in major teaching units and those in other types of institutions; (3) USMGs and FMGs play different roles and have different duties even in similar types of institution; (4) at least part—or perhaps most—of these differences are attributable to factors in the American health care system.

The role of the "entry hospital" should also be noted as an important element for socializing new FMGs. As nonaffiliated programs are given affiliation and/or are reduced in number, these "buffer" functions will have to be performed increasingly by affiliated units that have so far been protected from a less sophisticated and less homogeneous group of graduate entrants. The screening process of entry hospitals—effectively, the breaking-in of new recruits—deserves much more attention than has been given.

ON MYTHS AND MYTH MAKING

Our study calls to question a number of myths about foreign medical graduates. One issue that has been rife with premature statements are attributions of incompetence to foreign-trained physicians practicing medicine in the United States.

In other studies we found that the relationship between licensure and competence is problematic and complex.[4] Here we stress that perceived competence is the product of two types of competence. We show that it is important to distinguish cultural from technical competence. It is widely recognized in the literature that foreign-trained physicians usually have some difficulties adjusting to American culture and that for those trained in languages other than English the difficulties are particularly serious. Our studies indicate the importance of separating these variables and, if one hopes to work a solution that improves the quality of training received by FMGs and the quality of services they provide, the necessity for devising effective institutions for orienting FMGs to American culture—including orientation to the American medical care system.

Our studies indicate that foreign-trained physicians have substantially more clinical experience than is normally attributed to them in the literature. It is noted that in many of their formal school experiences very little clinical experience is built in. However, many of the foreign medical graduates in our sample have had substantial amounts of clinical experience between graduation from medical school and their assumption of positions in the United States. This background overlooked by senior American physicians in assigning duties to FMGs.

Another myth our study calls to question is that foreign-trained physicians are vastly overworked in the United States. We found that USMGs report somewhat longer hours of work per week and greater numbers of patients seen. However, our data do indicate substantial differences in informal experiences in the hospital, with USMGs treated more as "full physicians" with fuller interactions with non-FMG peers and superiors. It follows that it is important to focus on informal relations if improvements are to be worked in the quality of FMGs' training experiences and provision of medical services. At the practical level this means deliberate encouragement of discussions and consultations between American physicians and FMGs, designed to overcome the barriers of shyness, embarrassment, ignorance, and hostility that too often exist on both sides of the fence.

Another finding challenges the myth that most FMGs intend to stay in the United States when they first arrive here. Rather, a change in intention happens gradually throughout the FMG's experience in the United States related to changes in perceptions and knowledge about situations in the United States and in home countries, and is intimately related to FMG career decisions and their attempts to minimize discomfort and maximize personal benefit throughout their careers. From the point of view of theory, if social scientists desire better to understand the process of migration, it is important to abandon the traditionally used push-pull models that focus on characteristics of nations and predict migration behavior on that basis, and to develop models that are based on career patterns and predict migratory behavior as functions of career choices of migrants such as FMGs.

A further finding that contradicts a myth is the urban background and elite status of FMGs who come to the United States. Although our study only examines FMGs who did come to the United States, and we cannot make comparisons with nonmigrants, FMGs who come to the United States are almost entirely from major cities and they claim to be drawn from the highest ranks in their medical school classes. FMGs are physicians seeking specialist status, and it is unrealistic to expect them to seek primary practice in American rural areas. Like USMGs, their backgrounds have prepared them for practice in major cities.

Examination of Immigration and Naturalization Service data for physician migration from 1965 to 1973 uncovered some additional myths about FMG migration to the United States.[5] The data indicated that the pace of FMG migration did not increase markedly during that period, as is often reported by professional associations through the use of unadjusted INS data. In addition, proper examination of the data showed that the regional composition of migrants did not change over this period.

We found that the Immigration and Naturalization Service, in counting new entries to the United States, counted FMGs twice if they entered on an exchange visitor visa and switched, at a later date, to a permanent resident visa. Since this practice occurred with increasing frequency after the 1965 change in the immigration law, double counting rather than increased migration has accounted for the apparent but artifactual rise in migration reported through the 1970s. When the data are properly adjusted, the high year for migration of FMGs to the United States is 1968, with migration levels remaining relatively constant through 1975.

Furthermore, when proper adjustment is made, the proportion of migrants trained in European countries remains constant during that period, as does the portion of migrants trained in Asian countries. (Unadjusted data had indicated that the proportion of European migrants has declined whereas the proportion of Asian migrants has increased.)

Thus through analysis of Immigration and Naturalization Service data we were able to learn that the allegations of (1) a rapid increase in the pace of FMG migration, (2) rapid increases in the percentage of Asian migrants, and (3) a corresponding decline in Western European migrants were incorrect.

At least in these areas there are substantial misunderstandings about the process of migration and the role of foreign medical graduates in the American medical system. One might attribute this situation to difficulties of obtaining accurate information and communication breakdowns. Myths are, however, often useful devices. We argue, rather, that these misunderstandings have their origin in the role of foreign medical graduates within the structure of the American system. Foreign medical graduates basically fill gaps in existing American medical manpower needs. The substantial medical migrations of recent years are a result of the fact that there is a high demand for physicians in American hospitals. However, these physicians are channelled into specialties, hospitals, and states that American-trained physicians are less desirous of filling. To establish mechanisms of social control that allow for this kind of stratification, a complex process of "stigmatization" must take place. The stereotype of the foreign-trained physician who goes to great lengths to study in the United States and who practices substandard medicine fits very well with the need to place FMGs in permanent positions less desired by American-trained physicians. The stereotypes contribute to an ideology that makes it easy to continue to use FMGs as a buffer and to place them in less desired situations in the American medical manpower market or to discontinue their use entirely on grounds of "quality" when the supply of American graduates changes, as it is now promising to do.

These findings are not particularly surprising within the general study of immigration.[6] A host country usually has substantial "reasons" for allowing immigration, and migrants are often used very purposefully by the society they enter. We stress, however, that FMGs see themselves as both "immigrants" and "exchange students"; some one, some the other, and some, uneasily, both. Much of the complaining by FMGs over treatment in and by the American system derives from these FMGs, conflicting perceptions, paired with the American health care system viewing FMGs predominantly as a strategic manpower reserve.

In terms of policy-making, however, it is important that the myths be recognized for what they are: *as myths*. Much of what is generally claimed about FMGs is patently untrue.

WAYS OF THINKING ABOUT PHYSICIAN MIGRATION: IMPLICATIONS FOR SOCIAL SCIENCE THEORY

The research reported in the preceding chapters has approached the subject of physician migration in a somewhat heterodoxical manner. Although largely based on aggregated survey data, it attempts to reflect the experiences of the migrants as individuals, casting their experiences and decisions within the context of their medical careers. This perspective has a bearing on both the attribution of causes of physician migration and the concepts useful for analyzing the phenomenon. This approach highlights the shortcomings of the commonly used "push-pull" model of migration. Studies that contrast factors in one locale "pushing" a migrant to those in another locale "pulling" him or her are more useful for characterizing these locales than for understanding how migration decisions reflect the career and family situations of migrants. "Push-pull" theories are not useless, but they must be complemented by an analysis of the decisional processes of the individual actors if a migration process is to be satisfactorally understood. Its most basic limitation is that, used alone, the "push-pull" model suggests that societal forces operating on a collective level are reproduced in the decision processes of individuals. To clarify the migration decisions of individuals, the analytic focus must be on personal and career choices.

Physician migration exhibits interesting similarities and differences compared to the migration of other groups. Apart from the "international jet set" and their peregrinations, physicians are the most privileged contemporary international migrants. This elite migration is of particular interest because more data are routinely collected for this group than for migrants in other social strata. Furthermore, migration for physicians is less likely to be disruptive of personal plans than for individuals pursuing other occupational lines. The high demand for physicians in the United States, the relative ease of adjustment of visa status in the study period, and the availability of training-socializing postgraduate positions (with all their deficiencies) make the physician's plight quite distinct from that of the middle class shopkeeper, the contracted field hand, or the illegal manual laborer.

Physician migrants, despite their collective elite character, and despite their differences in treatment from USMGs, are well integrated within the market for American medical manpower. If one views the national labor market as a set of segmented labor markets,[7] as indicated previously, migrant physicians play a role distinct from, yet inextricably related to, the roles played by groups of American-trained physicians. Since World War II migrant physicians have been the "buffer" that blunted the impact of manpower shortfalls in certain specialties and types of hospital. We argue that in doing this the migrants gave other physicians a far freer choice of specialty and locale and removed short-term pressure from the American health care system to alter its means of training and allocating health personnel.

Finally, the migration of physicians must be viewed in its international context. From the point of view of the "donor" nations, this migration is seen as a brain drain, preventing highly trained individuals from serving their national interest. This view is somewhat complicated by the fact that, as health care systems are currently constituted in most Western and Third World nations, there tends to be an oversupply of physicians in national capitals. Out-migration simultaneously removes this source of upper-middle-class discontent and the corresponding pressure to re-organize these health care systems to better serve the poor and rural populations. Furthermore, in some nations (e.g., India and the Philippines) cash remittances from migrant professionals may be an important source of foreign exchange.

These complications all reflect the ways in which international physician migration buttresses existing sociopolitical arrangements. From the standpoint of international organizations such as The World Bank,[8] the major problem for Third World nations is to devise ways of responding to the needs of the poorer segments of their populations—and health needs are among those in most need of attention. The international migration of physicians is a symptom of this larger problem; adjustment of national goals is an important part of the solution, both in the United States and in other nations.

POLICY DEVELOPMENTS IN THE UNITED STATES

The survey on which this study is based was conducted in 1974. We are concluding this book in 1977. In the intervening period interest in the role of FMGs has accelerated and become of active concern in American legislative and professional arenas. In both cases the message is restrictive. The Health Professions Educational Assistance Act of 1976 (Public Law 94–484) amended the Immigration and Nationality Act to make it more difficult for foreign physicians to enter the United States. The reasoning behind this is clear: Congress "finds and declares that there is no longer an insufficient number of physicians and surgeons in the United States such that there is no further need for affording preference to alien physicians and surgeons in admission to the United States . . .'"[9] In less tortuous prose, we shall need fewer foreign physicians in future as resources to provide needed care for our own people. A reduced role is seen for the physician as *immigrant*.

Concurrently, various bodies representing the American medical profession have pressed for a decreasing reliance on foreign doctors as staff for the American health care system. The most notable report, from the Coordinating Council on Medical Education, also notes that the United States should be self-sufficient in its production of physicians for its own needs, thus reducing the demand for immigrants. It goes on to develop a series of recommendations designed to define the future role of the foreign physician as *exchange student*. Such students should, it is declared, "be assured high quality graduate medical education especially designed to improve their medical knowledge and skills for teaching and practice in their own country".[10] Specific recommendations to do this dovetail with those of the new legislation. Emphasis lies on restricting exchange visitors to programs with written commitments to provide training, and on ensuring that the beneficiary of such training will indeed return home when training is completed.

The profession's report includes recommendations for United States aid in international exchange more broadly defined—including the establishment of binational cost-sharing agreements and support of international agencies to encourage international exchange on a basis more firmly linked with the perceived needs of countries other than the United States. Yet the overall tone remains xenophobic. FMGs are to be admitted, grudgingly, to the United States. The specter of "competence" is raised in concern about the equivalency of their educational preparation with that available to American medical graduates, performance in the delivery of health care, and English language abilities—subjects of more appropriate concern to the acceptance of immigrants, than to the special educational needs of future teachers in foreign cultures where educational and performance norms may be quite different.

Yet for both exchange students and immigrants the old rules, while modified, continue to prevail. The dual regulatory barriers for entry to the United States (described in chapter 4), visa regulations and proficiency screening through a special test, are supposedly to be developed as more effective controls on the quantity (supply) and quality (competence) of those FMGs who continue to enter. Much, if not most, of the recent debates on FMG roles and responsibilities relate to number games. In the process, loopholes in existing visa law, including the relative ease of converting from an exchange visitor to an immigrant visa while in the United States, are being closed. Policies toward the reduction, return, and exclusion of FMGs are much more firmly developed than policies designed to meet the expectations of the *individuals* whose experiences we have described in these pages, or the articulated wishes of foreign governments or schools.

The new legislation makes these points quite clearly. While it is too early to state with any certainty how far the various provisions of the law will be fully implemented—and in which areas trade-offs will be made—the intention is to stem the flow of physician entrants irrespective of their career expectations, and to ensure that those entering as exchange visitors remain in the general category of international students with few options to remain in the United States.

As of January 10, 1977 alien physicians wishing to enter the United States as immigrants and exchange visitors must pass a new examination, supposedly more difficult than the ECFMG. The law actually states that FMGs must pass the test commonly taken by American medical students during medical school, Parts I and II of the test given by the National Board of Medical Examiners, or an equivalent examination. The National Board is in the process of developing such an "equivalent" in a new Visa Qualifying Examination, specifically designed for foreign physicians. This test will be administered cooperatively by the National Board and the ECFMG abroad through United States embassies and consulates. Canadian graduates and USFMGs are exempt from this test, as are immigrant aliens of "national or international renown in the field of medicine." Excluding the latter, prospective entrants must also pass tougher English language tests, demonstrating proficiency in oral as well as written English.

Other requirements in the legislation require exchange visitors, beginning January 10, 1978 to demonstrate that they will be "able to adapt to the educational and cultural environment" in the United States and have "adequate prior education and training." These requirements are delegated to accredited American medical schools or other health professional schools, which also have to assume responsibility in writing for appropriate training here. Exchange visitors must also be committed to return to their country (although "commitment" is not clearly defined at the time of writing), and the country must give written assurance that there is a need for persons with the skills that the individual would acquire. The legislation suggested that the country ensure that there would be an actual job waiting for the physician, but this has disappeared in subsequent debates. Finally, the new exchange visitor will be able to stay in the United States for no more than two years unless additional training (one year maximum) is requested specifically by his or her country. Those exchange visitors who wish to convert to permanent resident (immigrant) status must first return to their country for a two-year period, a situation that existed in earlier years of the exchange visitor arrangements.

The findings and conclusions of our study suggest that, even if all these requirements were fully implemented, these policies may have less impact than apparently intended. We have observed that tests have provided little barrier to those physicians who actually come to the United States. Given the large pool of physicians who consider coming here at some point in their career, there will continue to be a substantial number who will overcome any "barrier effects" of the Visa Qualifying Examination as readily as their predecessors passed the ECFMG. The examination may, however do such physicians a service by being designed as a test of readiness for American graduate education which is more appropriate to those a year or so out of medical school than the ECFMG.

Tougher oral and written screening examinations for English language may be inhibiting factors to many prospective migrants, particularly those trained in languages other than English (e.g. Latin American countries, Japan, certain European nations). Our findings have shown, however, that while English abilities were of concern to many successful migrants, while communication caused difficulty with staff and patients to some extent in American hospitals from the FMG's point of view, our study group was rated quite highly in English ability by our American interviewers. The great majority of our study group were rated as excellent or good English speakers.[11] While more stringent English language tests will undoubtedly screen out some physicians who would otherwise migrate, and will serve to emphasize the need for better communication skills both here and in foreign testing centers, such tests alone will probably have a minimally inhibiting effect.

The requirement that medical schools agree to provide training or asssume responsibility for training poses little additional responsibility on existing arrangements, since virtually all graduate training hospitals are now affiliated with university medical schools. We have stressed that foreign physicians need clarification of the differences between a major teaching unit and a hospital with less rigorous forms of medical school affiliation. However, it remains true that of the 18,115 FMGs (excluding Canadians) who were on duty as interns and residents in September 1974, the latest figures available, 15,181 (84 percent) were in hospitals with some formal affiliation agreement with an American medical school. Since then the percentage has undoubtedly risen, as affiliation agreements have proliferated.

Probably the biggest potential changes in the legislation relate to the "return home" requirements of exchange visitors after two, or at most three, years of stay. Such a requirement allows for the continuing entry of exchange students, while preventing them from becoming competitors in the American marketplace with USMGs, with respect to private practice and other permanent positions.

It says much about the domestic purposes of the legislation that in all probability two of the exchange visitor requirements, those relating to school affiliations and passage of examinations, will be waived for individual aliens until December 31, 1980, where American hospitals can show that they would suffer "substantial disruption" of services should the supply of new house staff be withdrawn. Hospitals in the "FMG States" we described in chapter 6 will undoubtedly rush to seek such waivers; the process is now beginning. The "return home" provisions, which could benefit the individual careers and protect the career choices of thousands of potential new entrants, are not subject to such waivers. FMGs in the American health care system as of January 1977 remain covered by the earlier provisions.

The message, then, is clear. Alien physicians will continue to be welcome in American hospitals for a short period of training, providing jobs continue to be available. The new visa and testing systems may act as delaying mechanisms for new entrants. Until they are fully in place prospective entrants must wait, and a backlog of applications may be expected. At the same time an unknown number of prospective migrants who would otherwise have come to the United States as exchange visitors with the option of adjusting to immigrant visas and remaining, may decide not to come to the United States. Applications for immigrant visas will probably rise; those for exchange visas may fall or at least stabilize. The number of FMGs actually entering the United States may not drop substantially, at least until the supply of American graduates more nearly matches the number of residency positions available. The number of FMGs remaining in the country after training will, however, drop considerably because of the "return home" provisions for exchange visitors.

Whether and how far these changes will aid other countries—let alone individuals such as those we have studied—remains at this point an open question. Our study group of 690 FMGs produced a mere 129 individuals who were considering returning to jobs in Asia or the Far East, 87 expecting to go back to Central or South America, 50 to the Middle East, and 25 to British Commonwealth countries or Africa. Whether they will return or not we cannot predict, although we expect far fewer to leave the United States than now expect to. Case studies of countries which have leaned heavily on American graduate education, including those whose migrants have *not* returned, as well as those with relatively high return rates, are indicated as a high priority research area. If the United States is in fact planning to continue to train thousands of foreign physicians and *send them back to their own countries* rather than absorb them here, those countries may face unexpected difficulties as hundreds of migrants, American-trained and with American expectations, begin to reappear. Here the domestic and international contexts of migration heavily inter-mesh. How far the "new" exchange program will press for serious com-mitments by foreign countries of future employment of their citizens may be a critical element in both domestic and international negotiations over international exchange, determining whether the future program is truly an "exchange" or a mechanism for the temporary influx of staff into the American health care system.

There is a tendency in policy-making in the United States to search for apparently simple "solutions." Yet the migration of physicians, as we have shown, is a complex mix of individual motivations, formal mechan-isms such as visa legislation and professional testing, conditions in the job markets for physicians around the world, and other more subtle con-siderations. The newest American solution to the "FMG problem" is to accept the idea of too many FMGs in the United States, and attack the problem by straightforward cutbacks in the future entry and retention of FMGs. From the domestic point of view, few would argue that there is something out of balance in a medical profession with one fifth of its members immigrants, while thousands of Americans are turned away from American medical schools (27,000 in 1975). Yet, as our findings have shown, concentrating on straight reductions in the inflow and retention of FMGs obscures the heterogeneity of backgrounds, goals and ex-pectations of FMGs coming for graduate medical education in the United States; while the stress on tighter testing requirements diverts serious discussion to the mythology of FMG competence, and away from the practical difficulties that individuals face.

We have shown FMGS as individuals who, even as trainees, make considerable contributions to the medical care of Americans. As private practitioners and hospital–based physicians, FMGs serve all types of populations, in all types of areas in the United States. Despite the stig-matization we have shown of FMGs in training, FMGs are perhaps the most adaptable, upwardly-mobile, and successful immigrant occu-pational group that has ever entered the United States. In focussing on a political solution to the "FMG problem" solely in the context of national domestic physician supply, there is danger that the "FMG benefit" side of the scale will be neglected.

Of perhaps more importance to the individuals who are foreign phy-sicians, it is evident that the exchange visitor program will only work effectively as an educational program if enormous efforts are made by American and foreign governments and schools to meet the special needs of individuals, taking into account each individual's cultural background, stage of career, and future expectations. We trust that in the process the rather different roles of physician immigrants will not be overlooked, including those physicians who enter the United States as dependents. Much of the discussion on FMGs has arisen from the articulated demands of institutions: hospitals, medical schools, professional groups, Congressional committees, State departments and other Federal agencies. If the American role in international medical education is to be truly educational, the focus must shift to the peculiar needs of the individuals who exist under the umbrella rubric of "alien doctors" or FMGs. It is to clarify their experiences and expectations that this study has been undertaken.

NOTES

1. From *Annual Report, United States Immigration and Naturalization Service, 1975*, Washington, D.C.: U.S. Department of Justice.
2. Unless otherwise indicated, the statistics that follow were taken from *JAMA, Medical Education in the United States*, December 12, 1976.
3. See Association of American Medical Colleges, "Graduates of Foreign Medical Schools in the United States," *The Journal of Medical Education*, (August 1974), 49: 821.
4. See Arlene Goldblatt, Louis Wolf Goodman, Stephen S. Mick, and Rosemary Stevens, "Licensure, Competence and Manpower Distribution," *New England Journal of Medicine, op. cit.*
5. See Stevens et al., "Physician Migration Re-examined," *Science, op. cit.*
6. See, for example, Michael Piore, "The Economic Role of Migrants in the U.S. Labor Market," paper presented at the Research Institute in Immigration and Ethnic Status, Smithsonian Institution, Washington, D.C., November 15, 1976.
7. For a discussion of the relationship between primary and secondary labor markets, see Peter B. Doeringer and Michael J. Piore, *Internal Labor Markets and Manpower Analysis*, Lexington, Mass. Heath, 1971.
8. World Bank, *Health Sector Policy Paper*, Washington, D.C.: World Bank, 1975.
9. *Health Profession Educational Assistance Act of 1976*, Public Law 94–484, Findings and Declarations of Policy, sec. 2 (c).
10. *Physician Manpower and Distribution, The Role of the Foreign Medical Graduate*, June 1976, reprinted in JAMA, December 27, 1976. Members of the Coordinating Council include the American Board of Medical Specialties, American Hospital Association, Association of American Medical Colleges, and Council of Medical Specialty Societies.
11. English rated Excellent, 41.0 percent; Good, 38.9 percent; Fair, 18.5 percent; Poor, 1.6 percent.

Appendix A

METHODOLOGY_____

What follows is a detailed explanation of the methodology used in completing this study. The organization of this section attempts to recapitulate the various logical steps we took as the study evolved. The principal data needed to carry out the aims of this study were obtained through personal interviews with house staff gathered over a 2-month period. The study design required a representative sample of all interns and residents in American Medical Association (AMA)-approved training programs in American hospitals to be interviewed at the end of the training year 1973–1974. Respondents were normally interviewed in the hospitals in which they worked by interviewers employed by the National Opinion Research Center (NORC) of the University of Chicago. They followed a prescribed procedure and a fixed schedule of questions. Details of the study's methodology, including sampling, research design, data collection, and data analysis, follow.

THE SAMPLE DESIGN

The population universe sampled in this study was the total number of interns and residents in AMA-approved training programs in American hospitals. Among this population were excluded physicians in research positions chiefly because the focus of the study was on physicians receiving postdoctoral training and engaged in clinical activities and the delivery of health care. The sample obtained included 865 medical graduates of whom 690 were foreign medical graduates (FMGs), 42 were American-born foreign medical graduates (USFMGs), and 133 were American medical graduates (USMGs).

AMA Physician Biographical File

Through the Center for Health Services Research and Development of the American Medical Association (AMA) we obtained a complete listing from the Physician Biographical Masterfile (as of year-end December 31, 1973) of all interns and residents in AMA-approved training programs in the United States for fiscal year 1973–1974. The procedure followed by the AMA in its development of the list is documented in detail elsewhere.[1] The principal method employed by the AMA is tabulating information contained in the "Physician's Practice Activities" (PPA) questionnaire, sent out on a continuing basis to physicians throughout the country. Data are collected on interns and residents primarily through the information that hospitals with approved house staff programs are required to send to the AMA soon after the beginning of each new training year, which begins on July 1. This basic information is then supplemented by data gathered through the PPA.

The number of interns and residents was 58,252.

Individuals in research fellow positions were excluded from the file, although, as will be discussed, our survey revealed that approximately 12.4 percent of those in the file held duties other than intern and resident, including research fellows. This must have been due largely either to incorrect coding by the AMA or individual changes from one activity to another. For each individual, there was information on the following characteristics: (1) medical education number, which includes a medical school code and its state or country of location, year of graduation, and a specific identifying number, (2) primary specialty choice, if any, (3) year of birth, (4) training position, that is, intern or resident status, (5) individual addresses.

The initial sampling frame consisted of all individuals in this file. Although doubts have been raised about the accuracy, the inclusiveness, and the thoroughness of the Physician Biographical Masterfile,[2] it nevertheless stands as the single best source of information available to researchers. Furthermore, most criticisms of the AMA's masterfile have been aimed at its weaknesses in including non-ECFMG-certified foreign medical graduates, medical graduates not in training positions, and individuals not in approved training programs. Our study is specifically directed toward medical graduates in approved training programs, and on the basis of earlier studies, we have reason to believe the AMA to have a high degree of accuracy when it comes to data from approved programs.[3]

The National Opinion Research Center: Use of its Multistage Probability Sample

Since our interest was to make generalizations about all interns and residents in training in the United States, we decided, on the advice of the National Opinion Research Center (NORC) of the University of Chicago, to draw a probability sample of house staff on the basis of a multistage sampling scheme designed by NORC.

Using the NORC's primary sampling units (PSUs) of counties and standard metropolitan statistical areas (SMSAs) as representative of the general population of the United States, we determined which individuals on the AMA physical biographical masterfile fell into these 101 PSUs. Of the original individuals on the AMA file, 40,379 names were located in the NORC PSUs and thus were potential respondents. Although this is a 30.7 percent reduction in the size of the sampling frame, the NORC PSUs are representative of the general population of the United States, and the statistical results are generalizable to all 1973–1974 house staff.[4]

Stratification Variables

In drawing the sample, it was our desire to have enough FMGs outside the major urban areas of the United States to permit statistical analyses determining what effects, if any, could be traced to FMG location in and outside the largest metropolitan areas in the country. To this end, we included as our first stratification variable the medical graduate's geographic location of training at the time of the survey. There are two strata: (1) location in one of the eight largest urban centers of the country[5] or (2) location elsewhere.

The second variable on which the sample was stratified was the medical graduate's country of medical education. Although it can be argued that other variables such as country of birth, country of citizenship, or even country of last permanent residence might be more appropriate, we rejected these options because (1) the country of medical education variable is the most complete and accurate country-related data on the AMA masterfile, (2) there is a high degree of correlation among the country-related variables,[6] and (3) from the point of view of the country underwriting undergraduate medical education, this variable is perhaps the most meaningful one substantively in terms of finance, costs, and international policy making, and (4) our problem is to compare foreign training and American training and, as such, to center our attention on the locale of training.

The strata of countries of medical education reflected that the main focus of our project is to assess the experiences of FMGs in the American health care system. They included the United States, the Philippines, India, South Korea, and all other countries. As Table A.1 demonstrates, the most drastic effect of stratification was to reduce the population proportion of USMGs from about two-thirds to a sample proportion of about one-seventh. The constraints on the three Asian nations were designed to assure that the final sample would not be so disproportionately Asian that all other areas of the world would be weakly

TABLE A.1 POPULATION AND SAMPLE DISTRIBUTIONS COMPARED BY SAMPLING STRATA

	Population strata	Percentage	Sample strata	Percentage
USMG				
Other locales	11,636	28.8	87	10.1
Large urban	13,416	33.2	46	5.3
FMG				
Other locales	3,427	8.5	416	48.1
Large urban	5,767	14.3	199	23.0
Philippines				
Other locales	654	1.6	35	4.0
Large urban	1,334	3.3	12	1.4
India				
Other locales	887	2.2	28	3.2
Large urban	2,132	5.3	12	1.4
South Korea				
Other locales	363	0.9	20	2.3
Large urban	763	1.9	10	1.2
Total	40,379	100.0	865	100.0

represented and thus not analyzable in a statistical sense. In the case of the USMGs, the relatively small sample size increases the standard error of estimate for generalizations to this group. This is a consequence of the goals of the study: (1) having a robust enough sample size of FMGs to permit internal FMG comparisons to emphasize our hypothesis of FMG heterogenerity and (2) permitting appropriate comparisons of FMGs against USMGs. This resulted in the final choice of permitting no more than 15 percent of the sample to be USMGs. Therefore, we are not in a position to make precise internal comparisons among groups of USMGs, but we are able to realize the two primary goals of the study.

Weighting of Data

The disproportionate stratified random sampling used in the construction of the sample of this study necessitates the use of weights whenever population estimates or inferences are to be made.[7] Whenever our data were used to make inferences, we employed those weights which corresponded to the particular purpose of the analysis. One result of this procedure is that the individual cell Ns, the marginal Ns, and the total table Ns vary from table to table, depending on the set of weights used as well as the number of missing cases or values that may be represented in any given table.

The most general set of weights (WTALL) adjusted the data on the basis of American locality and country of medical education to restore the sample distributions to an approximation of the actual population distribution. Thus, for example, USMGs were treated as if they were two-thirds of the sample, recapitulating their two-thirds representation in the population. Similar adjustments were accordingly introduced for other FMGs' countries of medical education.

By far the most commonly used set of weights (WTEACH) is one that maintains the proportion of USMGs as actually sampled (approximately 15 percent of the total) while correcting for the large urban and other urban distribution. This was employed whenever comparisons were made among sub-sets of FMGs. Thus the FMGs, although internally corrected for American location and country of medical education, continue to be represented as they are in the sample in any population estimate. But, since population estimates here reflect only FMGs (including USFMGs), no distortion is carried over into estimates of USMG proportions.

Two other sets of weights used in some analyses in this volume are URBWT and CMEWT. URBWT is a univariate adjustment for the effects of disproportionate sampling in the American location strata. This set of weights is employed whenever proportions within countries of medical education are examined. CMEWT adjusts for the effects of disproportionate sampling within the countries of medical education whenever proportions within large urban and other urban strata are analyzed.

As a result of the weighting procedures, however, the reader is cautioned against attempting to recalculate cell or marginal percentages on the basis of cell or marginal frequencies where given. Our standard procedure has been to present the unweighted cell or marginal frequencies and the weighted proportional results. Thus, the reader may see both the generalized proportions for the total FMG population and the actual number of individuals on whom the calculations have been based.

Sources of Error due to Sampling

Sampling Error: A familiar source of error in research that uses samples to estimate some larger universe or population is sampling error.[8] This is the tendency for any particular sample to deviate in some measure from the real or "true" population. Specifically, it is the risk that any value, attribute, characteristic, or whatever term one wishes to use, which is estimated from the sample, no matter how carefully drawn according to the canons of scientific sampling procedures, will deviate or "be off" from the actual population value (generally unknown) simply because of uncontrolled randomness or chance.

Within given probability limitations, the amount of error can be estimated, and the ability to perform these calculations rests on the Central Theorem.[9] Most data presented in this report are expressed in percentages, and we calculated standard errors of estimate and converted them into confidence intervals at the 95 percent level (Table A.2).

Because of the complex nature of our sample and the attendant difficulties in computing population estimates and measures of the amount of error of these estimates, we adjusted our estimates of confidence intervals using a procedure suggested by Kish.[10] Simply stated, the effect of stratifying the sample is compared to what would have happened had the sample not been stratified. This comparison, a factor called design effects (Deff) is the ratio for any particular variable of the variance computed within each stratum and summed across all sample strata to the variance calculated under the assumption of simple random sampling, disregarding the actual sampling strata.

The ratio indicates how much loss or gain occurs in terms of variance when the sample is stratified. These calculations were made for 14 selected variables that span the major areas of interest in the study; for example, proportions of males, non-Whites, medical graduates with physician relatives, first and current hospital characteristics, hospital-based specialists, and so on. To produce a more stable measure, the square root of the Deff for each variable was obtained. Then, for all medical graduates, USMGs, and FMGs,[11] separately, the average Deff was computed, and this produced values of 1.65, 1.06, and 1.53 respectively. These figures mean that, on the whole, stratifying the sample as we did had the effect of increasing the variance most for estimates made for all medical graduates, second most for estimates made for FMGs, and least for estimates made for USMGs. Stratification is usually accomplished to reduce variation on specific independent variables, and we achieved this goal in increasing the number of FMGs vis à vis USMGs, that is, by stratifying on country of medical education. However, in so doing we increased variation on other variables, the price we had to pay to have enough FMGs to do analyses within categories of FMGs.

The next step in our calculations was to compute a t_{deff} which was the 95 percent two-tailed level of the t distribution (1.96) multiplied by the relevant deff. This adjusted t value (t_{deff}) was then introduced in the usual formula for the computation of confidence limits for proportions. The adjusted confidence intervals in Table A.2 are therefore slightly wider than one would have expected. Consulting this table, the reader can judge the probable significance of a variety of percentage differences between USMGs and FMGs: maximally, a 14.56 percent difference will be significant at the .05 level.

Executing the Sample: An additional source of error may be introduced in estimations of population characteristics because of (1) individual physicians selected for the sample but not interviewed for one reason or another and (2) differential response rates for individuals within one stratum compared to others. The latter aspect is really a part of the first.

TABLE A.2   STANDARD ERROR OF ESTIMATES EXPRESSED IN PERCENTAGES AT THE 95 PERCENT CONFIDENCE INTERVAL LEVEL, ADJUSTED FOR DESIGN EFFECTS OF STRATIFIED SAMPLING

	Standard error in percentages for confidence interval estimates						
	2 or 98	5 or 95	10 or 90	20 or 80	30 or 70	40 or 60	50
All medical graduates	1.54	2.40	3.30	4.40	5.00	5.40	5.50
USMG	2.52	3.93	5.40	7.20	8.30	8.83	9.02
FMG[a]	1.55	2.45	3.33	4.44	5.10	5.43	5.54

[a] Includes USFMGs in estimates.

The original sample contained 963 names.[12] The NORC completed 865 usable interviews, a response rate of 89.8 percent. The distribution of reasons for nonresponse is given in Table A.3. The largest reason for nonresponse was refusal. This and repeated broken appointments, both indications of interviewee indifference or animosity toward the survey, formed the bulk of nonrespondents. A broad category consisting primarily of "unavailable" physicians rounded out the remaining nonrespondents.

The characteristics of nonrespondents as contrasted to respondents are displayed in Table A.4. Significantly different response rates appear for some variables. In the case of hospital position, the absence of any nonrespondents in the "other" category (for which there were 107 respondents) is a function of our reliance on the AMA's intern and resident code which did not list any other categories. Our survey revealed that of 865 respondents, 95 did not report being "interns or residents," but of these, 42 or 44.2 percent reported having resident responsibilities. If these 42 medical graduates are added to the "resident" category, the latter's proportion is raised to 74 percent, still more than 14 percent less than the nonrespondents. Interns are also overrepresented in the sample. Thus in general the National House Staff Survey contains a category of persons—fellows—we tried to exclude; residents were more likely to have been excluded from the sample than interns.

FMGs and USMGs were equally likely to respond to the survey, and this fact strengthens the reliability of comparisons between these two groups. On the other hand, our estimate of USFMG response rate shows their below-average willingness to participate in the study. The reasons for this may be complex, but more care must be taken when making estimates about USFMGs.

TABLE A.3 DISTRIBUTIONS OF INTERVIEW COMPLETION RATES AND REASONS FOR NONRESPONSE

	Percentage	N
Interview completed	89.8	(865)
Nonrespondents	10.2	(98)
Refusals	4.9	(47)
Broke appointments	2.1	(20)
Other (unavailable, vacationing, too busy)	3.2	(31)
Total	100.0	(963)

TABLE A.4 DISTRIBUTION OF RESPONDENT AND NONRESPONDENT
CHARACTERISTICS

Characteristic	Respondent Percentage	N	Nonrespondent Percentage	N
Hospital position				
Intern	17.7	(153)	11.2	(11)
Resident	69.9	(605)	88.8	(87)
Other	12.4	(107)	—	—
Type of medical graduate				
USMG	15.4	(133)	16.3	(16)
FMG	84.6	(732)	83.7	(82)
USFMG[a]	4.9	(42)	11.2	(11)
Country of medical education				
U.K., Europe, former Commonwealth	16.9	(146)	25.5	(25)
Asia, Far East	35.7	(309)	30.6	(30)
Middle East, Africa	11.2	(97)	14.3	(14)
Central and North America	9.0	(78)	10.2	(10)
South America	11.8	(102)	3.1	(3)
U.S.A.	15.4	(133)	16.3	(16)
Primary specialty				
General or family practice	4.3	(37)	2.0	(2)
Medical	25.1	(217)	24.5	(24)
Pediatrics	8.6	(74)	9.2	(9)
Ob/gyn	8.4	(73)	9.2	(9)
Surgical	22.6	(195)	22.4	(22)
Psychiatric	8.9	(77)	11.2	(11)
Hospital based	16.2	(140)	12.2	(12)
Other, unspecified	6.0	(52)	9.2	(9)
Total	100.0	(865)	100.0	(98)

[a] There was no way to determine from AMA data whether an individual was a USFMG; based on a conservative estimate of the nonrespondents with "American" names, we came up with 11 probable USFMGs.

Response rate did not vary significantly on the basis of the medical graduates' specialties. Sampling response does vary with country of medical education, although the differences are not significant. Asians and South Americans are somewhat overrepresented in the sample, whereas Her Majesty's current and former subjects and Europeans are underrepresented.

In sum, then, a certain margin of error of concern that may affect the generalizability of the data was introduced by differential response rates found by the greater reluctance of residents to respond to the survey. Other variables examined did not, in our opinion, discriminate any important characteristics of nonresponders. We therefore concluded that our sample does not suffer a serious weakness because of differential response rate. However, when focus is placed on interns versus residents, we exercise appropriate caution.

RESEARCH DESIGN

The basic research design of this study is one commonly referred to as a "static-comparison" group.[13] Its principal characteristics are (1) the study group is observed at a single point in time; (2) control or comparison groups are sorted out on the basis of some critical independent criterion or variable; that is, individuals are not and cannot (as is so often the case with survey or field research) be randomly assigned to one group or another. Some discussion of each of these characteristics is necessary to underline the strengths and weaknesses of the study.

First, studies such as this, insofar as they probe past events and states of mind, are retrospective and subject to the weaknesses of the human memory. For example, we asked the physicians to give us a complete work history since graduation from medical school. In addition to factual information like this, we asked attitudinal and motivational questions such as why each doctor decided to migrate, and when he or she made the decision. Despite methodological studies that show that retrospection introduces a certain amount of distortion,[14] the precision with which our respondents were able to recall the events after medical school graduation, for example, the dates, the places, and the specific activities, attests to the extraordinarily orderly career patterns of doctors. This orderliness and structure aid accurate recall, and we argue that as a consequence the retrospective data is generally improved.

An extensive list and treatment of the strengths and weaknesses of the static-comparison group is inappropriate in a volume of this type, and the interested reader is referred elsewhere.[15] However, apart from the recall problem, there are several technical problems arising from the design that deserve discussion because of their bearing on our analysis.

The issue of selection and "experimental mortality" are two important technical problems. Selection refers to the possibility that the two groups (FMGs and USMGs) would have differed without the occurrence of medical education abroad. For our purposes, this means that even without consideration of the principal independent variable, the fact that FMGs were not native-born American citizens would make them different from USMGs. This is, of course, a plausible hypothesis, and one we not only cannot eliminate, but also one we ourselves propose as an important explanation for the way in which FMGs are treated, taught, and placed within the American health care system.

There is very little influence one can exert experimentally over the country of birth and the past medical education of individuals. However, the inclusion in our sample of the USFMG (the American citizen educated abroad) effectively strengthens our research design because we can begin to assess the effect of foreign birth on a variety of dependent variables. We are nevertheless aware that, even in the case of USFMG–USMG comparisons, there is evidence that the groups differ in critical ways,[16] which underscores the formal nonequivalence of the two groups (equivalence is guaranteed only by random assignment).

"Experimental mortality" refers to differences in dependent variables between the group assumed to be "experimental" and that assumed to be the "control" or comparison group due to unequal dropout. Thus, even if, in some hypothetical manner, FMGs and USMGs were identical or equivalent at some point in time before the staging of our survey, they might differ now because of differential dropout or exclusion from one of the groups, rather than because of the effect of the independent variable, the country of medical education.

A related issue derives from an additional attribute of our study group, that is, the fact that it is, more or less, a cohort. These men and women were at a uniform level in their careers—graduate medical education. However, there was some variability in factors, such as year of arrival in the United States (Chapter 2, Table 2.2). This fact, combined with the retrospective nature of the design, means that the farther one moves back in time, the less likely it is that the individuals in our sample will form a full cohort at that earlier time. The reasons for this are simple: some medical graduates will not have begun training, others will not yet have left for the United States, and so on. This aspect of the methodology implies that caution is necessary in interpreting data that compares characteristics at the time of the survey with those at some earlier time. For example, in Chapter 7, which treats the institutional mobility patterns of medical graduates, the variable, "first hospital of training," is frequently compared to "current hospital of training." The distribution across the latter variable is representative of the 1973–1974 housestaff cohort, but it is not a substitute for the chronologically earlier variable, "first hospital," for the reasons mentioned. The implications of specific analyses would take too much space to develop here, but the reader is cautioned to consider this methodological constraint where relevant in the text.

DATA COLLECTION

Pilot Studies

Preceding the development of the survey instrument used in this study, we engaged in two separate but interlocking pilot studies to help establish appropriate research areas and to refine the study's eventual methodology.

Hospital field studies provided us with qualitative, on-the-scene observational materials from which to generate relevant questions that we ultimately incorporated in our final interview. Basic themes highlighted by this approach include issues surrounding an FMG's introduction to the first American hospital of training, recruitment to the hospital in the first place, the need to examine more closely the process through which an immigrant physician arrives at the decision to come to the United States, the manner in which this desire is implemented, and other topics.[17]

The Connecticut follow-up[18] proved to be valuable in pointing us to (1) the need to sample medical graduates in a larger geographical cross-section of the United States and (2) the desirability of using a face-to-face interview rather than a mail questionnaire or a telephone interview. The mail questionnaire we used in the study also pointed out good and poor ways of asking questions. One example of this was the imprecise way we gathered data on visa status and licensure information, two areas in which we subsequently improved our questioning technique (wording, precision, detailed specification, etc.).

Interview Schedule

In general, the information gleaned from the two pilot studies plus a review of existing materials used in house staff surveys, particularly those with special reference to FMGs, helped us devise the survey interview schedule, as presented in Appendix B. The basic sections of the interview reflect our research concerns:

Basic medical school training and other demographic information.
A complete career history.
Reasons for migration to the United States.

The mechanics or process of migration.
The hospital recruitment process.
Introduction to hospital life.
Duties, workloads, and graduate training.
Assessment of the training experience
Supervision
Responsibility
Life in the United States.
Career plans and migration intentions.
Feelings about medicine in general.

Closely connected with our inquiry into these areas of FMG life was a separate instrument used for the sample of 133 USMGs. The instrument was identical in all respects except for questions appropriately asked only of foreign-educated physicians, for example, differences between the medical needs of one's country of medical education and those of the United States, or questions related to the ECFMG examinations, reasons for migrating.

A preliminary instrument was devised, and with the help of the National Opinion Research Center (NORC) it was revised and then pretested on medical graduates (88 FMGs, 12 USMGs) listed on the AMA file and chosen randomly from 16 zip code areas in the New York City area. Divided into two stages, the first pretest produced a revised version of the survey instrument that was subsequently pretested during the second stage. On the basis of the pretest experience, final revisions were incorporated into the survey instrument, and it was used in the field during April/May 1974.

Measurement

In general, we employed straightforward measures of various attributes of individuals and the hospitals in which they were training. We refrained from using highly abstract constructs in our analysis because of our intention (1) to avoid using jargon and esoteric nomenclature and (2) to be as concrete as possible so that a wide audience might be reached. Thus we did not use scaling techniques, factor analysis, Guttman scaling, or other technical procedures (as we mention later, most techniques require statistical assumptions that would be unwarranted without considerable transformation of the data).

There are two areas, however, that need discussion: (1) determination of who falls into various categories of medical graduates and (2) categorization of hospitals.

The criterion variable we elected to use in delineating subgroups of medical graduates was a medical graduate's country of medical education. When we speak of foreign medical graduates, we have operationally defined them as men and women who received their medical education and their degree of medical doctor outside the boundaries of the United States.[19] We have done this for several reasons:

1. Any person who does not receive an MD degree from an American or Canadian medical school must pass the ECFMG examination before entering an AMA-approved intern or residency program.

2. Available data bases from which to generate adequate sampling frames usually have reliable listings of country of medical education but much poorer listings, if any, of other possible criterion variables: country of birth, citizenship, or country of last permanent residence.

3. The expenses of medical education are usually borne by the country in which a medical school is located. As such, from the standpoint of costs of physician manpower training, it makes the greatest sense to focus on country of medical education.

4. Country of medical education is the most invariant and stable variable (aside from country of birth) available. Although country of birth is even more stable than country of medical education, it can have only trivial importance in indicating the country most involved from the manpower training point of view. Citizenship and last permanent residence are unstable in that individuals can and may change either with relative ease, and neither of them may indicate directly the manpower "drain" or "gain" a particular country might undergo.

Nevertheless, we do not deny the importance of these other variables as indicators of other phenomena, most notably, mobility of physician manpower, and for classifying types of mobility and movers, topics covered in Chapters 3 and 4.

Comparing citizenship to country of medical education reveals a well-known but surprisingly little-studied group, the citizen of the United States who is a foreign medical graduate (USFMG).[20] Although the vast majority of the FMGs in our sample (92 percent) were citizens of foreign countries, a small group, 59 in number (8 percent) were citizens of the United States. Of these 36 (or 60 percent) were natural-born American citizens who went to medical school abroad and therefore fell into the FMG category.

In addition to this group, our study included 24 persons who had become American citizens through naturalization. Individuals in this group might be considered either American or foreign, depending on when their naturalization had taken place, how long they had lived in the United States, and the extent to which they had had an opportunity to absorb American customs and culture. Six of the group of 24 were found to have been naturalized before they graduated from medical school and, for the purpose of our study, were considered to be USFMGs.[21] The other 18 medical graduates were considered to fall into the bona fide FMG category, all having been naturalized after graduation from medical school and, in most cases, well after commencing graduate training in this country. Thus our sample contains 42 individuals we classified as USFMGs.

In Chapters 5–9 we discuss medical graduates in terms of their hospitals of training. Variables descriptive of the hospitals were derived from two sources, the annual issues of the *Directory of Approved Internships and Residencies* published by the American Medical Association and the *American Hospital Association Guide to the Health Care Field.*[22] For each medical graduate, each hospital in which he or she may have trained was matched with data extracted from these two sources. The variables included level of affiliation, size in beds, sponsorship, type of hospital, number of residency programs, necropsy rate, present FMG house staff.

The level of affiliation measures the extent to which a hospital's teaching program is linked to a university medical school. Four categories ranging from full affiliation to limited teaching to graduate programs only to unaffiliated programs were employed. Affiliation is a measure of the degree of commitment to teaching and research and is also used as a measure of prestige of the hospital.

The size of the hospital is self-evident, although other appropriate measures might have included number of personnel, amount in dollars of the annual budget, or the dollar value of the payroll. We elected to measure size in beds because of its face validity and of its ease of comprehension.

Sponsorship is merely descriptive and indicates whether the hospital is private for-profit, nonprofit, and/or church operated or government operated.

The type of hospital is another simple classification that mainly distinguishes between general, short-term hospitals and other varieties. Most hospitals fall into the former classification.

The number of residency programs is a measure of the complexity of the hospital.[23] The more specialty training programs, the more complex, organizationally speaking, the hospital is assumed to be.

The necropsy rate is the ratio of the number of autopsies performed and the total number of deaths in the hospital. It has been assumed that the larger the ratio, the more the hospital is committed to teaching and research activities.

Finally, the "percent" FMGs house staff variable is simply a ratio of the number of FMGs and the total number of house staff in a hospital. This allows the researcher to determine the house staff environment and estimate the possibilities of FMG–USMG interaction.

Data Preparation

The interviews were conducted in the field by the National Opinion Research Center and forwarded to our research team at Yale University. On receipt of the interviews, a coding manual was developed for all closed-ended questions. A random selection of schedules was used to develop coding frames for open-ended questions; once developed, it was incorporated into the coding manual. All interviews were then coded in separate code sheets, and the data were then punched onto computer cards and eventually transferred to magnetic tape and disk storage.

The major computer programming scheme employed batch processing via remote terminal using the Time Sharing Option (TSO) to generate programs within the (then) current version of the Statistical Package for the Social Sciences (SPSS).[24]

Other data analyses involved culling through the original questionnaires according to critical variables of interest, for example, the interviews of all Filipino FMGs were read for information on their work histories.

DATA ANALYSIS

Cross-Tabulation Techniques

Statistical analyses in this study were intentionally limited to tabular presentation. Our reasons for this are several. First, most of our data is categorical or nominal. With the exception of some attitudinal data that has a natural order (ordinal) and other data characterized by interval qualities (age, income, years in training, etc.), most assumptions of parametric statistical analyses—normality of distributions, homoscedascity—are not fulfilled.

Second, because the sample is a stratified random sample using disproportionate sampling fractions, population estimates must be computed using weighted data. Although the weighting process does not entail special technical procedures for tabular presentation, the problems encountered with more sophisticated interval multivariate statistics are considerable and are still at the frontier of knowledge awaiting solution.[25]

Third, our desire is to present a portrait of the FMG presence in the United States for a broad, knowledgable group of scholars, professionals, and policy makers. It is our feeling that advanced statistical techniques are not easily understood by the audience; thus we avoided their use in presenting our findings.

For these reasons, we elected to present our data in table form. For the reader unaccustomed to the general logic of statistical verification at this level, brief perusal of standard texts should suffice.[26]

NOTES

1. C. N. Theodore and G. E. Sutter, *Distribution of Physicians, Hospitals, and Hospital Beds in the U.S., 1966*, Volume 1, Chicago: American Medical Association, 1967, pp. 7–21.

2. T. C. Kleinman, R. J. Weiss, and D. S. Felsenthal, "Physician manpower data: the case of the missing foreign medical graduates," *Medical Care* (November 1974), 12, pp. 906–917.

3. Our error estimates of the AMA Masterfile range around 5 percent. See R. A. Stevens, L. W. Goodman, and S. S. Mick, "What happens to foreign trained doctors who come to the United States?" *Inquiry* (June 1974), 11, 112–124. For an independent assessment of the accuracy of the AMA Masterfile, see A. Lowin, *FMGs? An Evaluation of Policy-Related Research*, Minneapolis: Interstudy, 1975, pp. 221–235.

4. For a technical explanation of the NORC sample, see B. F. King and C. Richards, "The 1972 NORC National Probability Sample," Chicago: NORC, mimeo.

5. These include the following SMSAs: New York, Boston, Philadelphia, Washington, D.C., Chicago, Detroit, San Francisco, and Los Angeles.

6. Chapter 2 contains empirical evidence showing the interrelationship of these variables.

7. A brief discussion of the problems involved is found in M. Parten, *Surveys, Polls, and Samples: Practical Procedures*, New York: Cooper Square Publishers, 1966, pp. 235–236.

8. See H. M. Blalock, *Social Statistics*, 2nd ed., New York: McGraw-Hill, 1960, Chapter 20.

9. See W. L. Hays, *Statistics for Psychologists*, New York: Holt, Rinehart and Winston, 1963, pp. 238–244.

10. L. Kish, *Survey Sampling*, New York: Wiley, 1965, pp. 574–582.

11. Our practice in this volume is to examine FMGs separately from USFMGs. The data presented on sampling errors combines these two subgroups because there was, at the sampling stage, no way to discriminate between the two groups and consequently no independent means to stratify each separately. Computation of variances and standard errors with appropriate weights is therefore done only for USMGs and the total FMG pool. The effect of adding USFMGs to the FMGs in calculating sampling error and confidence bands is to decrease slightly the confidence band one would actually expect were FMGs considered alone because of the larger sample N, 732 versus 690. Thus the reader should keep in mind that the confidence bands are approximations, but not unrealistic ones.

12. The original list of randomly produced names numbered 1029. It soon became appar-

ent that 66 of the names should not have been included on the AMA Physician Masterfile as interns and residents, and they were excluded from the obtained sample. These 66 medical graduates were distributed thus: doctors in private practice (15), respondents included in the pretest (2), people who were "out of scope," that is, those who had left in the middle of training (8), those who had left the country (14), and those who were unknown or had never arrived at the hospital. Analyses of these nonrespondents against the other 98 "legitimate" nonrespondents (refusals, broken appointments, on vacation) failed to produce significant Chi-square values beyond the .05 level according to country of medical education, specialty, and type of position.

13. D. T. Campbell and J. C. Stanley, *Experimental and Quasi-Experimental Designs for Research*, Chicago: Rand McNally, 1963, pp. 12–13.

14. For a general review of problems of accurate recall, see S. Sudman and N. M. Bradburn, *Response Effects in Surveys: A Review and Synthesis*, Chicago: Aldine Publishing Co., 1974, Chapter 3, "Effects of Time and Memory Factors in Response," pp. 67–92.

15. D. T. Campbell and J. C. Stanley, *op. cit.*, pp. 12–13.

16. Data presented in Chapter 2 and elsewhere show that USFMGs and USMGs differ.

17. S. S. Mick and E. Hoffman, "Introduction to the Hospital Case Studies," FMG Project Working Paper, Yale University, 1973, mimeo.

18. The results of this study are reported in R. A. Stevens, L. W. Goodman, and S. S. Mick, *op. cit.*

19. Despite customary practice to exclude Canadians from this definition, we include them among FMGs.

20. For a brief review of pertinent literature on the USFMG, see A. Lowen, *op. cit.*, pp. 305–326 and S. S. Mick, R. A. Stevens, and L. W. Goodman, "The U.S. Foreign Medical Graduate: How he Compares with the Foreign Medical Graduate," *Medical Care* (June 1976).

21. All but one of the six appeared to have come to the United States and been naturalized in the wake of events in post-World War II Europe. They were naturalized at relatively early ages, between 12 and 24, and, since generally a person seeking naturalization must have lived in the United States as a permanent resident for 5 years before applying for naturalization, they had all probably lived in this country more than 15 years, from the time they were 7 years old, at one extreme, to 19 years, at the other, before they were naturalized. Of the two who were naturalized when they were over 21 years of age, one graduated from medical school 9 years and the other 17 years after naturalization.

22. Assorted volumes were used, such as *Directory of Approved Internships and Residencies, 1972–73*, Chicago: The American Medical Association, 1973 and *Guide to the Health Care Field, 1972*, Chicago: The American Hospital Association, 1972.

23. The number of residency programs reflects the complexity of the social organization of the hospital, not the technological complexity. However, these two variables are correlated. See W. V. Heydebrand, *Hospital Bureaucracy*, New York: Dunellen Publishing Company, 1973.

24. N. H. Nie, D. H. Bent, and C. H. Hull, *SPSS: Statistical Package for the Social Sciences*, New York: McGraw-Hill, 1970.

25. Leslie Kish, *op. cit.*, pp. 582 ff.

26. H. M. Blalock, *op. cit.*; M. Rosenberg, *The Logic of Survey Analysis*, New York: Basic Books, 1968, particularly Appendix A, pp. 251–258.

Appendix B

MEDICAL GRADUATE SURVEY _____

Survey 4182
April, 1974

NATIONAL OPINION RESEARCH CENTER
University of Chicago

MEDICAL GRADUATES SURVEY

for

YALE SCHOOL OF MEDICINE
Department of Epidemiology
and Public Health

BEGIN DECK 01

RESPONDENT ID #: ☐☐☐☐   01-04/

| TIME | _____ | AM |
| BEGAN: | | PM |

SUGGESTED INTRODUCTION

Hello, I'm _____ from the National Opinion Research
Center at the University of Chicago. We are doing the survey
for Yale University School of Medicine--the survey we mentioned
in the letter we sent you. The survey is about various aspects
of medical training and your personal reasons for being trained
at this hospital.

F/

1. Are you an intern, a resident, a research fellow or a post-doctoral fellow?

                                        Intern . . . .   (GO TO Q. 2) 1   05/
                                        Resident . . .   (GO TO Q. 2) 2
                                        A research fellow . . .   (ASK A) . . . 3
                                        A post-doctoral fellow .   (ASK A) . . . 4
                    (IF VOLUNTEERED):   Resident and research fellow
                                          combined . . (GO TO Q. 2) 5
                                        Other (SPECIFY AND ASK A) _____

                                        _____ 6

        A. IF CODES 3, 4, OR 6: Are you also a resident or do you have any
                                  residents' duties?
                                        Yes   . . . (GO TO Q. 2) 1   06/
                                        No . . . (SKIP TO Q. 30) 2

2. What (IF INTERN: will be   )
         (IF OTHER THAN INTERN: is) your primary specialty? RECORD RESPONSE VERBATIM.

                                                                             07-08/
                                                                             ☐☐

                    (IF VOLUNTEERED)   Undecided, don't know . . . 00

IF INTERN, ASK Q. 3. ALL OTHERS, SKIP TO Q. 4.

3. Are you taking a straight or rotating internship?

                        A straight internship . . . . . (ASK A)   1   09/
                        A rotating internship . . . (GO TO Q. 4) 2
                        Other (SPECIFY AND GO TO Q. 4) _____

                        _____ 3

        A. IF CODE 1: What type of internship are you in?
                        Medical 01   10-11/
                        Surgical 02
                        Pediatrics 03
                        Obstetrics/Gynecology 04
                        Psychiatry 05
                        Other (SPECIFY) _____ 88

300

ASK EVERYONE:

4. In this year of your training, are you doing all of your training at <u>one</u>
    hospital, or are you in a program which involves <u>more</u> than one hospital?

                    One hospital . . . . (GO TO Q. 5) 1   12/

                    More than 1 hospital . . .(ASK A, B, & D) 2

    IF CODE 2, ASK A, B, & D:

    A. What is the name of your training program?   13-14/

        ENTER NAME OF PROGRAM: _____

    B. Is there <u>one</u> hospital which serves as the main hospital for your
        training this year?

                            Yes . . . (ASK C) 1   15/

                            No   . . (GO TO D)   . . 2

    C. IF YES: What is the name of <u>that</u> hospital?

        ENTER NAME OF HOSPITAL: _____ (BE SURE   16-18/
                                                         TO GO ON
                                _____   TO D)

    D. What is the name of the hospital to which you are assigned at the
        present time? IF R IS <u>PRESENTLY</u> ASSIGNED TO MORE THAN ONE HOSPITAL,
        PROBE FOR NAME OF HOSPITAL AT WHICH HE SPENDS THE MOST TIME.

                                                                               19-21/

        ENTER NAME OF HOSPITAL: _____

5. A. During the past four weeks, about how many nights were you on call--
        not counting weekends?
                            No nights 0   22/
                            1-4 nights 1
                            5-8 nights 2
                            9-12 nights 3
                            13-16 nights 4
                            17-20 nights 5

    B. Out of the past 4 weekends, about how many weekends were you on call?
                            No weekends 0   23/
                            1 weekend 1
                            2 weekends 2
                            3 weekends 3
                            4 weekends 4

6. In general, about how many hours a week do you work, including "on call" time
   and study time?

                              60 hours or less 1   24/
                              61-70 hours 2
                              71-80 hours 3
                              81-90 hours 4
                              91-100 hours 5
                              101 hours or more 6

---

7. In this year of your training, have you ever worked in a department that served
   as <u>both</u> an Emergency Room (ER) and an Outpatient Department (OPD)?

                              Yes   . . . (ASK A)   1   25/
                              No . . . .(GO TO Q. 8) . . . 2

   A. <u>IF YES</u>: During this training year, about how often do you work there?
      RECORD RESPONSE VERBATIM.

                                                                    26-28/

                                             ┌───┬───┬───┐
                                             │   │   │   │
                                             └───┴───┴───┘

---

8. In this year of your training, have you ever worked in an Emergency Room (ER)
   (IF YES TO Q. 7: not counting the combined Emergency Room-Outpatient Department
   you just told me about)?

                              Yes . . . . (ASK A) 1   29/
                              No . . . . (GO TO Q. 9) . . 2

   A. <u>IF YES</u>: During this training year, about how often do you work there?
      RECORD RESPONSE VERBATIM.

                                                                    30-32/

                                             ┌───┬───┬───┐
                                             │   │   │   │
                                             └───┴───┴───┘

---

9. In this year of your training, have you ever worked in an Outpatient Department (OPD)
   (IF YES TO Q. 7: not counting the combined Emergency Room-Outpatient Department
   you already told me about)?

                              Yes . . . . (ASK A) 1   33/
                              No . . . . (GO TO Q. 10) . . 2

   A. <u>IF YES</u>: During this training year, about how often do you work there?
      RECORD RESPONSE VERBATIM.

                                                                    34-36/

                                             ┌───┬───┬───┐
                                             │   │   │   │
                                             └───┴───┴───┘

10. At the present time, to which service, or section of a service, are you assigned within the hospital? RECORD RESPONSE VERBATIM AND CODE BELOW WITHOUT READING CATEGORIES TO R.

                Outpatient Department . . . . (ASK A) . 1   37/
                Emergency Room . . . . (ASK A) . 2
                Combined Outpatient Department-Emergency Room (ASK A) . 3
                Other . . . . (ASK B) . 4

A. IF CODES 1, 2 OR 3:   About how many patients do you see there
                          on an average day?

                ENTER # OF PATIENTS: [| |] ⎤ NOW GO
                                                     ⎬   TO   38-40/
                                                     ⎦ Q. 11

B. IF CODE 4:   At the present time, to about how many
                 beds are you assigned?

                ENTER # OF BEDS: [| |]   41-43/

    (IF VOLUNTEERED:) N.A.: Do not work with bed patients 000

_____

11. During the day shift, about how many (READ EACH ITEM, A-I) are usually assigned to your service or section of service? Just your best estimate.

                                                NUMBER ASSIGNED

A. Interns . . . . [|]   44-45/

B. Residents . . . . [|]   46-47/

C. Medical students--for example, clinical clerks or
        externs . . . . [|]   48-49/

D. Nurses--registered and LPNs . . . . [|]   50-51/

E. Technicians . . . . [|]   52-53/

F. Student nurses . . . . [|]   54-55/

G. Aides, attendants and orderlies . . . . [|]   56-57/

H. Private attending physicians
        (IF VARIES WIDELY: How many are working there today?) . [|]   58-59/

I. Hospital attending physicians . . . . [|]   60-61/

12. We would like to ask some questions about the kinds of meetings that are held in your hospital or training program this year.

X. To your knowledge, are the following meetings conducted? (READ ITEMS A-D.) FOR EACH "YES," ASK Y BEFORE GOING ON TO NEXT ITEM.	FOR EACH "YES" TO X, ASK Y: Y. About how many times a month do you attend (READ ITEM)? CODE BELOW WITHOUT READING CATEGORIES TO R.

A. Record and Fatality Meetings?

    Yes . (ASK Y) . . . 1   62/

    No . (GO TO B) . . 2

Less than 1 a month . . . 1	
1-3 times a month 2	BE SURE
4-6 times a month 3	TO GO 63/
7-9 times a month 4	ON TO B
10 times a month or more . 5	

B. Clinical-Pathological Conferences (CPC)?

    Yes . (ASK Y) . . . 1   64/

    No . (GO TO C) . . 2

Less than 1 a month . . . 1	
1-3 times a month 2	BE SURE
4-6 times a month 3	TO GO 65/
7-9 times a month 4	ON TO C
10 times a month or more . 5	

C. Tissue Committee Meetings (Histopathology)?

    Yes . (ASK Y) . . . 1   66/

    No . (GO TO D) . . 2

Less than 1 a month . . . 1	
1-3 times a month 2	BE SURE
4-6 times a month 3	TO GO 67/
7-9 times a month 4	ON TO D
10 times a month or more . 5	

D. X-Ray Conferences?

    Yes . (ASK Y) . . . 1   68/

    No . (GO TO Q. 13). 2

Less than 1 a month . . . 1	
1-3 times a month 2	
4-6 times a month 3	69/
7-9 times a month 4	
10 times a month or more. 5	

70 71 72 73 74

75-76/01
77-80/4182

304

13. Are there other meetings, conferences, seminars, or such that you attended
    during this training year?

Yes . . (ASK X & Y) 1   05/

No . . (GO TO Q. 14) . . . 2

IF YES, ASK X & Y:

X. What kinds of meetings--what are they called? RECORD UP TO FIVE MEETINGS. AFTER YOU HAVE RECORDED ALL OF THE MEETINGS UP TO 5 THAT R MENTIONS, ASK Y FOR EACH MEETING.	FOR EACH MEETING LISTED IN X, ASK Y: Y. About how many times a month did you attend ...? (READ NAME OF MEETINGS, LINES 1-5.) CODE BELOW WITHOUT READING CATEGORIES TO R.	
(1) _____ ⬜⬜ 06-07/	Less than 1 a month . . . . 1 1-3 times a month. . . . . . 2 4-6 times a month . . . . . 3 7-9 times a month . . . . . 4 10 times a month or more . . 5	08/
(2) _____ ⬜⬜ 09-10/	Less than 1 a month . . . . 1 1-3 times a month . . . . . 2 4-6 times a month . . . . . 3 7-9 times a month . . . . . 4 10 times a month or more . . 5	11/
(3) _____ ⬜⬜ 12-13/	Less than 1 a month . . . . 1 1-3 times a month . . . . . 2 4-6 times a month . . . . . 3 7-9 times a month . . . . . 4 10 times a month or more . . 5	14/
(4) _____ ⬜⬜ 15-16/	Less than 1 a month . . . . 1 1-3 times a month . . . . . 2 4-6 times a month . . . . . 3 7-9 times a month . . . . . 4 10 times a month or more . . 5	17/
(5) _____ ⬜⬜ 18-19/	Less than 1 a month . . . . 1 1-3 times a month . . . . . 2 4-6 times a month . . . . . 3 7-9 times a month . . . . . 4 10 times a month or more . . 5	20/

14. Are there any other meetings that are held that you consider important for you
    to attend but that you don't attend because you don't have the time?

                                        Yes . . . .(ASK A) . . . 1   21/

                                        No . . . (GO TO Q. 15) . 2

    A. IF YES: What kinds of meetings--what are they called?
                 RECORD UP TO FIVE MEETINGS.

        (1) _____ [   ] 22-23/

        (2) _____ [   ] 24-25/

        (3) _____ [   ] 26-27/

        (4) _____ [   ] 28-29/

        (5) _____ [   ] 30-31/

---

15. We would like to ask everyone some questions about how often they do certain
    tasks. We know that some of these tasks may not be relevant to what you have
    been doing during this year of training. If that is the case, just let me know.
    FOR EACH ITEM, A-J, ASK:
    How often do you ... (READ ITEM)--often, sometimes, or never?

		Often	Some-times	Or never? CODE FOR NA HERE)	
A.	Have access to information on patient's economic and social circumstances--READ CATEGORIES.	3	2	1	32/
B.	Manage patients from their admission all the way through to discharge or to the Outpatient Department--READ CATEGORIES.	3	2	1	33/
C.	Start up I.V.s	3	2	1	34/
D.	Attend Grand Rounds	3	2	1	35/
E.	Attend daily patient rounds	3	2	1	36/
F.	Use your hospital's medical library	3	2	1	37/
G.	Administer electroshock treatments	3	2	1	38/
H.	Teach interns, residents or medical students	3	2	1	39/
I.	Talk over cases with consultants	3	2	1	40/
J.	Teach other health personnel such as nurses and paraprofessionals	3	2	1	41/
K.	Decide when patients are ready to be discharged from the hospital inpatient department	3	2	1	42/
L.	Do "scut" work such as daily blood counts, urines and stool exams	3	2	1	43/

306

16. Do you ever do work other than daily blood counts, urines or stool exams that you consider "scut work?"

Yes . . . . (ASK A & B) 1   44/

No . . . (GO TO Q. 17) 2

    IF YES, ASK A & B:
    A. What kinds of work?   RECORD RESPONSE VERBATIM.   45-46/
                                                                ☐☐

                                                               47-48/
                                                                ☐☐

                                                               49-50/
                                                                ☐☐

    B. About what per cent of your working time are you doing what you consider "scut work?"

                                ENTER PER CENT ☐☐   51-52/

17. In this year of training, about what per cent of all patients that you see are admitted by private attending physicians?

None 0   53/

1-25% 1

26-50% 2

51-75% 3

76% or more . . 4

18. We would like to ask a few more questions about what you have been doing during this year of your training.

		Often	Some-times	Or never?	
A.	How often is an attending physician present or available to work with you or to give instruction--(READ CATEGORIES).	3	2	1	54/
B.	How often do you work as an assistant to an attending physician	3	2	1	55/
C.	How often do you work alone but with previous instruction	3	2	1	56/
D.	How often do you work alone with no previous instruction and no instruction available	3	2	1	57/

19. I'm going to read a list of different activities that may have been involved in your work during this training year. Please tell me whether you were given a great deal of responsibility, a fair amount of responsibility, a small amount of responsibility, or no responsibility at all for each activity I read.

	A great deal of responsibility	A fair amount of responsibility	A small amount of responsibility	Or no responsibility	(IF VOLUNTEERED) Not applicable to my work	
A. Decisions on admittance to the hospital--would you say you are given (READ CATEGORIES) for this?	5	4	3	2	1	58/
B. Decisions on release of patients from the hospital--would you say you are given (READ CATEGORIES) for this? .	5	4	3	2	1	59/
C. How about dealing with the relatives of patients--how much responsibility are you given for this?	5	4	3	2	1	60/
D. How about decisions about outpatient care?	5	4	3	2	1	61/
E. How about the supervision of medical staff such as nurses and aides?	5	4	3	2	1	62/
F. How about the management of patients on nights and weekends?	5	4	3	2	1	63/

20. During this training year, are there any areas of your work or training in which you feel that you are not given enough responsibility?

Yes . (ASK A) 1   64/

No . (GO TO Q. 21) . 2

A. IF YES: Which areas are those?   RECORD RESPONSE VERBATIM.   65-66/

67-68/

69-70/

71 72 73 74   75-76/02
77-80/4182

308

21. During this training year, are there any areas of your work or training in which you feel that you are given <u>too much</u> responsibility?

Yes . . (ASK A) . . 1   05/

No . (GO TO Q. 22) 2

    A. <u>IF YES</u>: Which areas are those? RECORD RESPONSE VERBATIM.

▭▭ 06-07/

▭▭ 08-09/

▭▭ 10-11/

---

22. In general, during this training year, how much would you say you have learned from . . . ? (READ ITEMS, A-F.) A great deal, a fair amount, a small amount, or nothing at all?

	A great deal	A fair amount	A small amount	Nothing at all	(IF VOLUNTEERED) Not applicable to my work	
A. the private attending physicians	5	4	3	2	1	12/
B. the resident physicians .	5	4	3	2	1	13/
C. the chiefs of service . .	5	4	3	2	1	14/
D. the technicians	5	4	3	2	1	15/
E. the nurses	5	4	3	2	1	16/
F. the patients	5	4	3	2	1	17/

23. Are there <u>other</u> persons around the hospital from whom you learned a great deal or a fair amount?

Yes (ASK A) . . . 1   18/

No . (GO TO Q. 24) 2

    A. <u>IF YES</u>: What positions do these persons hold? RECORD RESPONSE VERBATIM.

▭▭ 19-20/

▭▭ 21-22/

▭▭ 23-24/

309

24. Are there any <u>other</u> persons around the hospital I have not mentioned from whom you expected to learn a great deal but from whom you learned only little or nothing?

                              Yes . (ASK A) . . . 1   25/

                              No   (GO TO Q. 25) . 2

   A. <u>IF YES</u>: What positions do they hold? RECORD RESPONSE VERBATIM.

                                              ☐☐   26-27/

                                              ☐☐   28-29/

                                              ☐☐   30-31/

---

25. Are you formally evaluated by (READ ITEMS AND CODE)--

		Yes	No	(IF VOLUNTEERED) Don't know	
A.	chiefs of service?	1	2	9	32/
B.	private attending physicians? .	1	2	9	33/
C.	full-time hospital physicians?.	1	2	9	34/
D.	senior residents?	1	2	9	35/

---

26. Do any other persons formally evaluate your work?

                  Yes . . . . . (ASK A) 1   36/

                  No . . . (GO TO Q. 27) 2

                  (IF VOLUNTEERED): Don't know
                     (GO TO Q. 27) 9

   A. <u>IF YES</u>: What positions do the persons hold? RECORD RESPONSE VERBATIM.

                                              ☐☐   37-38/

                                              ☐☐   39-40/

                                              ☐☐   41-42/

---

27. Considering the year of training you are in, what procedures or techniques, if any, do you feel have not been adequately taught? RECORD RESPONSE VERBATIM.

                                              ☐☐   43-44/

                                              ☐☐   45-46/

                                              ☐☐   47-48/

28. Considering the year of training that you are in, in general, would you say that
    the quality of your training this year has been better, about the same, or not
    as good as the quality of your postgraduate training last year?

                                    Better 3   49/

                                    About the same 2

                                    Not as good 1

                                    (IF VOLUNTEERED): Not
                                      applicable--this is
                                      my first year of
                                      training 0

---

29. Which one of the arrangements listed here best describes the type of practice you
    would prefer to enter at the completion of your training? CODE ONE ONLY. YOU MAY
    HAVE TO PROBE TO GET R TO PICK THE ONE ARRANGEMENT THAT BEST DESCRIBES THE TYPE OF
    PRACTICE HE WOULD PREFER TO ENTER.

                          A. Solo private practice 1   50/

        ┌─────────┐   B. Private practice partnership with one
        │ HAND   │   other physician 2
        │ CARD   │
        │   A   │   C. Private practice with a group of physicians. 3
        └─────────┘
                          D. Faculty position in a medical school 4

                          E. Full-time, salaried, hospital physician .. . 5

                          F. A government position 6

                          G. A research position 7

                          H. Other (SPECIFY) _____ 8

                              (IF VOLUNTEERED): Don't know 9

ASK EVERYONE:

And now some questions about your background and training before working at this hospital.

30. In which country did you graduate from medical school?

COUNTRY _____ 51-53/

31. From which medical school did you graduate?

SCHOOL: _____ 54-56/

32. And in what year were you born?

19 [ ][ ]

57-58/

33. In which country were you born?

COUNTRY: _____ 59-61/

34. In which country or countries
did you live while you were
growing up?

COUNTR(Y)/(IES): _____ 62-64/

_____ 65-67/

_____ 68-70/

A. IF GREW UP IN MORE THAN ONE COUNTRY, ASK: In which one of these countries did you spend most of your secondary school years?

COUNTRY: _____ 71-73/

35. Which category listed on this card best describes the size of the community in which you (grew up/spent most of your secondary school years)?

| HAND |
| CARD |
| B |

a) A large city (over 100,000 in population) (ASK A) 4   74/

b) A medium sized city (10,000 to less than 100,000 in
    population) (ASK A) 3

c) A town or village (less than 10,000 in population) (GO TO Q. 36) . 2

d) A farm or rural area, outside of any town or village (GO TO Q. 36). 1

75-76/03
77-80/4182

BEGIN DECK 04

A. IF CODES 4 OR 3: What is the name of the city or town?

_____ 05-07/

36. A. Are you a United States citizen?   Yes   (ASK B) . . 1   08/
                                                    No (ASK D-F) . . 2

IF YES TO A, ASK B:

B. Are you a natural born United States citizen or a naturalized United States
    citizen?
                                    Natural born (GO TO Q. 37) . . 1   09/

                                    Naturalized . (ASK C) 2

    C. IF NATURALIZED: In what month and year did you become a United States
                         citizen?

                         MONTH: [ ][ ]   YEAR: 19 [ ][ ]   10-11/
                                                                   12-13/
                                    (NOW SKIP TO Q. 37)

IF NO TO A, ASK D-F: [ ][ ][ ]
                                                                   14-16/
D. What is your current citizenship? COUNTRY: _____

E. What visa do you currently hold--permanent resident, immigrant, exchange
    visitor, student, or what?
                         Permanent resident/immigrant visa . . . 1   17/

                         Exchange visitor visa ("J" visa) . . . 2

                         Student visa 3

                         Other (SPECIFY) _____ 4

F. Did you ever have a different visa status here in the United States?
                                    Yes (ASK G-I) . . 1   18/

                                    No (GO TO Q. 37). 2

IF YES TO F, ASK G-I:

G. What was the last visa status you held, before your current status?
                                                                  [ ]
                    _____   19/

H. When was it changed--during what month and year?
                    MONTH: [ ][ ]   YEAR: 19 [ ][ ]   20-21/
                                                              22-23/

I. Why was it changed? RECORD RESPONSE VERBATIM.
                                                          [ ][ ]
                                                              24-25/
                                                          [ ][ ]
                                                              26-27/

313

37. When did you graduate from medical school--in what month and year? - - - - - - - - - -

---

38. I am going to ask you about your work or study activities, in this country and elsewhere, from the time you graduated from medical school up to, and including, your
present position.

By work and study activities we mean those related to the practice of medicine as
well as those not related to the practice of medicine.

A. What was the first work or study activity you undertook after graduating medical school? KEEP PROBING WITH: And what did you do after that? UNTIL CURRENT TRAINING YEAR IS REACHED. INCLUDE CURRENT POSITION.	FOR EACH ACTIVITY IN "A," ASK B - D.	
	B. In what country did you (ACTIVITY)? IF U.S.A., RECORD CITY AND STATE.	C. What was the name of the (hospital/lab/clinic/ school/company/etc.)?
32-33/	34-36/	37-39/
48-49/	50-52/	53-55/
BEGIN DECK 05 05-06/	07-09/	10-12/
21-22/	23-25/	26-28/
37-38/	39-41/	42-44/
53-54/	55-57/	58-60/
BEGIN DECK 06 05-06/	07-09/	10-12/
21-22/	23-25/	26-28/
37-38/	39-41/	42-44/

314

- - - - ENTER ☐☐   YEAR: 19 ☐☐
        MONTH:
                              28-29/
                              30-31/

39. When did you arrive in the United States
    after your graduation--during the
    month and year?

    MONTH: ☐☐   YEAR: 19 ☐☐   53-54/
                                   55-56/

40. IF TIME PERIOD BETWEEN GRADUATION AND
    ARRIVAL IN U.S.A. IS 3 MONTHS OR MORE,
    AND NO ACTIVITIES ARE LISTED FOR ANY
    PORTION OF THIS PERIOD, ASK:

    What did you do in the time between
    your graduation and your arrival in
    the United States? RECORD RESPONSE
    VERBATIM.

                                   ☐☐
                                   57-58/

                                   ☐☐
                                   59-60/

                                   ☐☐
                                   61-62/

D.

From what date to what date did
you (ACTIVITY)?

FROM:		TO:	
MONTH	YEAR	MONTH	YEAR
40-41/	42-43/	44-45/	46-47/
56-57/	58-59/	60-61/	62-63/
13-14/	15-16/	17-18/	19-20/
29-30/	31-32/	33-34/	35-36/
45-46/	47-48/	49-50/	51-52/
61-62/	63-64/	65-66/	67-68/
13-14/	15-16/	17-18/	19-20/
29-30	31-32/	33-34/	35-36/
45-46/	47-48/	49-50/	51-52/

64-74/R
75-76/04
77-80/4182

69-74/R
75-76/05
77-80/4182

41. IF TIME PERIOD BETWEEN ARRIVAL IN U.S.A.
    AND BEGINNING DATE OF FIRST U.S. HOS-
    PITAL POSITION IS 3 MONTHS OR MORE,
    AND NO ACTIVITIES ARE LISTED FOR ANY
    PORTION OF THIS PERIOD, ASK:

    What did you do in the time between
    your arrival in the United States and
    your first hospital position? RECORD
    RESPONSE VERBATIM.

                                   ☐☐
                                   63-64/

                                   ☐☐
                                   65-66/

                                   ☐☐
                                   67-68/

    69 70 71 72 73 74
    ☐ ☐ ☐ ☐ ☐ ☐   75-76/06
                      77-80/4182

315

```
INTERVIEWER:   IS R A NATURAL-BORN U.S. CITIZEN OR NATURALIZED PRIOR
               TO GRADUATION?   (SEE QS. 36 AND 37.)
                                                   YES  . . . . .1
                                                   NO   . . . . 2
```

IF YES IN BOX ABOVE, SKIP TO INSTRUCTIONS ABOVE Q. 45.

42. Suppose you had stayed in _____ and not
                              (ENTER COUNTRY OF MEDICAL EDUCATION FROM Q. 30.)
     come to the United States--what would you be doing now in the field of medicine?
     RECORD RESPONSE VERBATIM.

                                                          ☐☐ 05-06/

                                                          ☐☐ 07-08/

                                                          ☐☐ 09-10/

43. Why did you choose to come to the United States rather than stay in (COUNTRY OF
     MEDICAL EDUCATION)?   RECORD RESPONSE VERBATIM.   PROBE FOR CLARITY ONLY.   DO NOT
     PROBE FOR OTHER REASONS.

                                                          ☐☐ 11-12/

                                                          ☐☐ 13-14/

                                                          ☐☐ 15-16/

44. When did you decide to come to the United States for medical training or research--
     was it before your medical school years, during your medical school years, or was
     it after medical school

                              Before medical school years (GO
                                TO Q. 45) 1   17/
                              During medical school years
                                (ASK A) 2
                              After medical school (ASK B) . . . 3

     A. IF DURING MEDICAL SCHOOL: Did you decide at the beginning of medical school,
         in the middle of medical school, or toward the end of medical school?

                                   Beginning 1   18/

                                   Middle 2

                                   Toward the end 3

     B. IF AFTER MEDICAL SCHOOL: Did you decide within the year after completing
         medical school, or after a year had elapsed since completing medical school?

                                   Within the year 1   19/

                                   After a year 2

316

REFER TO Q. 38 FOR NAME OF FIRST UNITED STATES HOSPITAL R WORKED IN AS AN INTERN
OR A RESIDENT. REFER TO THIS HOSPITAL IN Q'S 45-54.

RECORD HOSPITAL NAME HERE:_____

45. How did you first hear about (NAME OF HOSPITAL ABOVE)? RECORD RESPONSE VERBATIM.

□□□
20-22/

46. A. Before taking a position with (NAME OF HOSPITAL ABOVE) did you apply to other
         hospitals in the United States?

                              Yes . (ASK B) 1   23/

                              No . .(GO TO Q. 47). . 2

     B. IF YES TO A: How many other hospitals did you apply to before taking
                       a position at (NAME OF HOSPITAL)?

                       NUMBER OF HOSPITALS: □□] NOW 24-25/
                                                 >SKIP
                                                 ] TO Q. 48

IF NO TO Q. 46, ASK Q. 47

47. A. Why did you apply to only one hospital?

□□
26-27/
□□
28-29/

     B. Did someone help assure, in advance, that you would obtain the position?

                              Yes . (ASK C) 1   30/
                              No (GO TO Q. 48) . . . 2

     C. IF YES TO B: Who was it--not names, but their position or relation-
                       ship to you? RECORD RESPONSE VERBATIM.

□ 31/

□ 32/

□ 33/

317

48. In your search for a United States hospital position . . .

	a great deal	a fair amount	a small amount	or, not at all? CODE HERE FOR "DOES NOT APPLY"	
A. did information from friends of yours who had been in the United States help you (READ CATEGORIES)	4	3	2	1	34/
B. did information from the E-C-F-M-G help you (READ CATEGORIES)	4	3	2	1	35/
C. How much did professors or deans of your medical school help you (READ CATEGORIES).	4	3	2	1	36/
D. How much did United States government offices like the U-S-I-S or consulate help you?	4	3	2	1	37/

In your search for a United States hospital position . . .

	a great deal	a fair amount	a small amount	or, not at all?	
E. How much did the A.M.A. Directory of Approved Internships and Residencies-- the Green Book--help you (READ CATEGORIES)	4	3	2	1	38/
F. How much did advertisements or notices in the American medical journals help you (READ CATEGORIES)	4	3	2	1	39/
G. How much did the intern matching program help you	4	3	2	1	40/

49. Did anything or anyone <u>else</u> help you a great deal or a fair amount in your search for a United States hospital position?

                              Yes . . . (ASK A) . . . 1   41/

                              No . (GO TO Q. 50) . . 2

A. <u>IF YES</u>: Please tell me about it--how were you helped? RECORD VERBATIM.

                                        42-43/

                                        44-45/

                                        46-47/

50. ASK A-G IN X BEFORE ASKING Y.

X. As it turned out, once you began working at (NAME OF HOSPITAL), did you feel you had been adequately informed... (READ ITEMS A-G.)

FOR EACH "NO" TO X, ASK Y.

Y. What do you feel you should have been told about (ITEM)? RECORD RESPONSE VERBATIM.

	Yes	No	

A. whether or not (NAME OF HOSPITAL) had an affiliation with a university medical school?   1   2   48/

☐☐ 49-50/

☐☐ 51-52

B. about the quality of (HOSPITAL)'s teaching program?   1   2   53/

☐☐ 54-55

☐☐ 56-57,

C. about its location? . .   1   2   58/

☐☐ 59-60/

☐☐ 61-62,

D. about its size?   1   2   63/

☐☐ 64-65,

☐☐ 66-67,

E. about the duties of your position?   1   2   68/

☐☐ 69-70,

☐☐ 71-72,

73-74/RR
75-76/07
77-80/418

BEGIN DECK 08

F. about the working conditions in general .   1   2   05/

☐☐ 06-07

☐☐ 08-09

G. about the social and economic characteristics of the patient population?   1   2   10/

☐☐ 11-12

☐☐ 13-14

51. Was there anything _else_ about which you felt you were not adequately informed?

                                    Yes . (ASK A) 1   15/

                                    No . (GO TO Q. 52) . . 2

      A. IF YES: What do you feel you should have been told?

                                                            ┌─────┬─────┐
                                                            │   │   │ 16-17/
                                                            └─────┴─────┘
                                                            ┌─────┬─────┐
                                                            │   │   │ 18-19/
                                                            └─────┴─────┘

---

52. Did you go through a formal orientation program at (NAME OF HOSPITAL) before you
     began to work?

                                    Yes . . (ASK X) 1   20/

                                    No . (SKIP TO Q. 55) . 2

      IF YES, ASK X:

      X. During the orientation program . . . (READ ITEMS, A-H)

		Yes	No	
A.	were you introduced to your chief?	1	2	21/
B.	were you informed about your daily schedule?	1	2	22/
C.	were you formally introduced to any fellow house staff?	1	2	23/
D.	were you informed about procedures for the ordering of drugs?	1	2	24/
E.	were you informed about procedures for the ordering of diagnostic tests?	1	2	25/
F.	was there an explanation of the rules and regulations of the hospital?	1	2	26/
G.	was there an explanation of United States medical terminology and abbreviations?	1	2	27/
H.	were you informed about the city or town?	1	2	28/

---

53. During the program, were you informed about the housing situation in the city or
     town? CODE AND RECORD RESPONSES VERBATIM.

                                    Yes 1   29/

                                    No 2

54. Did the orientation program fail to provide you with any information which you
    felt was needed?

                                    Yes . . (ASK A) . . . 1   30/

                                    No (GO TO Q. 55) . . 2

    A. IF YES: What kind of information?

                                                    [   ] 31-32/

                                                    [   ] 33-34/

                                                    [   ] 35-36/

IF R IS A NATURAL BORN U.S. CITIZEN OR WAS NATURALIZED PRIOR TO GRADUATION (SEE
INSTRUCTION BOX, TOP OF PAGE 18), SKIP TO INSTRUCTIONS ABOVE Q. 60, PAGE 25.

55. I am going to mention some reasons medical graduates often give for their decision
    to come to the United States. For each reason I mention, please tell me how much it
    influenced your decision, if at all.

	a great deal	a fair amount	a small amount	or, not at all? CODE HERE FOR "DOES NOT APPLY"	
A. Advice you received from teachers and professors in (COUNTRY OF MEDICAL EDUCATION-- Q. 30)--did that influence you in coming to the United States (READ CATEGORIES) . . .	4	3	2	1	37/
B. There were not enough training positions in (COUNTRY OF MEDICAL EDUCATION--Q. 30)-- did this influence you in coming to the United States (READ CATEGORIES)	4	3	2	1	38/
C. Americans place greater emphasis on specialization--how much did this influence you in coming to the United States?	4	3	2	1	39/
D. The higher salaries of training positions in the United States--how much did this influence you in coming to the United States? . .	4	3	2	1	40/
E. Service in the armed forces of (COUNTRY OF MEDICAL EDUCATION) is required--how much did this influence you in coming to the United States?	4	3	2	1	41/
F. There are restrictions of your freedom to practice medicine as you would wish in (COUNTRY OF MEDICAL EDUCATION)--how much did this influence you in coming to the United States?	4	3	2	1	42/
G. Political and social problems in (COUNTRY OF MEDICAL EDUCATION)--how much did this influence you in coming to the United States?	4	3	2	1	43/

56. Medical graduates who made the final decision to come to the United States for training sometimes mention personal and professional considerations which had weighed against their decision to come here.

I'll mention some of these considerations. For each one, please tell me to what degree it weighed against your decision, if at all.

		a great deal	a fair amount	a small amount	or, not at all CODE HERE FOR "DOES NOT APPLY"	
A.	Separation from your family and friends--did this weigh <u>against</u> your decision to come to the United States (READ CATEGORIES)	4	3	2	1	44/
B.	The possibility of losing contact with the professional job market in (COUNTRY OF MEDICAL EDUCATION)--how much did this weigh against your decision to come?	4	3	2	1	45/
C.	The illegal use of drugs in the United States--how much did this weigh against your decision to come?	4	3	2	1	46/
D.	The fast pace of life in the United States--how much did this weigh against your decision?	4	3	2	1	47/
E.	The competitiveness of work in the United States--how much did this weigh against your decision? . .	4	3	2	1	48/

IF R IS A NATIVE OF THE UNITED STATES, CANADA, GREAT BRITAIN, OR AUSTRALIA, SKIP TO INSTRUCTIONS ABOVE Q. 60, PAGE 25.

57. The necessity of speaking English in United States hospitals--how much did this weigh <u>against</u> your decision to come--

A great deal 4   49/

A fair amount 3

A small amount 2

Or, not at all?
(CODE HERE FOR "DOES
NOT APPLY") 1

58. Overall, since you came here for your postgraduate training, to what extent has
    difficulty with English caused you problems with professional staff--would you
    say to a great extent, to a moderate extent, to a small extent, or not at all?

                              To a great extent . (ASK A) . 1   50/

                              To a moderate extent (ASK A) . 2

                              To a small extent . (ASK A) . 3

                              Not at all (GO TO Q. 59) . . . 4

                              (IF VOLUNTEERED): I have no
                                dffficulty with English
                                (SKIP TO Q. 60) 5

    A. IF CODES 1-3: Which professional staff--what positions do they hold?

                                                    ☐☐   51-52/

                                                    ☐☐   53-54/

                                                    ☐☐   55-56/

59. Overall, since you came here for your postgraduate training, to what extent has
    difficulty with English caused you problems with patients--would you say to a great
    extent, to a moderate extent, to a small extent, or not at all?

                              To a great extent 1   57/

                              To a moderate extent 2

                              To a small extent 3

                              Not at all 4

    REFER TO Q. 2 FOR R'S SPECIALTY OR PLANNED SPECIALTY AND ENTER BELOW.   IF R HAS NO
    ACTUAL OR PLANNED SPECIALTY, SKIP TO INSTRUCTIONS ABOVE Q. 64.

60. You told me earlier that (your specialty is) _____ .
                            (you plan to specialize in) (ENTER NAME OF SPECIALTY)
    Did you ever have a different specialty or special field of interest?

                              Yes . . . . (ASK A & B) . . . 1   58/

                              No . . . . (GO TO Q. 61) . . . 2

    IF YES, ASK A & B:

    A. Which specialty or special field of interest did you have?   ☐☐
                                                                         59-60/
        SPECIALTY/SPECIAL FIELD OF INTEREST: _____

    B. Why did you change? (PROBE: What other reasons caused you to change?)

                                                    ☐☐   61-62/

                                                    ☐☐   63-64/

                                                    ☐☐   65-66/

323

61. Is your present specialty the one you wanted, or did you have to change specialties
     in order to get this position?

                                     Present specialty is the one
                                     I wanted (GO TO Q. 62) . . . 1   67/

                                     Had to change specialties in
                                     order to get this position
                                     (ASK A & B) 2

     IF CODE 2, ASK A & B:

     A. Which specialty would you have preferred to be in? RECORD RESPONSE VERBATIM.

                                                          ☐☐   68-69/

     B. Do you plan to change your specialty in the future?

                                     Yes . . . . . (ASK C) 1   70/

                                     No . . . . (SKIP TO INSTRUC-
                                     TIONS ABOVE Q. 64) 2

        C. IF YES: To which specialty do you plan to change? RECORD RESPONSE VER-
                     BATIM AND SKIP TO INSTRUCTIONS ABOVE Q. 64.

                                                          ☐☐   71-72/

                                                    73 74
                                                    ☐☐   75-76/08
                                                             77-80/4182

324

62. I am going to mention some reasons graduates often give for their choice of specialty.
    For each of the reasons I mention, please tell me how much it influenced your choice of (ACTUAL OR PLANNED SPECIALTY), or if it influenced your choice at all.

	a great deal	a fair amount	a small amount	or, not at all? CODE HERE FOR "DOES NOT APPLY"	
A. Your hospital has an excellent program in (ACTUAL OR PLANNED SPECIALTY)--did this influence your choice (READ CATEGORIES) . .	4	3	2	1	05/
B. Encouragement from others already training in this specialty -- did this influence your choice (READ CATEGORIES)	4	3	2	1	06/
C. Encouragement from the chief of medicine at (NAME OF CURRENT HOSPITAL)--did this influence your choice (READ CATEGORIES) .	4	3	2	1	07/
D. This specialty is more intellectually stimulating than some other specialties-- how much did this influence your choice? .	4	3	2	1	08/
E. You like the close patient contact this specialty brings--how much did this influence your choice?	4	3	2	1	09/
F. Specialists in (ACTUAL OR PLANNED SPECIALTY) are needed in the United States-- how much did this influence your choice? .	4	3	2	1	10/

IF R IS A NATURAL BORN U.S. CITIZEN OR NATURALIZED PRIOR TO GRADUATION (SEE INSTRUCTION BOX ABOVE Q. 42, TOP OF PAGE 18), SKIP TO Q. 63.

| G. Specialists in this field are needed in (COUNTRY OF MEDICAL EDUCATION--SEE Q. 30)-- did this influence your choice (READ CATEGORIES) . . . . | 4 | 3 | 2 | 1 | 11/ |

63. Are there any <u>other</u> reasons which influenced your choice of specialty?

Yes . .(ASK A). .1   12/

No (GO TO Q. 64) 2

A. <u>IF YES</u>: Please tell me about the reasons.

☐☐ 13-14/

☐☐ 15-16/

☐☐ 17-18/

IF R IS NATURAL BORN U.S. CITIZEN OR NATURALIZED <u>PRIOR TO</u> GRADUATION (SEE BOX ABOVE Q. 42, TOP OF PAGE 18), SKIP TO Q. 65.

64. Have you definitely decided to leave the United States after your training, or have you definitely decided to remain in the United States?

Definitely decided to leave (SKIP TO Q. 71) 1   19/

Definitely decided to remain (GO TO Q. 65) 2

Don't know, no decision, no definite decision (RECORD VERBATIM AND ASK A) 3

A. <u>IF CODE 3</u>: The way things look right now for you, what do you think your eventual decision will probably be--to leave the United States or to remain? (PROBE: Just your best guess as of today.)

Probably leave the United States (SKIP TO Q. 71) . . 1   20/

Probably remain (GO ON TO Q. 65) 2

Don't know, can't decide (RECORD VERBATIM AND SKIP TO Q. 78) 3

ASK Q. 65 IF R IS A NATURAL-BORN U.S. CITIZEN OR NATURALIZED PRIOR TO GRADUATION, OR IF R WILL DEFINITELY OR PROBABLY REMAIN (CODE 2 IN Q. 64 OR CODE 2 IN Q. 64A):

65. Where in the United States would you settle if you had your choice--in what town or city and state?

U.S. TOWN/CITY: _____   21-22/

STATE: _____   23-24/

IF R HAS NO SPECIFIC TOWN/CITY OR STATE IN MIND, BUT A GENERAL AREA OR TYPE OF AREA, RECORD VERBATIM RESPONSE.

25-26/

27-28/

IF R HAS NO IDEA AT ALL, CHECK BOX ☐ AND SKIP TO Q. 69. ALL OTHERS GO ON TO Q. 66.

66. Realistically, do you think you will actually be able to settle where you would like?

Yes . . . (SKIP TO Q. 69) . . . 1   29/

No . . . . . (ASK A) 2

Don't know. (SKIP TO Q. 69) . . 3

A. IF NO: Realistically, where do you think you actually will settle--in what town or city and state?

U.S. TOWN/CITY: _____
30-31/

STATE: _____
32-33/

IF R HAS NO SPECIFIC TOWN/CITY OR STATE IN MIND, BUT A GENERAL AREA OR TYPE OF AREA, RECORD VERBATIM RESPONSE.

34-35/

36-37/

No idea at all 00

(GO ON TO Q. 67)

327

67. I am going to mention some reasons physicians often give for not being able to
     settle where they would like.

     For each of the reasons I mention, please tell me how much it contributes to keep-
     ing you from settling where you would like in the United States.

	a great deal	a fair amount	a small amount	or, not at all? CODE HERE ALL "DOES NOT APPLY"	
A. Difficulty in obtaining an unrestricted state license to practice medicine-- how much does that contribute to your not being able to settle where you would like, would you say (READ CATE-GORIES)	4	3	2	1	38/
B. No positions available in your speci-alty--how much does that contribute (READ CATEGORIES)	4	3	2	1	39/
C. IF R IS NOT A U.S. CITIZEN (SEE Q. 36) ASK: Prejudice shown against foreign-ers--how much does that contribute to keeping you from settling where you would like?	4	3	2	1	40/
D. No positions available in top-rated hospitals--how much does that contribute to your not being able to settle where you would like?	4	3	2	1	41/
E. Difficulty in establishing a private practice--how much does that contribute to your not being able to settle where you would like?	4	3	2	1	42/

68. Are there any other reasons which contribute to keeping you from settling where you
     would like in the United States?

                                        Yes . . . (ASK A) . 1   43/
                                        No (GO TO Q. 69) . . 2

     A. IF YES: Please tell me about the reasons.

                                                          ☐☐ 44-45/

                                                          ☐☐ 46-47/

                                                          ☐☐ 48-49/

328

IF R IS U.S. CITIZEN (SEE Q. 36), SKIP TO Q. 78.

69. I'll mention some reasons physicians offer for remaining in the United States after training.

For each reason I mention, please tell me how much influence it has, if any, on your remaining here.

	a great deal	a fair amount	a small amount	or, not at all? CODE HERE FOR "DOES NOT APPLY"	
A. Economic prospects are better in the United States--does this influence your remaining here (READ CATEGORIES)	4	3	2	1	50/
B. Research opportunities are better in the United States--does this influence your remaining here (READ CATEGORIES)	4	3	2	1	51/
C. There is no state or socialized medicine in the United States--how much does this influence your remaining here?	4	3	2	1	52/
D. Your family likes it in the United States--how much does this influence your remaining here? .	4	3	2	1	53/
E. Your children's educational possibilities--how much does this influence your remaining here? .	4	3	2	1	54/
F. There are better chances of establishing a private practice here--how much does this influence your remaining here?	4	3	2	1	55/
G. There is political unrest in the country you would return to--how much does this influence your remaining here?	4	3	2	1	56/
H. You prefer the culture and life of the United States--how much does this influence your remaining here? . . .	4	3	2	1	57/

329

69. Continued

	a great deal	a fair amount	a small amount	or, not at all? CODE HERE FOR "DOES NOT APPLY"	
I. The physical facilities for the practice of medicine are superior in the United States--how much does this influence your remaining here?	4	3	2	1	58/
J. You would like to become a United States citizen--how much does this influence your remaining here?	4	3	2	1	59/

---

70. Are there any <u>other</u> reasons which have an influence on your remaining in the United States?

Yes . (ASK A) . . . 1   60/

No (SKIP TO Q. 78). 2

A. IF YES: Please tell me about them.

☐☐
61-62/

☐☐
63-64/

SKIP NOW TO Q. 78.

☐☐
65-66/

IF DEFINITELY OR PROBABLY LEAVE (CODE 1 IN Q. 64 OR CODE 1 IN Q. 64A, ASK QS. 71 & 72:

71. (When/If) you leave the United States after training, in which country will you settle? RECORD RESPONSE VERBATIM.

IF R MENTIONED MORE THAN ONE COUNTRY ABOVE, PROBE: In which <u>one</u> of these countries are you <u>most</u> likely to settle?

☐☐☐
67-69/

COUNTRY: _____

(DEFINITE OR MOST LIKELY DESTINATION)

No definite or most likely
destination (SKIP TO Q. 78) 000

70 71 72 73 74
☐☐☐☐☐
75-76/09
77-80/4182

72. Where would you settle in (COUNTRY NAMED ABOVE IN Q. 71)--in an urban area, a rural area, or what?

Urban area . . . 1   05/

Rural area . . . 2

Other (SPECIFY)

_____ 3

INTERVIEWER: IS R'S COUNTRY OF DESTINATION (Q. 71) THE SAME AS R'S COUNTRY OF MEDICAL EDUCATION (Q. 30)?

YES 1   06/

NO 2

IF NO, SKIP TO Q. 76.
IF YES, GO ON TO Q. 73.

73. I'll mention some reasons physicians often give for returning to their countries of medical education.

For each reason I mention, please tell me how much it influences your return, if at all.

	a great deal	a fair amount	a small amount	or, not at all? CODE HERE FOR "DOES NOT APPLY"	
A. Your family is in (COUNTRY OF MEDICAL EDUCATION)--does this influence your return (READ CATEGORIES).	4	3	2	1	07/
B. You are legally required by (COUNTRY OF MEDICAL EDUCATION) ro return--how much does this influence your return (READ CATEGORIES)	4	3	2	1	08/
C. You are legally required by the United States to return--how much does this influence your return (READ CATEGORIES)	4	3	2	1	09/
D. You feel a moral obligation to return-- how much does this influence your return?	4	3	2	1	10/
E. You would not wish to be drafted into the United States Armed Services--how much does this influence your return?	4	3	2	1	11/
F. You have not found adequate employment opportunities here--how much does this influence your return?	4	3	2	1	12/
G. You would have trouble obtaining a full unrestricted license to practice medicine here--how much does this influence your return?	4	3	2	1	13/

331

73. Continued

	a great deal	a fair amount	a small amount	or, not at all? CODE HERE FOR "DOES NOT APPLY"	
H. You feel you should serve the people of your country of medical education <u>first</u>--how much does this influence your return?	4	3	2	1	14/
I. You dislike aspects of life in the United States--how much does this influence your return?	4	3	2	1	15/

IF CODES 4-2 IN ITEM I ABOVE, ASK Q. 74. ALL OTHERS GO TO Q. 75.

74. Which aspects of life here do you dislike?


```
┌──┬──┐
│  │  │   16-17/
└──┴──┘

┌──┬──┐
│  │  │   18-19/
└──┴──┘

┌──┬──┐
│  │  │   20-21/
└──┴──┘
```

75. Are there any <u>other</u> reasons which influence your return to your country of medical education?

                                  Yes . (ASK A) 1   22/
                                  No (SKIP TO Q 78)   2

A. <u>IF YES</u>: Please tell me about them.

```
┌──┬──┐
│  │  │   23-24/
└──┴──┘

┌──┬──┐
│  │  │   25-26/
└──┴──┘

┌──┬──┐
│  │  │   27-28/
└──┴──┘
```

| NOW SKIP TO Q. 78. |

IF COUNTRY OF DESTINATION IS <u>NOT THE SAME</u> AS COUNTRY OF MEDICAL EDUCATION ("NO" IN INSTRUCTION BOX ABOVE Q. 73, PAGE 33), ASK QS. 76 & 77.

ALL OTHERS SKIP TO Q. 78.

76. I'll mention some reasons physicians often give for <u>not</u> returning to their countries of medical education.

For each of the various reasons I mention, please tell me how much it influences your not returning to your country of medical education, or if it has any influence at all.

	a great deal	a fair amount	a small amount	or, not at all? CODE HERE FOR "DOES NOT APPLY"	
A. The country of your medical education is not your country of nationality or where you grew up--how much does this influence your <u>not</u> returning--(READ CATEGORIES)	4	3	2	1	29/
B. There are better opportunities in (COUNTRY OF DESTINATION-SEE Q. 71) to practice medicine the way you wish--how much does this influence your <u>not</u> returning--(READ CATEGORIES).	4	3	2	1	30/
C. You do not like the way medicine is organized in your country of medical education--how much does this influence your <u>not</u> returning--(READ CATEGORIES)	4	3	2	1	31/
D. The medical system of (COUNTRY OF DESTINATION) is more like that of the United States--how much does this influence your <u>not</u> returning to your country of medical education?	4	3	2	1	32/
E. Your family lives in (COUNTRY OF DESTINATION)--how much does this influence your <u>not</u> returning?	4	3	2	1	33/
F. There is less political turmoil in (COUNTRY OF DESTINATION)--how much does this influence your <u>not</u> returning to your country of medical education?	4	3	2	1	34/
G. There is less discrimination or prejudice against you in (COUNTRY OF DESTINATION)--how much does this influence your <u>not</u> returning to your country of medical education?	4	3	2	1	35/

76. Continued.

	a great deal	a fair amount	a small amount	or, not at all? CODE HERE FOR "DOES NOT APPLY"
H. The standard of living in (COUNTRY OF DESTINATION) is higher than in your country of medical education--how much does this influence your <u>not</u> returning?	4	3	2	1 36/

---

77. Are there any <u>other</u> reasons which influence your returning to (COUNTRY OF DESTINA-TION) rather than to your country of medical education?

Yes . . (ASK A) . . . 1   37/

No . (GO TO Q. 78) . . 2

A. <u>IF YES</u>: Please tell me about them.

☐☐	38-39/
☐☐	40-41/
☐☐	42-43/

<u>ASK EVERYONE</u>:

78. In what month and year did you take the E-C-F-M-G examination on which you received a passing score?

ENTER MONTH: ☐☐   AND YEAR: 19 ☐☐   44-45/
                                           46-47/

---

79. In what country did you take this examination in which you received the passing score?

ENTER NAME OF COUNTRY: _____   ☐☐   48-50/

80. How many times altogether did you take the examination--including the time you re-
    ceived the passing score?

                    ENTER NUMBER OF TIMES . . [|]   51-52/

---

81. Do you hold any full, unlimited state licenses to practice medicine in the United
    States--not counting any temporary or hospital license or permit?

                              Yes . (ASK A-C) . . . 1   53/
                              No (GO TO Q. 82) . . 2

    IF YES, ASK A-C:

    A. In what state did you obtain the first unlimited license?   [|]

              ENTER STATE: _____   54-55/

    B. And in what month and year did you obtain your first unlimited license?

                    ENTER [|]   AND   [|]   56-57/
                    MONTH: YEAR: 19   58-59/

    C. How did you obtain this license--through the FLEX Examination or some other
    way?
                    The FLEX Examination . . . . . 1 ⎤ NOW   60/
                    Some other way (SPECIFY)   ⎬ SKIP
                                                     ⎥ TO
                    _____ 2 ⎦ Q. 83   61/

335

IF NO TO Q. 81, ASK Q. 82:

82. Have you ever taken an examination for a full, unlimited state license?

                                                        Yes (ASK A-C) . 1   62/
                                                        No (ASK D) . . 2

        IF YES, ASK A-C:

        A. When was the first time you took this type of licensing examination?

                    ENTER   [ ][ ]   AND   [ ][ ]   63-64/
                    MONTH: YEAR: 19   65-66/

        B. Was it the FLEX Exam or some other exam?

                                        The Flex Exam 1   67/
                                        Some other exam
                                        (SPECIFY) _____ 2

        C. For which state did you hope this exam would qualify you for a license?

                                                            NOW SKIP TO
                            ENTER NAME OF STATE _____ Q. 83.
                                                                    [ ][ ]
        IF NO, ASK D: 68-69/

        D. Do you intend to take an exam for a state license?

                                        Yes (ASK E & F) 1   70/
                                        No (GO TO Q. 83) . . . 2

            IF YES TO D, ASK E & F:

            E. Which exams do you intend to take? RECORD RESPONSE VERBATIM.
                                                                         [ ]
                                                                          71/
                                                                         [ ]
                                                                          72/
                                                                         [ ]
                                                                          73/

                                                                          74/R
                                                                       75-76/10
                                                                       77-80/4182

            F. For which state or states do you hope (this/these) exam(s) will qualify
                you for a license? RECORD RESPONSE VERBATIM.   BEGIN DECK 11
                                                                         [ ][ ]
                                                                          05-06/
                                                                         [ ][ ]
                                                                          07-08/
                                                                         [ ][ ]
                                                                          09-10/

336

83. I'll read some statements about United States medical training and the practice of
     medicine in general. For each statement, please tell me how much you agree or dis-
     agree with it.

	agree strongly	agree somewhat	disagree somewhat	or disagree strongly?	(IF VOLUNTEERED): Don't know	
A. In general, on the whole, United States medical training programs are the best in the world--do you (READ CATEGORIES)	1	2	3	4	9	11/
B. In general, foreign medical graduates are not given training equal to that of United States graduates--do you (READ CATEGORIES)	1	2	3	4	9	12/
C. In general, United States training programs are really excuses for staffing hospitals and are not really for training--how do you feel about this statement?	1	2	3	4	9	13/
D. In general, medicine is a science which can be practiced anywhere in the world regardless of social and cultural differences--	1	2	3	4	9	14/
E. In general, medical care can be delivered best by teams of physicians trained in subspecialties.	1	2	3	4	9	15/
F. In general, it is the responsibility of society, through its government, to provide everyone with the best available medical care, whether the individual can afford it or not. .	1	2	3	4	9	16/
G. In general, the physician who bases his diagnosis mainly on clinical signs is more likely to give better medical care than the physician who bases his diagnosis mainly on laboratory tests.	1	2	3	4	9	17/

83. Continued.

	agree strongly	agree somewhat	disagree somewhat	or disagree strongly?	(IF VOLUNTEERED): Don't know	
H. In general, the physician's responsibility is to his patients rather than to the community as a whole--	1	2	3	4	9	18/
I. In general, the United States needs a complete restructuring of its medical care system.	1	2	3	4	9	19/

IF R IS NATURAL BORN U.S. CITIZEN OR NATURALIZED PRIOR TO GRADUATION (SEE INSTRUCTION BOX, PAGE 18), SKIP TO Q. 89, PAGE 42.

	agree strongly	agree somewhat	disagree somewhat	or disagree strongly?	(IF VOLUNTEERED): Don't know	
J. In general, (COUNTRY OF MEDICAL EDUCATION) needs a complete restructuring of its medical care system.	1	2	3	4	9	20/

84. Would you say that the primary health needs of (COUNTRY OF MEDICAL EDUCATION-Q. 30) and those of the United States are about the same, somewhat different, or very different?

About the same 1	21/
Somewhat different 2	
Very different 3	

---

85. In your opinion, what are the primary health needs of (COUNTRY OF MEDICAL EDUCATION)?

☐☐	22-23/
☐☐	24-25/
☐☐	26-27/

---

86. In what ways is your United States training preparing you to meet the needs of (COUNTRY OF MEDICAL EDUCATION)?

☐☐	28-29/
☐☐	30-31/
☐☐	32-33/

---

87. To what extent is your United States training providing you with skills usable in (COUNTRY OF MEDICAL EDUCATION) -- would you say to a great extent, to a moderate extent, to a small extent, or not at all?

To a great extent 1	34/
To a moderate extent 2	
To a small extent 3	
Not at all 4	

339

88. As you see it, to what extent <u>should</u> your United States training provide
    you with skills usable in (COUNTRY OF MEDICAL EDUCATION) -- to a great
    extent, to a moderate extent, to a small extent, or not at all?

                                    To a great extent 1   35/

                                    To a moderate extent 2

                                    To a small extent 3

                                    Not at all 4

ASK EVERYONE:

89. In your opinion, what are the primary health needs of the United States?

                                    [|]   36-37/

                                    [|]   38-39/

                                    [|]   40-41/

90. In your opinion, in what ways is your training preparing you to meet the health
    needs of the United States?

                                    [|]   42-43/

                                    [|]   44-45/

                                    [|]   46-47/.

91. To what extent is your training providing you with skills usable in United
    States medical practice -- would you say to a great extent, to a moderate extent,
    to a small extent, or not at all?

                                    To a great extent 1   48/

                                    To a moderate extent 2

                                    To a small extent 3

                                    Not at all 4

92. How would you rate your medical school training for its relevance in preparing
    you for graduate medical training <u>in the United States</u> -- would you say it was
    (READ CATEGORIES) --

                                    Excellent 1   49/

                                    Good 2

                                    Fair 3

                                    Or, poor. 4

340

93. On the whole, do you find that you personally are treated better, about the same, or not as well as <u>most</u> (READ ITEMS, A-C AND CODE).

	Better	About the same	Not as well as	(If Vol.) don't know	
A. other foreign medical graduates? (PROBE: just your impression). .	3	2	1	9	50/
B. United States citizens who studied medicine outside the United States?	3	2	1	9	51/
C. United States citizens who studied medicine <u>in</u> the United States . .	3	2	1	9	52/

94. Have you joined . . .

	Yes	No	
the American Medical Association?	1	2	53/
the (STATE) Medical Association?	1	2	54/
a Medical Specialty Association?	1	2	55/
any medical associations representing (COUNTRY OF MEDICAL EDUCATION) doctors?	1	2	56/

95. Do you belong to any clubs, organizations or church groups here in (NAME OF CITY OR TOWN), or around here?

    Yes (ASK A)   1   57/
    No (GO TO Q. 96)   2

A. <u>IF YES:</u> What kinds of organizations or groups have you joined here? RECORD RESPONSE VERBATIM.

                                        58-59/

                                        60-61/

                                        62-63/

96. Are, or were, any of your relatives physicians?

                                    Yes (ASK A & B) 1   64/
                                    No (GO TO Q. 97) 2

IF YES, ASK A & B:

A. How many of your relatives are, or were, physicians?

                                    NUMBER . . . . [ ]   65/

B. Which relatives? PROBE FOR RELATIONSHIP TO R.

_____ 66/   _____ 69/

_____ 67/   _____ 70/

_____ 68/   _____ 71/

                                            72 73 74
                                          [| |]   75-76/11
                                                        77-80/4182

---

97. Are you currently married, separated, widowed, divorced,   BEGIN DECK 12
    or have you never been married?

                                    Married (ASK A-C) 1   05/
                                    Separated (ASK A-C) 2
                                    Widowed (GO TO Q. 98) . . . 3
                                    Divorced (GO TO Q. 98) . . 4
                                    Never been married. 5
                                            (GO TO Q. 99)

IF CURRENTLY MARRIED OR SEPARATED (CODES 1 OR 2), ASK A-C:

A. What is your spouse's citizenship?

    COUNTRY: _____ [| |] 06-08/

B. In what country is your spouse living now?

    COUNTRY: _____ [| |] 09-11/

C. What kind of work does your spouse mainly do -- what does your spouse
   actually do on (his/her) main job?

    OCCUPATION: _____ [| |] 12-14/

    C[1]. In what kind of industry or business is that -- what do they make
          or do?

    INDUSTRY: _____ [| |] 15-17/

342

98. IF EVER MARRIED (CODES 1-4 IN Q. 97). ASK: How many children do you have?

                                    None (GO TO Q.99) . . . 00
                                                                    18-19/
                            NUMBER: [ ][ ]   (ASK A)

    A. IF ANY CHILDREN: In what country or countries do your children live?

            COUNTRY(IES):_____ [ ][ ][ ] 20-22/

                         _____ [ ][ ][ ] 23-25/

                         _____ [ ][ ][ ] 26-28/

---

99. IF NOT CURRENTLY MARRIED (CODES 3 - 5 IN Q. 97), ASK: Are you engaged to be
    married?
                                    Yes (ASK A-C) 1   29/
                                    No (GO TO Q. 100) . . 2

    IF YES, ASK A-C:

    A. What is your fiancé's citizenship?

            COUNTRY: _____ [ ][ ][ ] 30-32/

    B. What country is your fiancé living in now?

            COUNTRY: _____ [ ][ ][ ] 33-35/

    C. What kind of work does your fiancé mainly do -- what does your
        fiancé actually do on (his/her) main job?

            OCCUPATION: _____ [ ][ ][ ] 36-38/

        C [1]. In what kind of industry or business is that -- what do
                they make or do?

            INDUSTRY: _____ [ ][ ][ ] 39-41/

343

100. What is your religious preference?

☐☐ . 42-43/

101. In which country was your mother born?

COUNTRY: _____ ☐☐☐ 44-46/

102. A. What kind of work (does/did) your mother mainly do -- what (does/did) she do on her <u>main</u> job?

OCCUPATION: _____ ☐☐☐ 47-49/

B. In what kind of industry or business is that -- what do they make or do?

INDUSTRY: _____ ☐☐☐ 50-52/

103. What was the highest grade or year of school that your mother completed?

```
┌──────┐
│ HAND │
│ CARD │
│  C   │
└──────┘
```

No formal schooling	1
Some primary school	2
Completed primary school	3
Some secondary school	4
Completed secondary school	5
Some college, university	6
Completed college, university	7
Some or completed graduate or professional school	8
Other (SPECIFY) _____	9

53/

104. In which country was your father born?

COUNTRY: _____ ☐☐☐ 54-56/

105. A. What kind of work (does/did) your father mainly do -- what (does/did) he do on his <u>main</u> job?

OCCUPATION: _____ ☐☐☐ 57-59/

B. In what kind of industry or business is that -- what do they make or do?

INDUSTRY: _____ ☐☐☐ 60-62/

106. What was the highest grade or year in school that your father completed?

<table>
<tr><td rowspan="4">HAND
CARD
C</td><td>No formal schooling . . . . 1</td><td>63/</td></tr>
<tr><td>Some primary school . . . . 2</td><td></td></tr>
<tr><td>Completed primary school . . . . . . 3</td><td></td></tr>
<tr><td>Some secondary school . . . . 4</td><td></td></tr>
</table>

                        Completed secondary school 5

                        Some college, university 6

                        Completed college, university 7

                        Some or completed graduate or
professional school 8

                        Other (SPECIFY) _____ 9

---

107. When you graduated from medical school, were you in the upper third, the middle third, or the lower third of your graduating class?

                        Upper third 1   64/

                        Middle third 2

                        Lower third 3

                        Other (SPECIFY) _____ 4

108. In __addition__ to your yearly salary, do you receive any benefits such as
      financial bonuses, housing, or board?

                                    Yes (ASK A) 1   65/

                                    No (GO TO Q. 109) 2

      A. __IF YES:__ Which benefits?   ⬜
                                                                                66/
                                                                                ⬜
                                                                                67/
                                                                                ⬜
                                                                                68/

---

109. Which one of the categories on this card best describes your yearly salary
      from the hospital -- before taxes and __not__ including additional benefits such
      as financial bonuses, housing or board?

      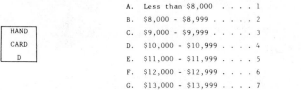

                          A. Less than $8,000 1   69/
                          B. $8,000 - $8,999 2
      ┌─────────┐   C. $9,000 - $9,999 3
      │ HAND   │   D. $10,000 - $10,999 4
      │ CARD   │   E. $11,000 - $11,999 5
      │   D   │   F. $12,000 - $12,999 6
      └─────────┘   G. $13,000 - $13,999 7
                          H. $14,000 or more 8

                              Refused (RECORD VERBATIM). 9

---

110. Do you now live in the same building with other interns and residents?

                                    Yes 1   70/

                                    No 2

---

111. In your life outside of work at the hospital, how often do you see house staff
      who are United States medical graduates -- would you say (READ CATEGORIES) --

                                    Daily 1   71/

                                    Once a week or more 2

                                    At least once a month 3

                                    Less often than that 4

                                    Or, never 5

346

112. In your life outside of work at the hospital, how often do you see house
      staff who are (COUNTRY OF MEDICAL EDUCATION) medical graduates -- would you
      say (READ CATEGORIES) --

                              Daily 1   72/

                              Once a week or more 2

                              At least once a month 3

                              Less often than that 4

                              Or, never 5

113. In your life outside of work at the hospital, how often do you see (other)
      house staff who are foreign medical graduates -- would you say (READ CATEGORIES)--

                              Daily 1   73/

                              Once a week or more 2

                              At least once a month 3

                              Less often than that 4

                              Or, never 5

        IF R IS A NATURAL BORN U.S. CITIZEN OR NATURALIZED PRIOR TO GRADUATION
        (SEE INSTRUCTION BOX, PAGE 18), SKIP TO Q. 119.

114. In your life outside of work at the hospital, how often do you have social
      contact with United States families -- would you say (READ CATEGORIES) --

                              Daily 1   74/

                              Once a week or more 2

                              At least once a month 3

                              Less often than that 4

                              Or, never 5

                                                        75-76/12
                                                        77-80/4182

347

115. Please think of three people who are your closest friends in the United
     States. What is their nationality? IF R CAN ONLY THINK OF ONE OR TWO,
     DO NOT PROBE FOR MORE.

                          No close friends   (SKIP TO Q. 117) 1   05/

FOR EACH FRIEND LISTED, ASK A:	FRIEND #1		FRIEND #2		FRIEND #3	
A. Off duty, how often do you see your friend whose nationality is (NATIONALITY) --would you say (READ CATEGORIES)--	(NATIONALITY) ☐☐ 06-07/		(NATIONALITY) ☐☐ 08-09/		(NATIONALITY) ☐☐ 10-11/	
Daily	1	12/	1	13/	1	14/
Once a week or more . .	2		2		2	
At least once a month .	3		3		3	
Less often than that .	4		4		4	
Or, never?	5		5		5	

116. Would you say that in your life outside of your work at the hospital, you have
     many Americans as friends, some, a few or none?

                                        Many 1   15/
                                        Some 2
                                        A few 3
                                        None 4

117. Would you like to have as neighbors (READ EACH ITEM) --

	Yes	No	No difference, doesn't matter	Depends (RECORD VERBATIM)	
A. White Americans	1	2	3	4	16/
B. Black Americans	1	2	3	4	17/
C. Spanish-speaking Americans	1	2	3	4	18/
D. Oriental Americans	1	2	3	4	19/

118. Would you like to have as personal friends (READ ITEM) --

	Yes	No	No difference, doesn't matter	Depends (RECORD VERBATIM)	
A. White Americans	1	2	3	4	20/
B. Black Americans	1	2	3	4	21/
C. Spanish-speaking Americans	1	2	3	4	22/
D. Oriental Americans	1	2	3	4	23/

119. Of all the patients that you usually see, approximately what percentage
      are (READ CATEGORIES) --

PER CENT

A. White? . . . . ☐☐☐   24-26/

B. Black? . . . . ☐☐☐   27-29/

C. Spanish-speaking or
    Latin descent?. . . . . ☐☐☐   30-32/

D. Oriental or of Oriental
    descent?. . . . . ☐☐☐   33-35/

120. Of all the patients that you usually see,
      approximately what percentage have low   ENTER   ☐☐☐   36-38/
      incomes?   PER CENT:

121. In terms of your training goals for your future medical practice, how would you
      rate the mixture of patients you now get to see -- would you say excellent,
      good, fair, or poor?

                      Excellent . . . . . . (ASK A) 1   39/
                      Good . . . . (ASK A) 2
                      Fair . . . . (ASK A) 3
                      Poor . . . . (ASK A) 4
                      Other . . . . (SPECIFY, AND GO TO Q. 122).
                      _____ 5

      A. IF CODES 1-4: Please tell me more about that.   ☐☐   40-41/

                                                                ☐☐   42-43/

                                                                ☐☐   44-45/

122. That concludes the interview. Thank you very much for your cooperation and time. You have been very helpful.

Are there any aspects of your training and responsibilities during this training year you would like to comment about?

	46-47/
	48-49/
	50-51/

52-74/R
75-76/13
77-80/4182

350

INTERVIEWER OBSERVATIONS -- TO BE COMPLETED <u>AFTER</u> YOU LEAVE THE RESPONDENT.

1. Please total the time you spent interviewing this respondent and convert
    to minutes:

                                    ☐☐☐   05-07/

                                  Minutes

---

2. Please rate the respondent's understanding of the questions . . .

                         No difficulty at all (GO TO Q. 3) . . . 1   08/
                         Some difficulty (ANSWER A) 2
                         A great deal of difficulty (ANSWER A) . 3

    A. <u>IF ANY DIFFICULTY</u>: Please give the numbers of the questions
                                which were especially hard for R to understand:

---

3. Rate the respondent's verbal use of English in answering the questions --

                         Excellent 1   09/
                         Good 2
                         Fair 3
                         Poor 4

351

4. As far as you could tell, how accurate were the respondent's answers --

        Accurate throughout the questioning (GO TO Q. 5) . . 1   10/

        Some inaccuracies (ANSWER A) 2

        Many inaccuracies (ANSWER A) 3

  IF ANY INACCURACIES:

  A. What do you think caused this? CODE AS MANY AS APPLY.

        Problems with English 1   11/

        Inability to think in the specific detail
        required by the questions 2   12/

        Inability to recall past events or past
        states of mind 3   13/

        Difficulty in thinking about the future 4   14/

        Fear of how data might be used (PLEASE
        ELABORATE IF YOU CAN) _____ 5   15/

        Other (SPECIFY) _____ 6   16/

---

5. Respondent (CODE ONE CATEGORY) --

        Showed high interest in survey 1   17/

        Showed mild interest 2

        Lacked interest in survey 3

        Interest varied within time of
        interview (PLEASE DESCRIBE) 4

---

6. Respondent (CODE ONE CATEGORY) --

        Was hostile toward survey 1   18/

        Suspicious 2

        Favorable 3

        Extremely favorable 4

        Attitude varied within time of
        interview (PLEASE DESCRIBE) 5

7. Code the R's sex.

                                    Male 1   19/

                                    Female 2

8. Code the racial background of respondent.

                                    White 1   20/

                                    Black 2

                                    Oriental 3

                                    Indian (from India) . . 4

                                    Other (SPECIFY)

                                    _____ 5

9. A few questions deal with the prejudice R feels in certain contacts.
    We would like to analyze such reports in terms of the light-dark vari-
    ations in skin color within nationality groups. Please circle one code
    which best describes your R in reference to the majority of people you
    have seen in the nationality or racial group of R --

                                    Light 1   21/

                                    Medium 2

                                    Dark   3

                                    Very dark 4

10. Privacy in interview situation --

    Other persons present or within earshot (CODE ONE) --

                         From time to time (ANSWER A & B) . . . 1   22/

                         Often (ANSWER A & B) 2

                         Continually (ANSWER A & B) 3

                         No one else present or within
                           earshot (GO TO Q. 11) 4

    IF CODES 1-3, ASK A & B:

    A. How many other persons?   ENTER # OF PERSONS: [| |]   23-25/

    B. How were they related to R? (Fellow interns, spouse, etc.)

                                                          [ ]   26/

                                                          [ ]   27/

                                                          [ ]   28/

353

11. Any comments or observations you feel we should know about this R or the
     interview situation? (IF YES, PLEASE DESCRIBE.)

---

12. Interview conducted in . . .

                          R's room, apartment, house
                          (within actual living quarters) 1   29/

                          Elsewhere (SPECIFY _____ 2
                          IF IN A HOSPITAL, SPECIFY NAME OF
                          HOSPITAL AS WELL AS PLACE WITHIN HOSPITAL

---

13. Date of completion of this interview.

              _____ _____ , 1974   30-31/
                  MONTH   DAY   32-33/

---

14. Interviewer signature:

                          _____

              Interviewer's Number: [ ][ ][ ][ ][ ]   34-38/

                                                               39-74/R
                                                               75-76/14
                                                               77-80/4182

INDEX